Cardiac Rehabilitation

Adult Fitness, and

Exercise Testing

THIRD EDITION

Cardiac Rehabilitation

Adult Fitness, and

Exercise Testing

THIRD EDITION

PAUL S. FARDY, PhD

Professor of Physical Education
Queens College, City University of New York
Flushing, New York

FRANK G. YANOWITZ, MD

Associate Professor of Medicine
Director, Cardiac-Rehabilitation
Medical Director, The Fitness Institute at LDS Hospital
University of Utah
Salt Lake City, Utah

With assistance from

PHILIP K. WILSON, EdD

Professor of Exercise and Sport Science
College of Health, Physical Education, and Recreation
University of Wisconsin-LaCrosse
LaCrosse, Wisconsin

Williams & Wilkins

BALTIMORE • PHILADELPHIA • HONG KONG
LONDON • MUNICH • SYDNEY • TOKYO

A WAVERLY COMPANY

Editor: Jonathan W. Pine, Jr.
Managing Editor: Molly L. Mullen
Copy Editor: Elizabeth Mahoney
Designer: Ashley Pound
Illustration Planner: Ray Lowman
Production Coordinator: Barbara J. Felton

Copyright © 1995
Williams & Wilkins
351 West Camden Street
Baltimore, Maryland 21201-2436, USA

Accurate indications, adverse reactions, and dosage schedules for drugs are provided in this book, but it is possible that they may change. The reader is urged to review the package information data of the manufacturers of the medications mentioned.

Printed in the United States of America

Chapter reprints are available from the Publisher.
First Edition 1981
Second Edition 1988
Library of Congress Cataloging-in-Publication Data
Fardy, Paul S.
    Cardiac rehabilitation, adult fitness, and exercise testing / Paul S. Fardy.
  Frank G. Yanowitz : with assistance from Philip K. Wilson.—3rd ed.
    p. cm.
  Includes bibliographical references and index.
  ISBN 0-683-03031-0
  1. Heart—Diseases—Patients—Rehabilitation.   2. Exercise tests.   3.
  Physical fitness.   4. Community health services—Planning.
  I. Yanowitz, Frank G.   II. Wilson, Philip K.   III. Title.
    [DNLM: 1. Heart Diseases—rehabilitation.   2. Exercise Test.   3. Physical
  Fitness.   WG 200 F221c 1995]
  RC682.F37   1995
  616.1'203—dc20
  DNLM/DLC
  for Library of Congress   94-37793   CIP

95 96 97 98 99
1 2 3 4 5 6 7 8 9 10

To our former teachers and professors who provided knowledge, insight and motivation; and to our students, past and present, who provide challenge, fun, and keep us on our toes.

– P.S.F. & F.G.Y.

Preface

SINCE THE PUBLICATION of the first edition of *Cardiac Rehabilitation, Adult Fitness, and Exercise Testing*, considerable change has occurred in both the business and service of cardiac rehabilitation and other preventive programs. Most of these changes have resulted in improved care, expanded patient numbers, and greater acceptance by both the medical and lay communities.

Unfortunately, some aspects of cardiac rehabilitation and prevention have changed little, in particular in the area of reimbursement. Financial constraints caused by lack of reimbursement have had and continue to have a serious limiting effect upon the delivery of programs. As a consequence, the broad-based armamentarium of services and expertise available at many centers are underutilized, thereby reducing the quality of care that the patient might have received. As the knowledge base grows in support of comprehensive multidisciplinary programs for long-term behavior modification, the importance of in-depth programs for the patient in areas such as nutrition, weight control, food selection and preparation, smoking cessation, motivation, and stress management is better understood. However, while health care professionals recognize the importance of these preventive services, it is not entirely clear **who will pay for them.**

The element of cost is a major factor in many facets of the health care industry. Nowhere has the concern for cost become more obvious than in the current debate about a **national health care plan**. The U.S. Department of Health and Human Services has fostered the development and publication of a health plan for the 1990s, **Healthy People 2000** (1), and more recently an update looking at the success in attaining the goals set forth in the original document (2). Much of the emphasis in these documents focuses on prevention of cardiovascular diseases, which remain the number-one cause of death and disability in our society. But, for all the rational intellectualism and intuitive common sense that the best and most economic approach is to prevent the occurrence of disease, the same question arises—**"Who will pay for these services?"** There is room for legitimate debate in health care cost concerning the role of the individual (the consumer) versus the role of government (the payer). Still, policy needs to be enacted that emphasizes disease prevention, whether primary, secondary, or tertiary, as the best approach to lowering costs and improving long-term health. Otherwise, potentially beneficial preventive programs will continue to be omitted from patient care because of lack of payment.

In structuring the third edition the authors have tried to accomplish three objectives: (a) to place greater emphasis on the importance of comprehensive preventive medicine, (b) to synthesize and update the knowledge base of cardiac rehabilitation and preventive programs because much has changed, and (c) to reorganize the presentation of material so that the different phases of cardiac rehabilitation are discussed in a comprehensive continuum from onset to implementation without having to go back and forth through different chapters in other sections of the book. As a result of reorganization the latest edition consists of 12 chapters, compared to 16 in the previous edition. The reorganization also includes an in-depth discussion of administrative concerns that has implications for all aspects of cardiac rehabilitation and prevention, an encompassing presentation of each of the three phases of cardiac rehabilitation and, in particular, an added comprehensive discussion of lifestyle management that focuses on early prevention.

The authors hope that the readers will find the third edition to be a logical progression of our earlier efforts. We especially hope that you may be stimulated to include some goals of primary prevention in your programs. The book continues to be designed for all professionals who are responsible for program planning, development, and implementation. We wish all of you the best and hope that the information contained herein will serve you well.

REFERENCES

1. Public Health Service. Healthy people 2000. DHHS Pub. No. 91–50213. Washington DC: U.S. Government, 1991.
2. National Center for Health Statistics. Healthy people 2000 review 1992; Hyattsville, MD: Public Health Service, 1993.

P.S.F., F.G.Y

Contents

I. FOUNDATIONAL INFORMATION

1

THE PREVENTION AGENDA

CARDIOVASCULAR DISEASES IN THE 1990s
DOMAINS OF PREVENTION
DISABILITY PREVENTION MODEL
CONCLUSIONS

AN ASTUTE OBSERVER OF THE 1990s health care reform debate might easily conclude that these were the best of times *and* the worst of times. Certainly the American medical industry is at an all-time pinnacle of productivity. From the depths of molecular biology to the heights of organ transplant surgery, Americans enjoy the most sophisticated and highly technologic advances in the diagnosis and treatment of complex human diseases. The incredible array of scientific tools and the vast medical knowledge available to physicians today enable the delivery of the finest medical care available anywhere in the world. Yet, unlike most other countries in the civilized world, millions of Americans are either uninsured or underinsured. As a result, many have inadequate health care or limited access to the wide array of health care services available to more fortunate Americans who have medical insurance. To make matters worse, the costs of health care in the United States are staggering and far greater than in any other country in the world, consuming over 14% of our gross national product (1). It has been suggested that the unrelenting upward spiraling of health care costs will reach into the *trillions* of dollars by the year 2000.

Many reasons have been suggested for this confusing paradox and the resulting crisis in American medicine. This book addresses one of the most important issues: the need to focus more attention on the delivery of preventive medical services. This is not just a challenge to the medical profession and other health care providers to become more involved in preventive medicine; it is also a societal challenge. We must take more responsibility for improving and maintaining our own health and the health of our families. Too much of the high cost of modern medical care is spent on end-stage, chronic diseases where the only choices left are highly expensive medical and surgical procedures, and where the resultant outcomes are barely noticeable in terms of added length or quality of

3

Figure 1.1. Leading causes of death in the United States by sex. **A**, Cardiovascular diseases and stroke; **B**, cancer; **C**, accidents; **D**, chronic obstructive pulmon-ary disease; **E**, pneumonia; **F**, Suicide; **G**, AIDS. (Adapted from American Heart Assoc-iation. 1992 heart and stroke facts, AHA Publication 55-0386 [com]. National Center, 7272 Greenville Avenue, Dallas, TX 75231-4596.)

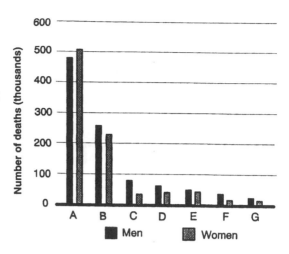

life. Nowhere is the saying "an ounce of prevention is worth a pound of cure" more applicable than in today's costly medical environment.

In this chapter we address the burden of cardiovascular disease in the 1990s and the ramifications for the health care professionals—physicians, nurses, exercise specialists, nutritionists, and others working in preventive medicine. A model for disability prevention pertinent to cardiovascular and other chronic diseases is discussed. This model has important implications for health care workers interested in cardiac rehabilitation and other preventive programs. The purpose of this discussion is to prepare the reader for the comprehensive prevention agenda that is necessary to influence our health care system and to improve the health and well-being of our population. In subsequent chapters in this book, we focus on more specific and practical aspects of prevention and rehabilitation, especially as they pertain to cardiovascular diseases.

CARDIOVASCULAR DISEASES IN THE 1990s

"A life every 34 seconds" is the warning from the American Heart Association (AHA) in their annual publication, "Heart and Stroke Facts" (2). Although cancer is the deadly disease most feared by millions of Americans, cardiovascular disease heads the list of leading causes of death and disability. Moreover, deaths from heart and blood vessel diseases overshadow cancer deaths by 2 to 1, as indicated in Figure 1.1. More bad news is that adults in this country have a 50% likelihood of dying from cardiovascular diseases, most often diseases related to atherosclerosis. Although coronary heart disease (CHD) is the most common cause of death and disability in older Americans, more than 170,000 people under the age of 65 die each year from this disease, often at the peak of their productive lives (2). The estimated cost for cardiovascular disease in 1992 is $108.9 *billion*, which includes physician and nursing services, hospital and nursing home

4

charges, medications, and lost productivity because of disability (2). The sad fact is that most of these costs are spent on advanced coronary heart disease, stroke, and other complications of hypertension, diseases that could have been prevented or minimized by risk factor modification and lifestyle changes. Clearly this is a catastrophic and unnecessary crisis for the American health care system.

The risk factors for atherosclerotic vascular disease are well known and widely prevalent in our population (2). The AHA estimates that 102.7 million adults in the United States have "borderline high" blood cholesterol levels (200 to 239 mg/dl), and 48.7 million Americans have "high" levels, ≥240 mg/dl (Fig. 1.2). More alarming is the estimated 36% of American children and teenagers who have elevated cholesterol levels for their age (i.e., >170 mg/dl). Guidelines for treating hypercholesterolemia and other lipid abnormalities have been widely publicized by the American Heart Association (3) and the National Cholesterol Education Program (4). Although public and professional awareness of the dangers of hypercholesterolemia is increasing, considerable controversy still exists as does a large gap between the national guidelines and the actual delivery of cholesterol-lowering services by health care professionals (5, 6).

Cigarette smoking, a second major cardiovascular risk factor, accounts for more than one out of every six deaths in the United States; i.e., approximately 400,000 premature deaths per year (7). These deaths are not just from heart disease but from a variety of other smoking-related conditions, including cancer, emphysema, pneumonia, and stroke. It has been estimated that 21% of all cardiovascular deaths and 30% of all cancer deaths can be attributed to cigarette smoking (7). Although the prevalence of smoking in the United States has declined by more than 32% in the last 20 years, the AHA estimates that 28,854,000 men and 26,358,000 women in the United States are current smokers (Fig. 1.3), and this includes 2.3 million young people aged 12 through 17 years (2). For smokers who quit, the risk of death from heart disease attributed to smoking decreases over 10 years to that of people who never smoked. Unfortunately, the

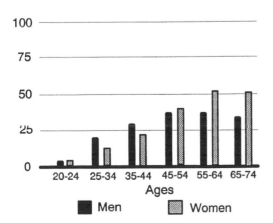

Figure 1.2. Estimated percentage of American adults with "high" cholesterol levels (240 mg/dl or more). (Adapted from American Heart Association. 1992 heart and stroke facts. AHA Publication 55 0386 [com]. National Center, 7272 Greenville Avenue, Dallas, TX 75231-4596.)

5

Figure 1.3. Prevalence of current cigarette smoking by age and educational level. (Adapted from American Heart Association. 1992 heart and stroke facts. AHA Publication 55-0386 [com]. National Center, 7272 Greenville Avenue, Dallas, TX 75231-4596.)

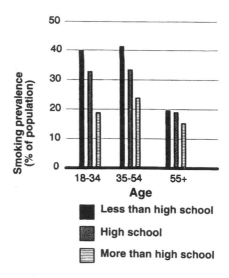

success rate of smoking cessation interventions is dismal (8).

Hypertension is the third major cardiovascular risk factor and affects almost 63 million Americans or approximately 40% of the population in the United States (2). Without a doubt, hypertension is one of the most common and treatable cardiovascular diseases encountered by physicians. This "silent killer" causes morbidity and mortality primarily as a result of target organ malfunction—stroke, heart disease, and renal failure. More than 50% of women over age 55 have significant hypertension, and this number increases to 66% by age 65 (3). The successful treatment of hypertension results in significant decreases in strokes, myocardial infarctions, and cardiovascular morbidity and mortality from all causes (9, 10).

High-fat diets and sedentary lifestyles are also implicated in the burden of chronic diseases experienced by modern society, accounting for at least 300,000 deaths each year in the U.S. from cancer, heart disease, diabetes, and strokes (7). The scientific data are now of sufficient strength to include these adverse behaviors in the list of *major* chronic disease risk factors.

The good news is that the age-adjusted mortality for major cardiovascular diseases has declined significantly in the last 30 years (Fig. 1.4). From the late 1960s through the mid-1980s, for example, mortality from coronary heart disease in the U.S. fell by more than 30%, which translates to a savings of more than 800,000 lives (2). The reasons for the decline are multifactorial and include healthier lifestyles, reductions in coronary risk factors, earlier diagnosis and treatment of heart disease, improved medications, and new interventional technologies. Although it is hard to determine the exact contribution of each of these surgical, medical, and public health strategies, considerable evidence suggests that preventive health behaviors and risk-factor modification have contributed to more than 50% of the decline in mortality (11). Primary care physicians have played an important role in these improved statistics by their more aggressive management of risk factors and restructuring of unhealthy lifestyles.

Public and professional interests in exercise training, physical fitness, wellness, and prevention have accelerated since the 1960s, creating an immense sports and fitness industry with far-reaching economic and health care implications. In 1980 the U.S. Department of Health and Human Services recommended that by 1990 all adults should participate in "exercise which involves large muscle groups in dynamic movement for periods of 20 minutes or longer, 3 or more days per week, and which is performed at an intensity of 60 percent or greater of an individual's cardiorespiratory capacity" (12). In spite of increasing interests in exercise and fitness, and the wealth of data documenting the health benefits of exercise, fewer than 10% of the adult American population are exercising at this level (13). Furthermore, less than 50% of adults exercise at any intensity for more than 20 minutes a day, 3 or more days per week (13).

The scientific evidence for the role of exercise and physical fitness in health maintenance and disease prevention continues to accumulate. The data are especially compelling for the prevention and management of coronary heart disease (14). Although studies of exercise in the primary prevention of coronary heart disease have been observational in design, a rigorous meta-analysis of 27

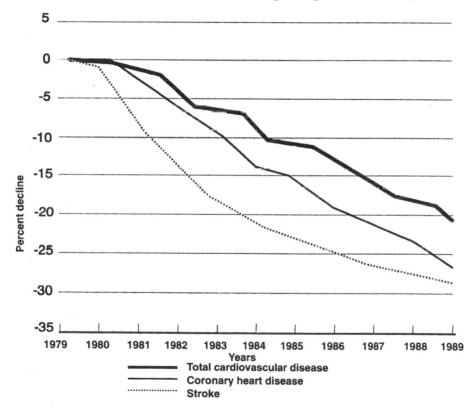

Figure 1.4. Decline in age-adjusted death rates for major cardiovascular diseases in the United States. (Adapted from American Heart Association. 1992 heart and stroke facts. AHA Publication 55-0386 [com]. National Center, 7272 Greenville Avenue, Dallas, TX 75231-4596.)

cohort studies revealed a CHD risk reduction of 35 to 55% in physically active as compared with sedentary individuals (15). In addition, a meta-analysis of previously reported, randomized, controlled trials of cardiac rehabilitation concluded that all-cause and cardiovascular mortality were significantly lower in the rehabilitation group than in the controls (16). The exercise hypothesis, although not entirely proven, is certainly credible enough to merit our serious attention. The prescription of exercise, whether carried out by increased leisure-time activity or more formal training programs, is the foundation for all successful comprehensive prevention programs.

DOMAINS OF PREVENTION

Services to prevent disease and disability can be subdivided into three domains: *primary, secondary*, and *tertiary* (13). Although specific interventions such as smoking cessation apply to all three categories, it is useful to consider each of these separately because they often involve different subsets of the population, they have different goals and objectives, and they differ in the range of treatment options.

Primary prevention refers to strategies and interventions that are recommended to apparently healthy individuals to prevent or reduce the *risk of disease onset.* Counseling to prevent or eliminate adverse lifestyles and behaviors, immunizations against common infectious diseases, and chemoprophylaxis (e.g., aspirin to prevent myocardial infarction) are the three types of preventive strategies in this domain. Although the primary focus is on children and young adults, these interventions often apply to all age groups, including the very old. A recent and influential report of the U.S. Preventive Services Task Force (USPSTF) has made a significant contribution to our understanding of the rationale for various preventive services based on age, sex, and other demographics (13). Specific lifestyle recommendations pertinent to the prevention of cardiovascular diseases are described in Chapter 11.

Secondary prevention includes those services that are recommended to *improve outcome in those with preclinical disease.* The major focus of this aspect of preventive medicine is on early detection of disease through screening before it has reached the stage of causing symptoms or illness. Examples recommended by the USPSTF and other national organizations include blood pressure screening to detect hypertension, cholesterol screening programs, and a variety of early cancer detection guidelines. Screening of asymptomatic individuals for coronary heart disease by exercise stress testing, although controversial, is also an important component of secondary prevention programs and is discussed in Chapter 5. Diseases detected early are usually more responsive to therapeutic interventions aimed at slowing, halting, or reversing the progression and thereby preventing the occurrence of chronic, disabling complications. In addition to screening and early detection, secondary prevention guidelines include similar recommendations as suggested for primary prevention such as lifestyle and behavioral counseling, diet, exercise, and chemoprophylaxis. Also, specific treatments for hypertension, hypercholesterolemia, and diabetes in asymptomatic individuals are considered to be secondary prevention strategies. Numerous scientific studies have documented the value of treating these common diseases in terms of preventing the onset of clinical manifestations and complications (14). An important aspect of health care reform in the 1990s is focused on secondary prevention strategies.

Tertiary prevention refers to intervention programs that are designed for patients with established and clinically significant disease to *prevent recurrences and slow the progression of disabling complications*. (This is sometimes called "secondary" prevention in the older rehabilitation literature.) The comprehensive rehabilitation of patients with cardiovascular disease is an excellent example of this domain of preventive medicine. Not only is cardiac rehabilitation focused on the restoration of function and confidence in patients recovering from cardiac illnesses and procedures, but it is also an effort to reverse or slow the progression of atherosclerosis and thereby prevent recurrence of disease manifestations. The process of cardiac rehabilitation is a major emphasis of this book and is discussed in Chapters 6 through 12.

The implementation of preventive services, whether primary, secondary, or tertiary, involves the participation of health care professionals from diverse disciplines: medicine, nursing, dietary and nutrition, physical therapy, psychology, exercise, and many others. The task is both *multi*disiplinary and *inter*disciplinary because of the need for these diverse professionals to work together in an integrated network of patient care services. This is especially important in the management of chronic diseases such as coronary heart disease where fragmented care provided independently by different health professionals in multiple care settings often leads to inefficient, costly, and unnecessary procedures or treatments with suboptimal outcomes.

DISABILITY PREVENTION MODEL

For almost 200 years the traditional framework for understanding the majority of medical problems encountered by health care professionals has been the *biomedical model* with its emphasis on disease diagnosis, treatment, and cure (17). In this mechanistic model the "patient" is conceptualized as a complex biologic organism, best studied from the reductionist perspective of organ systems, tissues, cells, and intracellular components. A "disease" represents a breakdown or malfunction in one or more of the body's component parts. The "diagnostic process" is analytic; that is, it is the search for abnormalities in measurable biologic parameters of structure and function. Finally, the "treatment" or "cure" of disease is

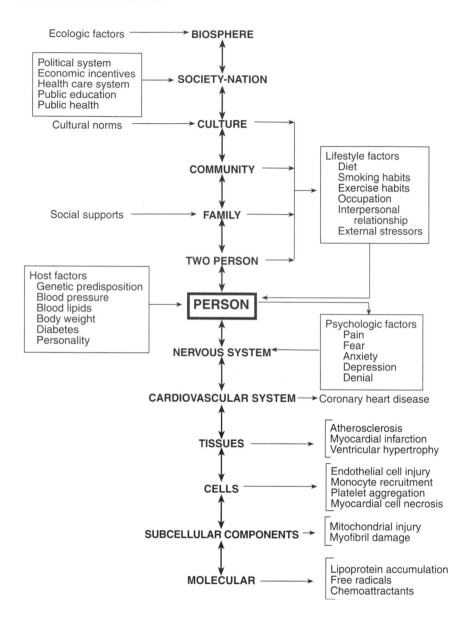

Figure 1.5. Hierarchy of biologic and nonbiologic systems in Engel's biopsychosocial model. The model is modified to illustrate the origins, processes, and clinical manifestations of coronary heart disease. (Adapted from Yanowitz FG. Atherosclerosis: processes versus origins. In: Yanowitz FG, ed. Coronary heart disease prevention. New York: Marcel Dekker, 1992.)

usually a physical intervention—chemical, electrical, or mechanical—designed to correct the particular abnormality in structure or function. The enormous progress in the diagnosis and treatment of cardiovascular diseases achieved in recent years serves to reinforce the biomedical framework as the only legitimate scientific model for medicine. In spite of impressive technologic successes, however, a crisis in health care exists as discussed previously. Many health care providers and medical scientists are beginning to question the ability of the traditional medical model to meet the needs of people with chronic diseases and disabilities (18).

Chronic diseases such as coronary heart disease can no longer be fully understood and managed from a purely biologic perspective. This was first articulated by George L. Engel who formulated the *biopsychosocial model* in 1977 (18). In this model the patient, conceptualized as a biopsychosocial entity, is viewed from the perspective of general systems theory where the "whole" person is a living system in a hierarchy of systems ranging from the molecular at the lowest level to the entire biosphere at the highest level. Figure 1.5 illustrates Engel's biopsychosocial model from the perspective of the origins, progression, and clinical manifestations of coronary heart disease (19). Systems below the "person" level are purely biologic systems, while those at or above the person are psychosocial systems. Each system in the hierarchy is an organized whole and contains all lower-level subordinate systems while, at the same time, being a component part of higher-level systems. The origins and processes of diseases such as atherosclerosis are influenced by events occurring at multiple levels (Fig. 1.5). Physicians and other health care providers working within the framework of general systems theory are better able to appreciate the importance of nonbiologic issues and the need to integrate all relevant information from various levels in the hierarchy in their diagnostic and therapeutic activities.

The implications of a biopsychosocial perspective for chronic diseases were persuasively stated by the Institute of Medicine in their publication, *Disability in America* (20). Chronic diseases were conceptualized in terms of four distinct stages (Fig. 1.6):

1. Pathology   The interruption or interference of normal bodily processes or structures as a result of cellular and tissue changes caused by disease, infection, trauma, congenital conditions, or other agents.

2. Impairment   A discrete loss and/or abnormality of mental, emotional, physiologic, or anatomic structure or function, including all losses or abnormalities caused by all forms of pathology, not just those attributable to active pathology.

3. Functional limitations   Restriction or lack of ability to perform an action or activity in the manner or within the range considered

11

normal. All functional limitations result from impairments, but not all impairments lead to functional limitations.

4. Disability   The inability or limitation in performing socially defined roles and tasks expected of individuals within a social and physical environment.

Consider, as an example, a 47–year-old male truck driver with a recent acute myocardial infarction, complicated by left ventricular dysfunction and congestive heart failure. The *pathologic processes* involving cells and tissues include severe coronary atherosclerosis, myocardial necrosis and fibrosis, and pulmonary congestion and edema. The resulting *impairments* at the organ system level are reduced left ventricular ejection fraction, left ventricular wall motion abnormalities, and recurrent chest pains caused by angina pectoris. In addition, pulmonary function abnormalities, manifested by dyspnea and cough, may be present because of the congestive heart failure. Emotional impairments might include depression, anxiety, anger, and denial resulting from his recent acute illness and the poor prospects for full recovery. *Functional limitations* secondary to these impairments occur at the whole person level and include decreased exercise tolerance, easy fatigability, and reduced ability to perform physically demanding tasks. *Disability* is the final stage and involves societal issues. The inability of this patient to perform his usual occupational and recreational activities prevents fulfilling his socially defined roles and often necessitates the involvement of other individuals and organizations to assist in these roles. If the functional limitations brought on by his heart disease are significant, there will be a need for his family, friends, neighbors, and/or social agencies to assist in managing the household activities, financial affairs, and community responsibilities, as well as a need for a substitute at work, until the patient is able to return to these activities.

It is not inevitable that chronic diseases such as coronary heart disease progress through all of these stages to the final stage of disability. The progression from stage to stage is strongly influenced by the presence or absence of *risk factors* from the three domains of the biopsychosocial model. These are illustrated

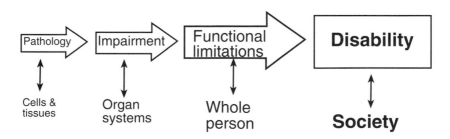

Figure 1.6. The four stages of disability.

in Figure 1.7 and listed in Table 1.1. Risk factors include those that may be causally related to the origins of disease (e.g., genetic abnormalities), as well as those that accelerate the progression of disease or increase the likelihood of functional limitations and disability. Many of the well-known coronary risk factors such as smoking, hypertension, and hypercholesterolemia interact at multiple stages. Also illustrated in Figure 1.7 is the interaction of a person's *quality of life* with the stages of disability. It is clear from this relationship that quality of life influences and is influenced by the outcomes of each stage of the chronic disease process. A disease as complex as atherosclerosis has its origins and subsequent manifestations influenced by the nonlinear interplay of many different risk factors occurring within the body, the mind, and the external physical and social environments. The risk factors, once identified, become the targets for the prevention and rehabilitation programs described in this book.

CONCLUSIONS

The concept of prevention when dealing with a chronic disease goes beyond just preventing the disease, but must also be extended to the prevention of disability. Primary prevention, for example, includes those measures designed to prevent the onset of pathology. Secondary prevention is directed at preventing the stage of impairment resulting from pathology. Tertiary preventive efforts focus on preventing functional limitations and disability. In all three domains the prevention agenda must be individualized for each patient. Strategies to be implemented

TABLE 1.1. Examples of Risk Factors for Chronic Disease and Disability

Biologic risk factors
  Genetic predisposition
  Comorbid diseases
  Adverse drug effects

Environmental risk factors
  Lack of support system
  Death of spouse
  Lack of access to health care
  Lack of transportation
  Exposure to pollutants

Lifestyle and behavioral risk factors
  Poor eating habits
  Tobacco, alcohol, drugs
  Sedentary lifestyle
  Stress and inadequate coping mechanisms

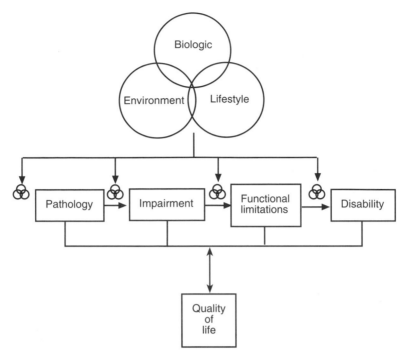

Figure 1.7. The disability prevention process. (Adapted from Pope AM, Tarlov AR, eds. Disability in America. Toward a national agenda for prevention. Washington, DC: The Institute of Medicine, National Academy Press, 1991.)

are derived from a knowledge of the biologic, environmental, and behavioral risk factors most closely implicated with the next stage of the disease. This has important implications for those health care professionals working in cardiac rehabilitation and disease prevention facilities. The patient who is at risk for coronary artery disease and its complications must be understood from the perspective of a "host inhabiting a particular biopsychosocial space" (21). The challenge to health care workers interested in prevention and rehabilitation is to broaden their world view to include the relevant data from all levels of organization.

REFERENCES

1. Fries JF. Reducing need and demand. Healthcare Forum J, November/December 1993;18–23.
2. American Heart Association. 1992 heart and stroke facts. AHA Publication 55-0386 (COM). National Center, 7272 Greenville Avenue, Dallas, TX 75231-4596.
3. Gotto AM (Conference Chairman). AHA conference report on cholesterol. Circulation 1989;80:715–748.
4. Expert Panel on Detection, Evaluation, and Treatment of High Blood Cholesterol in Adults. Summary of the second report of the National Cholesterol Education Program (NCEP) Expert Panel on Detection, Evaluation, and Treatment of High Blood Cholesterol in Adults. JAMA 1993;269:3015–3023.

5. Gotto AM. Diet and cholesterol guidelines and coronary heart disease. J Am Coll Cardiol 1989;13:503–507.

6. Fix KN, Oberman A. Barriers to following National Cholesterol Education Program guidelines. An appraisal of poor physician compliance. Arch Intern Med 1992;152:2385–2386.

7. McGinnis JM. Actual causes of death in the United States. JAMA 1993;270:2207–2212.

8. Fiore MC, Novotny TE, Pierce JP, et al. Methods used to quit smoking in the United States. Do cessation programs help? JAMA 1990;263:2760–2765.

9. Stamler J, Neaton JD. Blood pressure, systolic and diastolic, and cardiovascular risks. US population data. Arch Intern Med 1993;153:598–615.

10. Hebert PR, Moser M, Mayer J, et al. Recent evidence on drug therapy of mild to moderate hypertension and decreased risk of coronary heart disease. Arch Intern Med 1993;153:580–581.

11. Goldman L, Cook EF. The decline in ischemic heart disease mortality rates. Ann Intern Med 1984;101:825–836.

12. Public Health Service. Promoting health preventing disease: objectives for the nation. Washington, DC: US Department of Health and Human Services, 1980.

13. US Preventive Services Task Force. Guide to clinical preventive services: an assessment of the effectiveness of 169 interventions. Baltimore: Williams & Wilkins, 1989.

14. Manson JE, Tosteson H, Ridker PM, et al. The primary prevention of myocardial infarction. N Engl J Med 1992;326:1406–1416.

15. Berlin JA, Colditz GA. A meta-analysis of physical activity in the prevention of coronary heart disease. Am J Epidemiol 1990;132:612–628.

16. Oldridge NB, Guyatt GH, Fisher ME, et al. Cardiac rehabilitation after myocardial infarction. Combined experience of randomized clinical trials. JAMA 1988;260:945–950.

17. Capra F. The turning point. Science, society and the rising culture. New York: Simon & Schuster, 1982.

18. Engel GL. The need for a new medical model: a challenge for biomedicine. Science 1977;196:129–136.

19. Yanowitz FG. Atherosclerosis: processes versus origins. In: Yanowitz FG, ed. Coronary heart disease prevention. New York: Marcel Dekker, 1992.

20. Pope AM, Tarlov AR, eds. Disability in America. Toward a national agenda for prevention. Washington, DC: The Institute of Medicine, National Academy Press, 1991.

21. Foss L, Rothenberg K. The second medical revolution—from biomedicine to infomedicine. Boston: New Science Library, Shambhala, 1987.

2

Anatomic and Physiologic Concepts

FOR THE HEALTH PROFESSIONAL working in health promotion, adult fitness, cardiac rehabilitation, or exercise testing, an understanding of anatomy and physiology is essential. This chapter presents a basic review of anatomic and physiologic concepts relevant to exercise training and testing. In addition, the pathogenesis of atherosclerosis is discussed to prepare the reader for subsequent chapters dealing with various aspects of coronary heart disease. Readers interested in a more complete discussion of these issues will find many textbooks and review articles on these subjects (1–4).

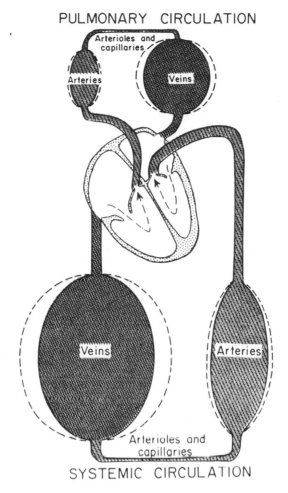

PULMONARY CIRCULATION

SYSTEMIC CIRCULATION

Figure 2.1. Schematic view of the pulmonary and systemic circulation. The heart serves as a four-chamber muscular pump to move the blood through these two circulations. (From Guyton AC. Textbook of medical physiology. 6th ed. Philadelphia: WB Saunders, 1981.)

CARDIOVASCULAR SYSTEM

The three fundamental functions of the cardiovascular system are (a) to deliver oxygen (O_2) and nutrients to the cells and tissues of the body; (b) to facilitate the removal of carbon dioxide (CO_2) and other waste products produced by these cells and tissues; and (c) to transport regulatory substances and cells between various regions of the body. A schematic view of the circulation is illustrated in Figure 2.1 (4). This system is a continuous circuit involving two major subdivisions, the pulmonary and systemic circulations, with the heart functioning as a muscular pump providing the necessary pressure to move the blood

17

Figure 2.2. Schematic view of the cardiac chambers and great vessels. (From Guyton AC. Textbook of medical physiology. 6th ed. Philadelphia: WB Saunders, 1981.)

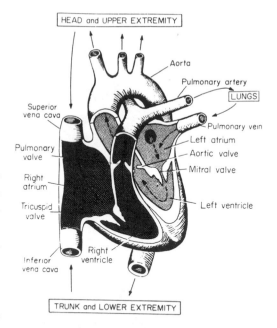

through these two circulations. Resistance to blood flow primarily occurs at the level of the arterioles and capillaries situated between the arteries and veins of each circulatory subdivision.

Cardiac Anatomy

From a structural perspective the heart consists of four separate muscular pumps: two primer pumps, the right and left atria, and two power pumps, the right and left ventricles (Fig. 2.2). Each "side" of the heart serves a major subdivision of the circulatory system. The right heart receives venous blood from the inferior and superior vena cavae and pumps blood into the pulmonary circulation where CO_2 is eliminated and O_2 is added. The left heart receives oxygenated blood from the pulmonary circulation and pumps blood into the systemic circulation to serve the cells, tissues, and organ systems of the body. The two atria primarily function as reservoirs for venous blood returning to the heart during ventricular systole and as conduits during ventricular diastole. In addition, atrial contraction just prior to ventricular systole provides a further increment of blood into the ventricles that augments the contractile force of ventricular systole.

The heart consists of two separate syncytia of cardiac muscle, the thin-walled atria and the thick-walled ventricles. The atria and ventricles, the four heart valves, and the two arterial trunks leaving the ventricles are fastened to the fibrous "skeleton" of the heart. Within this fibrous tissue are four dense connective tissue rings called *annuli fibrosi* (Fig. 2.3) (5). The atrial musculature, aorta, pulmonary artery, and semilunar valves are anchored to the superior surface of the fibrous skeleton, while the ventricular muscle syncytium and mitral and tricuspid valves originate from the inferior surface.

The two semilunar heart valves (aortic and pulmonary) each consist of three symmetric valve cusps that form perfect seals when closed, preventing regurgitation of blood back into the ventricles. Behind the valve cusps are

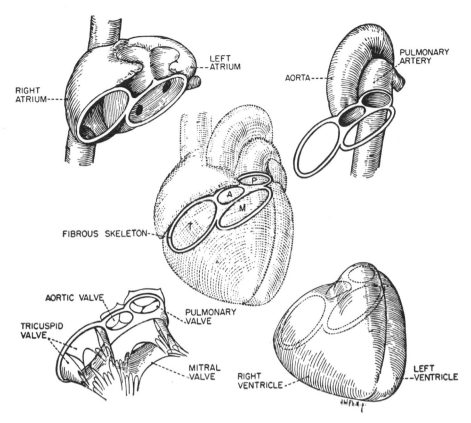

Figure 2.3. The fibrous skeleton of the heart and its relationships to the atrial and ventricular syncytia of cardiac muscle and the great arteries. (From Rushmer RF. Cardiovascular dynamics. 3rd ed. Philadelphia: WB Saunders, 1970.)

outpouchings called *sinuses of Valsalva*. The ostia for the right and left coronary arteries are located in the anterior two sinuses of Valsalva in the aorta.

The mitral and tricuspid valves are more complex structures. The proximal ends of these valves are attached to the annuli fibrosi of the fibrous skeleton, while the distal ends are connected to papillary muscles by fibrous strands called *chordae tendineae* (Fig. 2.4) (1). The tricuspid valve has three leaflets of unequal size; the mitral valve has two leaflets, also of unequal size.

Normal function of the mitral and tricuspid valves requires the intricate interaction of six anatomic structures: the atrial wall, the annuli fibrosi, the valvular tissue, the chordae tendineae, the papillary muscles, and the ventricular wall. Abnormalities of one or more of these components can lead to valvular regurgitation during ventricular systole. For example, in mitral valve prolapse, which affects approximately 6% of the general population, there is myxomatous degeneration of the valve leaflets resulting in their prolapse into the left atrium during ventricular systole. Depending on the severity of the degenerative

19

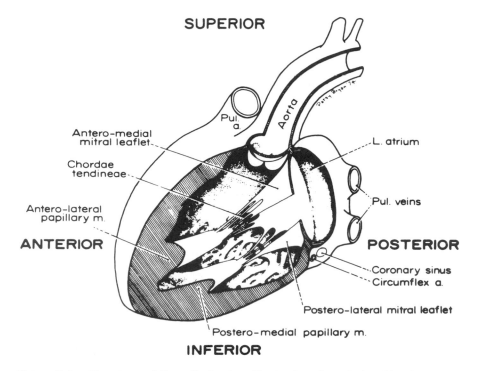

Figure 2.4. Structure of the mitral valve, illustrating the relationships between the papillary muscles, chordae tendineae, and the valve leaflets. (From Hurst JW, ed. The heart. 6th ed. New York: McGraw-Hill, 1986.)

process, there may or may not be concurrent valvular regurgitation. In contrast, mitral regurgitation may occur in coronary artery disease when the papillary muscles become ischemic or infarcted. Finally, in bacterial endocarditis, mitral regurgitation may occur if the chordae tendineae rupture as a result of the infectious process.

The mechanical activities of the heart are initiated and coordinated by an intrinsic electrical system called the *specialized conduction system* located within the chambers of the heart (Fig. 2.5) (6). Spontaneously derived electrical impulses originate in a region of pacemaker cells, the *sinoatrial (SA) node*, located at the junction of the superior vena cava and the right atrium. Electrical impulses in the SA node initiate wavefronts of electrical activation that spread through the atrial musculature to trigger atrial contractions. Poorly defined internodal tracts in the right atrium preferentially conduct the electrical signals to the *atrioventricular (AV) node* located in the AV junction in close proximity to the medial leaflet of the tricuspid valve. The electrical impulses conduct slowly through the AV node to allow time for atrial contraction to contribute to ventricular filling. Distal to the AV node is the *common bundle of His*, which divides into *right and left bundle branches* located in the right and left ventricles, respec-

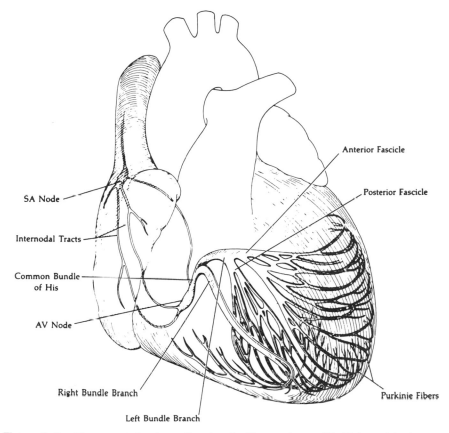

SA Node

Internodal Tracts

Common Bundle
of His

AV Node

Right Bundle Branch

Left Bundle Branch

Anterior Fascicle

Posterior Fascicle

Purkinje Fibers

Figure 2.5. The specialized cardiac conduction system. *AV*, Atrioventricular; *SA*, sinoatrial. (From Scientific American Medicine, Section 1, Subsection VI. © 1987 Scientific American, Inc. All rights reserved.)

tively. The left bundle branch further splits into an *anterior* and *posterior fascicle* before terminating in a complex network of specialized conducting cells called *Purkinje fibers*, which rapidly conduct the electrical impulses to all regions of the left ventricle. The right bundle branch terminates in a similar network of Purkinje fibers in the right ventricle. Electrical activity spreads from the endocardial surfaces of the ventricles to the epicardial surface and from apex to base to initiate an organized sequence of ventricular contraction. The sequence of electrical activation and the subsequent recovery of electrical activity in the myocardium can be recorded on the body surface as the electrocardiogram (ECG). Clinical aspects of electrocardiography are discussed in Chapter 3.

The heart is richly innervated by the sympathetic and parasympathetic divisions of the autonomic nervous system. Postganglionic sympathetic fibers originate in ganglia located along the right and left cervical sympathetic chains. Beta-1 sympathetic receptors are found in the atria, ventricles, and specialized

21

conduction system. Sympathetic stimulation of the heart results in increased contractility (*inotropic* effect), increased heart rate (*chronotropic* effect), and increased conduction velocity (*dromotropic* effect). Parasympathetic fibers travel in the right and left vagus nerves and are primarily distributed to the atria, the SA node, and the AV node. Parasympathetic activation results in slowing of the heart rate and AV conduction and in decreased contractile force in the atria. Sensory afferent fibers conduct from various locations in the heart back to the central nervous system. These fibers are activated under a variety of conditions, including distention of heart chambers and myocardial ischemia. They also mediate the sensations of chest discomfort caused by myocardial ischemia (angina pectoris) and infarction.

Systemic Circulation

The systemic or peripheral circulation distributes the output of the left ventricle to the cells and tissues of the body to maintain a biochemical environment for bodily functions at rest and during exercise (Fig. 2.1). Beginning with the *aorta*, the thick, muscular arteries transport oxygen-rich blood under high pressure to the various tissues and organ systems. The *arterioles*, or terminal muscular branches of the arteries, are the resistance vessels that serve as control valves regulating blood flow into various capillary beds depending on need. These arterioles are under the complex control of the autonomic nervous system, circulating hormones, and local chemical substances. An exchange of fluids, nutrients, oxygen, carbon dioxide, and regulatory substances between the interstitial space of tissues and the blood occurs in the *capillaries*, which are just distal to the arterioles. These are thin-walled tubules with pores through which substances can diffuse in both directions depending on chemical and hydrostatic gradients. Similar exchanges occur between the interstitial spaces and the cells. The *venules* begin at the distal end of the capillaries and join together to form veins that transport blood back to the heart under low pressure. The venous drainage from the various organ systems in the body empty into the *inferior and superior vena cavae*, which terminate in the right atrium (Fig. 2.2).

CORONARY CIRCULATION

The coronary circulation is an important component of the systemic circulation that is particularly relevant to workers in cardiac rehabilitation and preventive cardiology. The right and left *coronary arteries* (Fig. 2.6) originate from the ascending aorta immediately above the two anterior cusps of the aortic valve (7). The right coronary artery runs in the groove between the right atrium and right ventricle with branches to the right atrium and the anterior right ventriclar wall. In approximately 90% of individuals, the right coronary artery also provides the blood supply to the AV node, the posterior third of the interventricular septum, and the posterior walls of both ventricles. These individuals are defined as

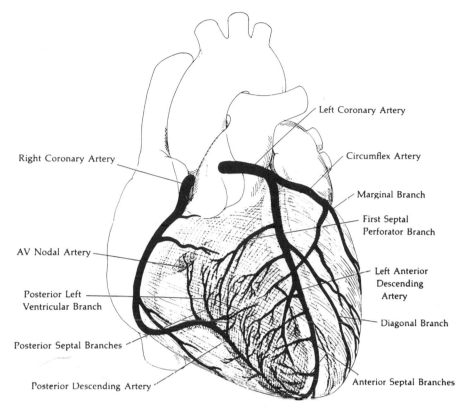

Left Coronary Artery

Circumflex Artery

Marginal Branch

First Septal
Perforator Branch

Left Anterior
Descending
Artery

Diagonal Branch

Anterior Septal Branches

Right Coronary Artery

AV Nodal Artery

Posterior Left
Ventricular Branch

Posterior Septal Branches

Posterior Descending Artery

Figure 2.6. The coronary circulation. (From Scientific American Medicine, Section 1, Subsection IX. © 1987 Scientific American, Inc. All rights reserved.)

having a *right dominant* coronary circulation (Fig. 2.6). The left coronary artery has a short *left main* segment before bifurcating into a *left anterior descending* artery, which runs in the anterior groove between the ventricles, and a *left circumflex* artery, which travels in the groove between the left atrium and left ventricle. In subjects with a right dominant circulation the circumflex artery and its branches are limited to the lateral left ventricular wall (Fig. 2.6). Approximately 10% of individuals, however, have a *left dominant* coronary circulation with a large left circumflex artery, which travels posteriorly between the left atrium and left ventricle supplying the AV node, the posterior interventricular septum, and the posterior walls of both ventricles. The anterior two-thirds of the septum, the right bundle branch, and the anterior division of the left bundle branch are supplied by septal perforating branches of the left anterior descending coronary artery.

PULMONARY CIRCULATION

The function of the pulmonary circulation is to provide a mechanism for gas exchange between the blood and the external environment. The pulmonary circulation is part of the respiratory system, which also includes the lungs and the skeletal muscles of respiration. The main pulmonary artery bifurcates into a right and left pulmonary artery branch to supply the right and left lung, respectively. These branches continue to divide providing smaller and smaller branches to all segments of the lungs. The volume of blood flowing through the lungs from the right heart is comparable to that in the systemic circulation. Unlike the systemic circulation, however, the pulmonary circulation is a low-pressure, low-resistance system with thin muscular walls and more distensible arteries than their systemic counterparts. This enables a high-volume pulmonary blood flow through the lungs with right ventricular systolic pressures that are only one-fourth that generated by the left ventricle. Oxygen uptake and carbon dioxide release take place in the pulmonary capillaries, which are adjacent to the terminal air sacs, the *alveoli*. At the distal end the pulmonary capillaries coalesce to form the pulmonary venuoles and veins, which join together to form two major pulmonary veins from each lung emptying into the left atrium.

Pathogenesis of Atherosclerosis

Atherosclerosis is the leading cause of death and disability in the Western world and accounts for the largest proportion of our health care expenditures (8). It is unfortunate that the financial burden of atherosclerosis is disproportionately spent during the final stages of the disease spectrum when patients are suffering from the complications of far advanced disease. There is now ample evidence that the complications of atherosclerotic diseases can be prevented by careful attention to lifestyle and risk factors (9). An understanding of the origins and mechanisms of this disease, therefore, is a necessary prerequisite for physicians and other health care professionals working in health promotion, preventive medicine, and cardiac rehabilitation. Although it is beyond the scope of this chapter to review in detail the complex mechanisms of atherosclerosis, many of which are only partially understood, a brief discussion of these processes is presented to acquaint the reader with potential targets for preventive action.

Figure 2.7 illustrates the fundamental lesion of atherosclerosis, the atherosclerotic plaque or *atheroma*, as it evolves in medium-sized blood vessels such as the coronary arteries, the carotid arteries, the renal arteries, and the arteries of the lower extremities (10). Atherosclerotic narrowing or occlusions in these different circulations can result in serious impairments in function, including myocardial infarction, stroke, hypertension, renal failure, and claudication.

The structure of the normal arterial wall is shown in Figure 2.7A, illustrating three morphologically distinct layers. The inner layer, or *intima*, consists of a

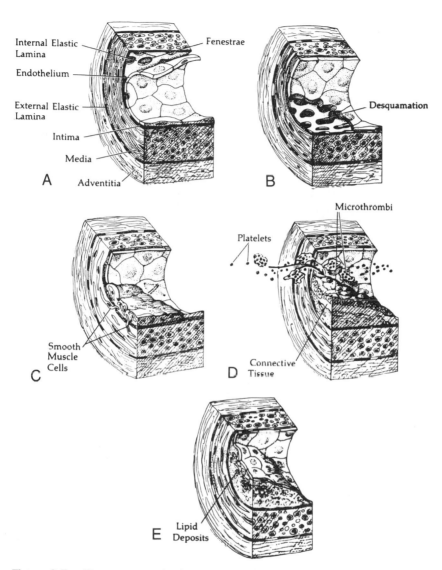

Figure 2.7. The process of atherogenesis. **A.** The structure of the normal artery. Endothelial injury is the primary stimulus leading to **(B)** desquamation and **(C)** smooth muscle cell migration and proliferation. **D.** Platelets adhere to the injured endothelium, releasing vasoconstrictive and thrombogenic substances. **E.** Lipid deposits, primarily LDL-cholesterol, accumulate in the lesions. (From Ross R, Glomset JA. The pathogenesis of arteriosclerosis. N Engl J Med 1976;295:369–420, 1976.)

single lining of endothelial cells bound to the middle muscular layer, the *media*, by the *internal elastic lamina*. The media, the largest component of the vessel wall, is made up of smooth muscle fibers and varies in thickness depending on the size of the artery. The outer layer of loose connective tissues is called the *adventitia* and provides protective and nutritive functions for the artery.

The development of the atherosclerotic plaque is illustrated in Figure 2.7, *B–E* and diagrammed in Figure 2.8 (11). The lesion primarily involves the intimal layer of the artery. From hypercholesterolemic animal studies it has been shown that the earliest lesion, the *fatty streak*, begins when circulating monocytes attach themselves to the surface of "injured" arterial endothelium

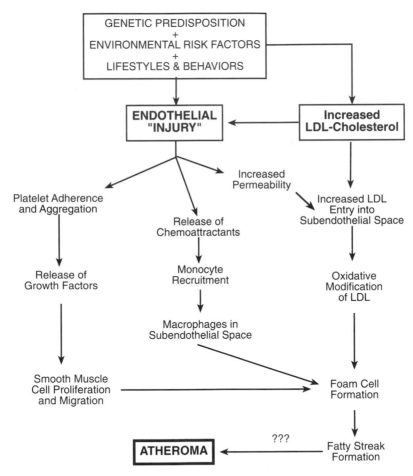

Figure 2.8. The process of atherosclerosis: interaction of circulating LDL-cholesterol with injured endothelial cells, monocyte/macrophages, and platelets in the evolution of the atherosclerotic plaque. (Adapted from Yanowitz FG. Atherosclerosis: process versus origins. In: Yanowitz FG, ed. Coronary heart disease prevention. New York: Marcel Dekker, 1992.)

and then migrate into the subendothelial space to establish residency as macrophages or phagocytic cells (3, 11). Various chemoattractants and growth factors produced by the injured endothelial cells are responsible for monocyte recruitment and also for causing smooth muscle cell proliferation and migration. Increased levels of circulating, low-density, lipoprotein cholesterol (LDL-C) are thought to be a source of endothelial injury. In response to injury the LDL molecules are oxidatively modified by the endothelial cells and rapidly taken up in the subendothelial space by macrophages and smooth muscle cells to become *foam cells* (12). Oxidative forms of LDL and foam cells are toxic to the tissues and lead to fatty streak formation, the initial lesion of atherosclerosis.

Although fatty streaks are ubiquitous in growing children, only some of these early lesions eventually evolve to become mature fibrous plaques or *atheroma*. It is likely that, as a result of recurrent endothelial injury in the presence of increased circulating LDL-C, the influx of oxidized LDL molecules into the subendothelial space exceeds the capacity of macrophages to remove them. The cytotoxic effects of these atherogenic particles in the interstitium lead to tissue destruction and the accumulation of more lipid and necrotic debris to form the atheromatous lesion. The atheroma is a raised lesion protruding into the lumen of the blood vessel and covered by a fibrous cap. At this stage, blood platelets are likely to become involved in plaque formation (Fig. 2.7D), as continued endothelial injury permits a direct interaction of circulating blood components and platelets with the subendothelial connective tissue. Under the appropriate atherogenic conditions the injured endothelial cells facilitate the disease process by attracting additional platelets, monocytes, and smooth muscle cells to participate in a proliferative response leading to lesion growth and narrowing of the vessel lumen.

It is only during the final phase of atherosclerosis that the atheromatous lesion reaches a critical size to significantly reduce coronary blood flow and cause the onset of clinical coronary disease manifestations. At least four scenarios can be envisioned that account for the major clinical syndromes of coronary heart disease (Fig. 2.9). In the first scenario the lesion slowly grows until symptoms of *angina pectoris* first appear and evolve into a stable clinical pattern. In stable angina pectoris, symptoms of chest discomfort arise only during periods of increased heart work, usually brought on by exercise or emotional stress. When stable, these symptoms are predictable and are relieved as soon as the work of the heart is reduced either by rest or by administration of a rapid-acting nitroglycerin preparation. The clinical recognition of angina pectoris is discussed further in Chapter 3.

The other three scenarios lead to the unstable coronary syndromes: *unstable angina, acute myocardial infarction*, and *sudden cardiac death*. All three of these acute syndromes are thought to arise from unstable or damaged atherosclerotic plaques. The initial event in each of these syndromes is a rupturing or fissuring

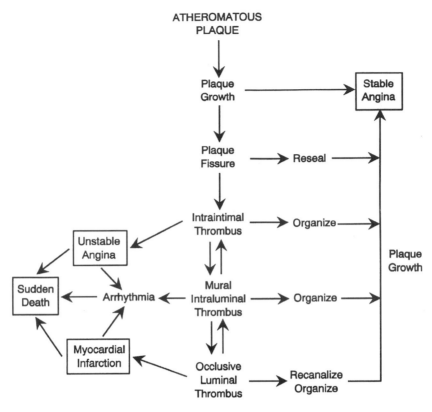

Figure 2.9. The pathogenesis of the coronary heart disease syndromes: stable angina pectoris, unstable angina, acute myocardial infarction, and sudden cardiac death. (Adapted from Davies MJ, Thomas AC. Br Heart J 1985;53:363–373.)

of the fibrous cap overlying the atheroma, often precipitated by hemodynamic stressors in the blood or spasm of the coronary artery wall (13). When this occurs, the contents of the lipid-rich plaque come in contact with circulating blood components, which results in acute thrombus formation. The fate of this fresh thrombus ultimately determines the subsequent clinical course (Fig. 2.9). If the thrombus is small, it may be dissolved by the body's own fibrinolytic processes or incorporated into the lesion. This leads to lesion growth with or without the appearance of clinical symptoms. Larger thrombotic occlusions may only partially resolve and then recur in a waxing and waning clinical picture, often accompanied by unstable anginal symptoms (new onset angina, accelerating angina, or angina at rest). A thrombus that totally occludes the vessel lumen is the most common cause of acute myocardial infarction. The complete absence of blood flow to a segment of myocardium leads to tissue necrosis and cell death. Finally, if a portion of the fresh thrombus breaks off and embolizes distally, it

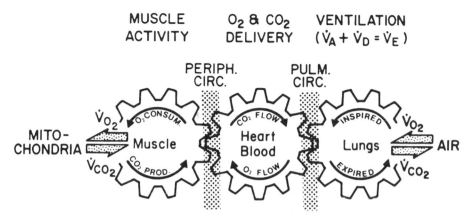

Figure 2.10. Homeostatic gas exchange between the outside environment and the skeletal muscle mitochondria. (From Wasserman K et al. Principles of exercise testing and interpretation. Philadelphia: Lea & Febiger, 1987.)

can lead to sudden electrical instability and cause ventricular tachycardia, ventricular fibrillation, and sudden death.

THE PHYSIOLOGY OF EXERCISE

The successful performance of endurance exercise requires the coordinated interaction of three major organ systems: (a) the skeletal muscles, (b) the cardiovascular system, and (c) the respiratory system. As illustrated in Figure 2.10, these three systems are closely coupled to provide homeostatic gas exchange (i.e., oxygen and carbon dioxide) between the external environment and the working muscle fibers (14). During exercise each system adjusts its function on a moment-to-moment basis, according to the metabolic needs of the body, primarily those of the exercising skeletal muscles. In addition to this acute response to exercise, the body also adapts to repeated exercise activities over a period of weeks and months to become *conditioned*.

It is important to appreciate that a disturbance or breakdown within one or more of these organ systems may result in exercise intolerance. The workup for suspected disability or limited exercise tolerance often requires a comprehensive assessment of all three organ systems to determine the specific mechanisms responsible for the patient's impairment. In the following sections the physiology of exercise is reviewed, beginning with skeletal muscle structure and function and, in turn, considering the cardiovascular and respiratory systems.

Skeletal Muscle Structure and Function

The contraction and relaxation of skeletal muscles provide the basis for all physical activities. Although an understanding of the structural and biochemical mechanisms for these processes is still incomplete, the significant contributions of H.E. Huxley (15, 16) and A.F. Huxley (17) and their coworkers have greatly expanded our knowledge of these complex phenomena. Only a brief and simplified description of skeletal muscle is presented here; a more detailed discussion can be found in several excellent textbooks (18, 19).

Figure 2.11 presents a schematic diagram of the intracellular structure of a skeletal muscle fiber (20). Voluntary muscle contractions are under the control of the central nervous system. Electrical impulses arriving at the myoneural junctions initiate the release of stored calcium ions, Ca^{++}, from the sarcoplasmic reticulum, an elaborate network of tubular sacs, vesicles, and channels surrounding the myofibrils. The Ca^{++} ions, in turn, trigger a chemical interaction between the thin actin and thick myosin filaments within the myofibrils. According to the *sliding-filament* or *cross-bridge theory* (19), muscle contraction and shortening occurs when the thin actin filaments, which are attached to the

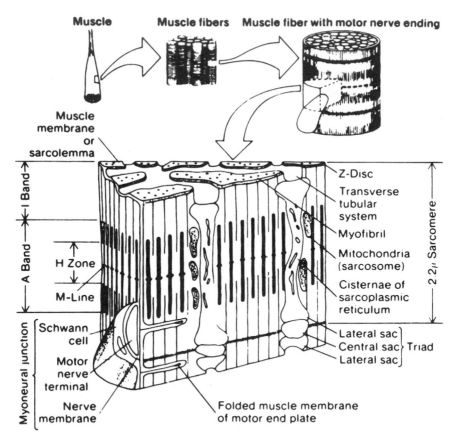

Figure 2.11. The intracellular structure of skeletal muscle. (From Carlson FD, Wilkie DR. Muscle physiology. Englewood Cliffs, NJ: Prentice-Hall, 1974.)

30

Z-disk (Fig. 2.11), are pulled inward by the sequential chemical interactions with myosin cross bridges. In an isometric contraction there is no change in muscle length, although tension is generated as actin reacts chemically with the myosin cross bridges.

The mechanical events responsible for muscle shortening and tension development require a continuous source of chemical energy in the form of high-energy phosphate compounds (19). The most important of these compounds, adenosinetriphosphate (ATP), releases energy when the phosphate bonds are broken during a series of reactions called *hydrolysis* (ADP, adenosinediphosphate; AMP, adenosine-monophosphate):

$$ATP + H_2O \rightarrow ADP + P + energy$$

$$ADP + H_2O \rightarrow AMP + P + energy$$

The free energy liberated in these reactions is used by the cells for muscle contraction and a variety of other biologic processes requiring energy.

In the muscle fibers ATP molecules are continuously resynthesized by several important chemical reactions. An immediate reservoir of high-energy phosphate compounds is available in the form of phosphocreatine (CP), which is in equilibrium with ATP and creatine (C) as indicated by the following reaction:

$$ADP + CP \leftrightarrow ATP + C$$

For sustained skeletal muscle work, however, an adequate supply of ATP can be provided by the oxidation of foodstuffs consumed in the diet or stored in the body as glycogen and triglycerides. The chemical reactions involved in the oxidation of glucose, glycogen, and fatty acids are part of a process called *oxidative phosphorylation* (18).

As indicated in Figure 2.12 (18), the main energy-yielding fuels for the resynthesis of ATP are carbohydrates (muscle glycogen, blood glucose) and fatty acids from stored triglycerides in the adipose tissue. In the resting state muscle tissue obtains virtually all of its fuel from circulating fatty acids. During the first several minutes of exercise, stored glycogen in the muscle is utilized for fuel. With continuous exercise, however, bloodborne fuels from glucose and fatty acids become increasingly important sources of energy for muscle contraction. Except in starvation states, proteins contribute very little to the total energy expenditure of working muscle fibers.

Oxidative phosphorylation involves an initial anaerobic sequence of reactions that take place in the cytoplasm of the muscle fibers. During this phase glycogen and glucose are metabolized to pyruvic acid by a process called *glycolysis*, yielding three moles of ATP for every glucose molecule in glycogen or two moles of ATP for every glucose molecule entering directly from the blood. The availability of oxygen enables pyruvic acid to enter the more productive aerobic phase of oxidative phosphorylation, which takes place in the

31

Figure 2.12. Anaerobic and aerobic metabolism (oxidative phosphorylation). Anaerobic metabolism takes place in the cytoplasm of the muscle cell where carbohydrates are metabolized to pyruvic acid by a process called glycolysis in the absence of oxygen. Lactic acid is the end product of anaerobic metabolism. Aerobic metabolism occurs in the mitochondria where the end products are CO_2 and water. (Adapted from Astrand P, Rodahl K. Textbook of work physiology. 2nd ed. New York: McGraw-Hill, 1977.)

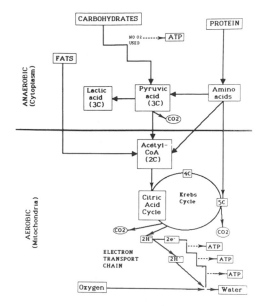

mitochondria. Initially, pyruvic acid is oxidized to acetyl-CoA, which is also the first step in the metabolism of fatty acids. Acetyl-CoA subsequently enters into a cyclic series of reactions called the *Krebs* or *citric acid cycle* (18, 19), yielding carbon dioxide and hydrogen. Electrons from hydrogen are transported down an electron-transport chain, releasing energy for the phosphorylation of ADP to ATP. At the end of the chain, the electrons are recombined with hydrogen ions and oxygen to form water. A total of 36 ATP molecules per glucose molecule are synthesized in the mitochondria during aerobic oxidation.

During muscle relaxation newly synthesized ATP molecules are taken up by the myosin filaments resulting in their detachment from actin and the subsequent release of tension in the muscle fibers. The Ca^{++} ions are actively pumped back into the sarcoplasmic reticulum; this turns off the chemical interactions between actin and myosin cross bridges and allows the actin and myosin filaments to return to their original position.

Skeletal muscle fibers in humans are predominately *twitch-type*, which refers to their ability to respond to nerve stimulation with fast shortening or tension development. Three distinct subclasses of twitch-type fibers have been described that have different metabolic and contractile properties (19, 21). *Slow fatigue-resistant* fibers, also known as type I or slow-twitch fibers, have highly developed oxidative enzyme systems and are rich in mitochondria and myoglobin. The myoglobin content makes the muscle fibers red in color. The contractile response of these fibers is slow, but they are well suited for prolonged aerobic exercise activities. *Fast fatigable* fibers, also known as type II or fast-twitch fibers, are better designed for strength (isometric) and brief bursts of high-speed activity. These fibers have a low myoglobin content (white color) and a well-developed glycolytic enzyme system with a small mitochondrial content and oxidative activity. They have a fast contractile response and fatigue rapidly. *Fast fatigue-resistant* fibers have an intermediate glycolytic enzyme system, large mitochondrial content, and high myoglobin content. The skeletal muscles in humans contain a mixture of these fiber types in varying percentages depending on the function of the particular muscles and whether they are trained. It is also possible that specific types of chronic exercise training may result in an actual transformation from one fiber type to the other (21). For the most part, however, the proportions of the three fiber subtypes are genetically determined for each individual (21).

Physiologic Aspects of Exercise

AEROBIC PARAMETERS

It is clear from the preceding discussion that there are two major metabolic requirements for sustained skeletal muscle work: (a) adequate gas exchange between the muscle fibers and the external environment (i.e., the delivery of O_2 and the removal of CO_2), and (b) the availability of combustible materials in the form of glycogen, glucose, and fatty acids (19). Since the ATP yield from aerobic metabolism is more than 10 times that provided by anaerobic glycolysis, the delivery of O_2 to working muscles becomes the single most important determinant of the maximal workload that can be achieved and sustained during exercise.

During dynamic, isotonic exercise, oxygen is taken in by the lungs and transported by the cardiovascular system in increasing amounts to the exercising skeletal muscles (Fig. 2.10). The carbon dioxide produced during aerobic metabolism is transported in the reverse direction and eliminated by the lungs. The *Fick equation* represents the relationship of parameters participating in this sequence of events. At rest the Fick equation for oxygen can be expressed as follows:

$$\dot{V}O_2 = \dot{Q} \times (CaO_2 - C\bar{v}O_2)$$

or

$$\dot{V}O_2 = (SV \times HR) \times (CaO_2 - C\bar{v}O_2)$$

Where $\dot{V}O_2$ is the oxygen uptake (ml O_2/min), $\dot{Q}$ is the cardiac output (L/min), SV is the stroke volume (L), HR is the heart rate (bpm), CaO_2 is the arterial O_2 content (ml O_2 per L of blood), and $C\bar{v}O_2$ is the mixed venous O_2 content. The combined term, $\dot{Q} \times CaO_2$, represents the quantity of oxygen transported to the tissues per minute. The term, $CaO_2 - C\bar{v}O_2$, is also called the a-v O_2 content difference and represents the amount of oxygen utilized by the tissues each minute. Oxygen uptake is often normalized for body weight and expressed in units of ml O_2/kg/min. One *metabolic equivalent* or 1 MET is the resting oxygen uptake in a sitting position and is approximately 3.5 ml O_2/kg/min.

Figure 2.13. Acute response to progressive exercise. The abscissa indicates the resting state and four incremental levels of exercise to maximal effort. Oxygen uptake increases linearly until reaching a plateau at maximal exercise. Heart rate also increases linearly to a maximal value of approximately "220 – age." Stroke volume increases only modestly during the first half of exercise and then levels off. The arteriovenous O_2 content difference widens from rest to maximal exercise. (Adapted from Mitchell JH, Blomqvist G. Maximal oxygen uptake. N Engl J Med 1971;284:1018–1023.)

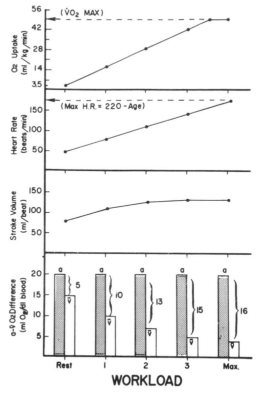

During an incremental exercise activity (e.g., a treadmill test) an increasing percentage of the oxygen uptake is redistributed to the exercising muscles until maximal exercise is reached (22). The Fick equation at maximal exercise,

$$\dot{V}O_{2max} = (SV_{max} \times HR_{max}) \times (CaO_{2max} - C\bar{v}O_{2min}),$$

reflects the maximal ability of the body to *take in, transport,* and *utilize* oxygen; this defines a person's *functional aerobic capacity*. $\dot{V}O_{2max}$ has become the "gold standard" laboratory measure of cardiorespiratory fitness and is the most important parameter measured during functional exercise testing (23). Techniques for measuring $\dot{V}O_{2max}$ are discussed in Chapter 5.

Figure 2-13 illustrates the changes in Fick equation parameters as a healthy person goes from rest to maximal exercise on a device such as a treadmill or cycle ergometer (23). Several important observations can be made from these relationships: (a) the $\dot{V}O_2$ response to exercise is linear until maximal $\dot{V}O_2$ is achieved; in many individuals there is a plateau at near-maximal exercise beyond which the $\dot{V}O_2$ does not change; (b) the SV response is curvilinear, increasing early in exercise with little change thereafter; (c) the heart rate response is linear up to a maximal heart rate that is approximately equal to "220 – age"; and (d) the a-v O_2 content difference widens as the mixed venous O_2 content decreases; arterial O_2 content does not change in normal subjects.

To illustrate further the parameters of the Fick equation as they change from rest to maximal exercise, Table 2.1 contrasts four hypothetical 30–year-old subjects: a world-class athlete, a trained normal, a sedentary normal, and a post-MI patient with mild congestive heart failure (CHF) (24). These four subjects are compared at rest, during submaximal exercise, and at maximal exercise. The data illustrate important differences between sedentary and trained persons, as well as the more serious functional consequences of congestive heart failure.

At rest all four subjects have the same $\dot{V}O_2$ (normalized for body weight), the same cardiac output, and the same a-v O_2 content difference and oxygen utilization. Major differences, however, are seen in the two components that determine cardiac output. The world-class athlete has the greatest stroke volume and slowest heart rate, while the other three subjects have progressively smaller stroke volumes and faster heart rates. End-diastolic volumes (EDV), end-systolic volumes (ESV), and ejection fractions (EF) also reflect these differences. The physiologic interpretation of these *central adaptations* to exercise training is that the resting cardiac output in trained individuals is more a function of a large stroke volume and is less dependent on heart rate. This implies an improved efficiency of cardiac work, since heart rate is a greater determinant of myocardial oxygen requirements than stroke volume. In sedentary individuals and in heart failure patients the lower stroke volumes necessitate higher rates and myocardial O_2 utilization to maintain the resting cardiac output. During submaximal exercise (e.g., 5 METS), the similarities and differences in Fick parameters measured in the four subjects are maintained (Table 2.1).

At maximal exercise significant differences are seen in all parameters of the Fick equation (Table 2.1). The wide range in $\dot{V}O_{2max}$ reflects the different maximal workloads achieved by each subject. Although heart rates are similar for the three normal subjects ($HR_{max} \approx 220 -$ age in years), the patient with CHF has a lower maximal heart rate for reasons that are not entirely clear. The stroke volumes are also significantly different at maximal exercise as are the maximal cardiac outputs and ejection fractions. Unlike the resting and submaximal exercise data, however, the maximal a-v O_2 content difference is greatest in the athlete and is progressively smaller in the other three subjects. These differences among normal subjects reflect the *peripheral adaptations* to exercise training. Increases in the number and size of skeletal muscle mitochondria, as well as in their aerobic enzyme content, are well-known training effects (25). In addition, exercise training results in a greater density of blood capillaries per unit mass of skeletal muscle. These changes enable aerobically trained individuals to extract and utilize more oxygen during exercise to achieve higher maximal workloads.

The post-MI patient with heart failure has an additional handicap during exercise that limits oxygen extraction by the muscle fibers and maximal widening of the a-v O_2 difference. Patients with heart failure appear to have an

35

TABLE 2.1. Four Hypothetical Cases: All Age 30 years

Resting Data

	VO_2 (ml/kg/min)	Heart Rate (BPM)	EDV (ml)	ESV (ml)	SV (ml)	Q (l/min)	CaO_2 (mlO$_2$/l)	CvO_2 (mlO$_2$/l)	a-v O_2D (mlO$_2$/l)	Q × CaO$_2$ (mlO$_2$/min)	O_2 extract (%)
World class	3.5	45	190	50	136	6.1	200	160	40	1220	20
Trained normal	3.5	55	160	54	110	6.1	200	160	40	1220	20
Sedentary normal	3.5	70	150	63	87	6.1	200	160	40	1220	20
Heart failure	3.5	90	160	92	68	6.1	200	160	40	1220	20

Submaximal Exercise at 5 METS

	VO_2 (ml/kg/min)	Heart Rate (BPM)	EDV (ml)	ESV (ml)	SV (ml)	Q (l/min)	CaO_2 (mlO$_2$/l)	CvO_2 (mlO$_2$/l)	a-v O_2D (mlO$_2$/l)	Q × CaO$_2$ (mlO$_2$/min)	O_2 extract (%)
World class	17.5	70	200	24	176	12.3	200	100	100	2460	50
Trained normal	17.5	90	170	33	137	12.3	200	100	100	2460	50
Sedentary normal	17.5	120	150	47	103	12.3	200	100	100	2460	50
Heart failure	17.5	160	160	83	77	12.3	200	100	100	2460	50

Table 2.1. Cont.

Maximal Exercise

	VO_2 (ml/kg/min)	Heart Rate (BPM)	EDV (ml)	ESV (ml)	SV (ml)	Q (l/min)	CaO_2 (mlO$_2$/l)	CvO_2 (mlO$_2$/l)	a-v O$_2$D (mlO$_2$/l)	Q×CaO$_2$ (mlO$_2$/min)	O$_2$ extract (%)
World class	80	190	200	16	184	35	200	40	160	7000	80
Trained normal	56	190	170	33	137	26.1	200	50	150	5220	75
Sedentary normal	35	190	150	57	93	17.7	200	60	140	3500	70
Heart failure	21	175	170	93	77	13.5	200	90	110	2680	60

EDV, End-diastolic volume; *ESV*, end-systolic volume; *SV*, stroke volume; *Q*, cardiac output; *CaO₂*, arterial O₂ content; *CvO₂*, mixed venous O₂ content; *a-v O₂D*, arterial-venous O₂ content difference.

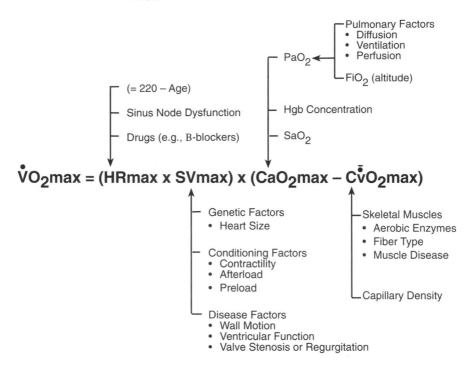

Figure 2.14. The Fick equation at maximal exercise and the determinants of maximal oxygen consumption. (Adapted from Yanowitz FG. CARDIO April 1993, pp. 56–64.)

impaired ability to maximally vasodilate during exercise, presumably because edema in the arteriolar wall limits the response to vasodilatory stimuli (26). As a result oxygen extraction and utilization is further compromised in these patients.

Figure 2.14 summarizes the various factors that have both positive and negative effects on the Fick equation parameters that determine $\dot{V}O_{2max}$ (24). In particular, functional aerobic impairment, or an abnormally low $\dot{V}O_{2max}$, can result from any factor or combination of factors that reduces maximal heart rate, maximal stroke volume, maximal arterial O_2 content, or maximal a-v O_2 content difference. A brief review of these parameters further illustrates the multitude of factors that may result in exercise intolerance.

HEART RATE RESPONSE TO EXERCISE

The heart rate is determined by the rate of discharge of the pacemaker cells in the SA node. Although pacemaker cells have an intrinsic frequency of impulse formation, the heart rate at any given moment is under extrinsic controls, including the autonomic nervous system, circulating catecholamines, and other biochemical substances produced in the body or administered as drugs and other chemicals. At rest the heart rate is normally betwen 50 and 90 beats per minute (bpm) and is predominately under the influence of the parasympathetic nervous system (right and left vagus nerves). During physical activities (Fig. 2.13) or emotional stress the heart rate increases as a result of withdrawal of parasympathetic tone, increases in sympathetic tone, and increases in circulating catecholamines. Although, as stated previously, the maximal rate of SA nodal discharge is approximately "220 – age," there is considerable variation in maximal heart rate among individuals of the same age (standard deviation = ±10 bpm) (18). Assuming all other parameters of the Fick equation remain unchanged, $\dot{V}O_{2max}$ will decline with age in proportion to the decline in maximal heart rate.

Several disease-related and drug-induced states can affect pacemaker activity in the SA node and further limit the heart rate response to exercise. Ellestad (27) has coined the term *chronotropic incompetence* to indicate an abnormally low heart rate maximum defined as below the 95th percent confidence limits for the age-determined normal values. This may be caused by coronary artery disease or other diseases involving the SA node. Atrioventricular nodal heart block may also limit the ventricular response to exercise by blocking some or all of the SA nodal impulses from reaching the ventricles. Finally, drugs used in the treatment of heart disease and hypertension, including the beta blockers and some of the calcium-channel blockers, can have a profound effect on exercise heart rates and exercise tolerance.

STROKE VOLUME RESPONSE TO EXERCISE

The stroke volume is the volume of blood ejected from the right and left ventricles during ventricular systole. It is a complex function depending on at least three different hemodynamic parameters: (a) preload, (b) afterload, and (c) inotropic state or contractility of ventricular muscle (28). In patients with previous myocardial infarctions, regional ventricular wall-motion abnormalities may further compromise the stroke volume response to exercise.

The *preload* represents the passive filling characteristics of ventricular muscle during diastole that determine the end-diastolic fiber length just prior to ventricular systole. Ventricular filling occurs in three phases. Early rapid filling takes place as soon as the AV valves open at the beginning of diastole when pressures in the atria exceed the ventricular pressures. In mid-diastole there is a second, slower phase of filling that is limited by the compliance characteristics of the ventricular muscle. Filling during this phase may be impaired by diseases that increase the stiffness of ventricular muscle such as occurs in coronary disease and conditions associated with ventricular hypertrophy. In late diastole there is a third component of filling resulting from atrial systole. This important contribution to ventricular filling is lost in atrial fibrillation, which may account for some of the symptoms associated with this common arrhythmia.

According to the *Frank-Starling Law of the Heart* (28), the greater the end-diastolic fiber length (or end-diastolic ventricular volume), the greater the contractile force of the subsequent ventricular contraction and the resultant stroke volume. A similar relationship exists between end-diastolic pressure and stroke volume, since ventricular filling pressures are related to both the diastolic fiber length and the compliance of the ventricular muscle. In the normal heart there is a near linear increase in stroke volume as end-diastolic volumes increase. One of the adaptive mechanisms that enable young athletes to generate enormous stroke volumes at rest and during exercise is enlargement of the ventricles ("the athlete's heart"), which increases preload and, by the Frank-Starling Law, the stroke volume. In congestive heart failure the ventricles also dilate in an attempt to take advantage of the larger preloads, but the weakened myocardium often defeats this compensatory mechanism and a vicious circle of declining cardiac function often results.

The *afterload* is a measure of the resistance against which the ventricles contract during systole. In the left ventricle this resistance is determined by several different factors, including the systemic vascular resistance, the stiffness of the aortic wall, the mass of blood in the systemic circulation, and the blood viscosity. The afterload affects the rate of ventricular contraction and the extent to which the ventricles empty with each contraction (i.e., end-systolic volume). Increases in stroke volume occur when the afterload is reduced, usually the result of factors that decrease systemic vascular resistance. When this occurs, there is more complete emptying of the ventricles during systole. To some extent the increase in stroke volume during exercise is the result of a decrease in the systemic vascular resistance caused by vasodilation within the exercising skeletal muscles. The treatment of congestive heart failure with vasodilating drugs (e.g., angiotensin-converting enzyme inhibitors) is another example of afterload reduction to enhance stroke volume and cardiac output.

The *inotropic state* or contractility is determined by the intrinsic contractile state of the myocardium, as well as by extrinsic inotropic stimuli from cardiac sympathetic nerves, circulating catecholamines, and in some patients, pharmacologic agents such as digitalis glycosides. The increase in stroke volume resulting from these factors is caused by an increase in the velocity of fiber shortening and more complete emptying of the ventricles. During exercise contractility is increased as a result of increases in sympathetic tone and circulating catecholamines.

The *ejection fraction* is a function that reflects all three parameters affecting stroke volume and is a clinically useful measure of global ventricular function. Conceptually it represents the fraction of blood ejected by the ventricles during each systole and is equal to the stroke volume divided by the end-diastolic volume. Clinically, this measurement is obtained by cine-nuclear or ultrasonic imaging of the ventricle during the cardiac cycle. Normally the ventricles eject 60 to 70% of the blood they receive. The ejection fraction is often reduced in heart disease as a result of decreases in contractility and/or increases in systemic vascular resistance (e.g., hypertension).

ARTERIAL OXYGEN CONTENT

The third important determinant of $\dot{V}O_{2max}$ in the Fick equation is the arterial oxygen content (CaO_2). At maximal exercise the quantity of oxygen delivered to the tissues each minute is calculated as the product of blood flow and arterial O_2 content:

$$\text{Max } O_2 \text{ transport (ml } O_2/\text{min)} = (\text{max HR} \times \text{max SV}) \times \text{max } CaO_2.$$

The oxygen content of arterial blood is a complex function that depends on (a) the arterial partial pressure of oxygen (PaO_2), (b) the hemoglobin concentration (g/100 ml), and (c) the affinity of hemoglobin for oxygen (29). Disturbances in one or more of these factors may significantly limit oxygen transport to the tissues and, in turn, reduce exercise tolerance.

PaO_2 is a function of several additional parameters, the first being the concentration of oxygen in the inspired air. Although the *fraction* of oxygen in the air is always 21%, the oxygen tension or partial pressure (PIO_2) falls with increasing altitude in proportion to the fall in barometric pressure (PB) according to the following equation:

$$PIO_2 = (PB - 47) \times 0.21$$

where 47 is the vapor pressure (mm Hg) of water at normal body temperature. As a result the concentration of oxygen in the inspired air, reflected by PIO_2, becomes significantly reduced when one goes from sea level to high altitude (Fig. 2.15). Individuals living at sea level often find significant exercise intolerance when traveling to altitudes above 5000 feet.

From the inspired air to the tissues and cells of the body, the oxygen tension or PO_2 drops in a series of steps called the *oxygen cascade*. The initial fall in PO_2 from inspired air to pulmonary alveoli ($PIO_2 - PAO_2$) is a function of the magnitude of pulmonary ventilation. The alveolar oxygen partial pressure, PAO_2, is calculated from PIO_2, $PaCO_2$, and the respiratory exchange ration (R), which is the ratio of CO_2 output to O_2 uptake ($\dot{V}CO_2/\dot{V}O_2$), according to the following equation:

$$PAO_2 - PIO_2 + PaCO_2/R$$

The importance of this relationship becomes apparent when considering the acute adaptations to high altitude. The reduced ambient oxygen pressure illustrated in Figure 2.15 at high altitude causes a stepwise reduction of PAO_2 and PaO_2. The fall in PaO_2 reduces the quantity of arterial oxygen (hypoxemia), which in turn stimulates increased ventilation via the carotid body chemoreceptors. This results in a decreased $PaCO_2$, an increase in the respiratory exchange ratio (i.e., CO_2 output), and from the preceding equation, an increase in PAO_2. This feedback mechanism compensates for the initial fall in PaO_2 by decreasing the drop in PO_2 from inspired air to alveoli.

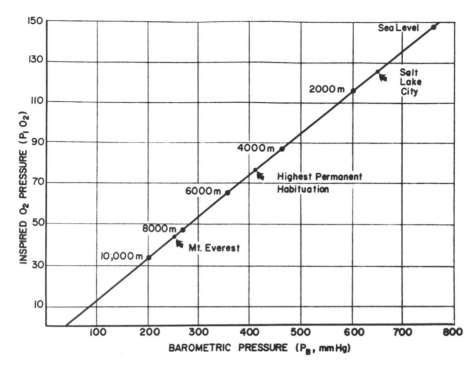

Figure 2.15. The effects of altitude on barometric pressure and inspired O_2 pressure.

The second step in the oxygen cascade is the drop in PO_2 from alveolar air to arterial blood, called the A-a PO_2 gradient. To a large extent this gradient reflects the adequacy of gas exchange in the lungs. In normal lungs where ventilation and perfusion are well matched and where diffusion across the air-blood barrier is not impaired, the A-a gradient ranges from 12 to 20 mm Hg. Factors that increase the A-a gradient and thereby reduce PaO_2 include right-to-left vascular shunts either in the lungs or the heart, ventilation-perfusion mismatch abnormalities found in various pulmonary parenchymal and vascular diseases, and possibly diseases that primarily affect diffusion across the alveolar-capillary membrane. The end result of these pathophysiologic disturbances is a reduction in PaO_2 (arterial hypoxemia).

The third step in the oxygen cascade concerns the actual mechanism by which O_2 is carried in the arterial blood (30). Oxygen molecules entering the pulmonary capillary blood quickly diffuse into red blood cells and chemically combine with reduced hemoglobin to form oxyhemoglobin. Since each gram of hemoglobin (Hb) can combine with 1.34 ml O_2, the oxygen-carrying capacity of arterial blood can be computed as follows:

$$O_2 \text{ capacity (ml } O_2/100 \text{ ml) = [Hb](g/100ml)} \times 1.34$$

In normal individuals with approximately 15 g of hemoglobin per 100 ml of blood, the O_2 capacity is 20 ml/100 ml, or 20 vol%.

Not all of the O_2 molecules entering the pulmonary capillary blood are able to combine with hemoglobin. The reversible chemical interaction between oxygen and hemoglobin is defined by the oxygen-hemoglobin dissociation curve, which is illustrated in Figure 2.16. A family of curves depending on pH, temperature, and other factors represent relationships between the partial pressures of O_2 (x-axis) and the percent hemoglobin saturation (So_2, y-axis). At sea level, for example, where the PaO_2 is approximately 100 mm Hg, the arterial oxygen saturation, SaO_2, is 97.5%, assuming normal body temperature of 37°C, pH 7.40. The curve's flat upper portion is physiologically advantageous, allowing high oxygen saturation to remain, despite falling arterial PO_2 values. The steep middle segment permits large quantities of O_2 to be released in the peripheral capillaries, where PO_2 values are much lower, enabling oxygen to diffuse into the cells and tissues of the body.

The affinity of hemoglobin for oxygen is conveniently defined by the $P50$, which represents the PO_2 value where hemoglobin oxygen saturation is 50%. Normally, the $P50$ is 26.6 mm Hg (curve A, Fig. 2.16). The oxygen affinity of hemoglobin is strongly influenced by a number of factors, including body temperature, hydrogen ion concentration (pH), carbon monoxide exposure, and abnormal hemoglobin molecules. Decreased body temperature, increased pH, and carbon monoxide exposure all shift the curve to the left (curve B, Fig. 2.16), enabling more oxygen to be bound to hemoglobin in the lungs but making it more difficult for oxygen to be released at the peripheral tissues (increased affinity, decreased $P50$). A rightward shift in the oxyhemoglobin dissociation curve (curve C, Fig. 2.16) occurs with increased body temperature and decreased pH (acidosis), allowing for a greater release of oxygen at the peripheral tissues where the PO_2 is approximately 40 mm Hg. This physiologically important mechanism is used during exercise to increase oxygen delivery to the working muscle fibers.

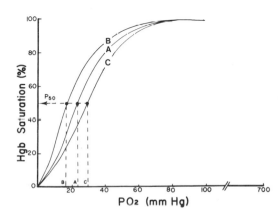

Figure 2.16. Oxygen-hemoglobin dissociation curves. **A.** The normal relationship between PO_2 and hemoglobin saturation. **B.** The curve shifts to the left as a result of decreased body temperature, increased pH, or carbon monoxide exposure. **C.** The curve shifts to the right as a result of increased body temperature or decreased pH.

43

Table 2.2. Causes of Low Arterial Oxygen Content

Reduced ambient O2 tension ($\downarrow$ F$_I$O$_2$)
  High altitude
Global alveolar hypoventilation ($\downarrow$ P$_A$O$_2$)
  Impaired central respiratory drive
    Primary central alveolar hypoventilation
    Pickwickian syndrome (massive obesity)
    Drug induced (barbiturates, morphine)
  Neuromuscular diseases affecting respiratory muscles
Ventilation-perfusion abnormalities ($\uparrow$ A-a PO$_2$ gradient)
  Parenchymal lung diseases
  Right-to-left pulmonary or cardiac shunts
  Pulmonary embolism
Hematologic abnormalities
  Anemia
  Abnormal hemoglobin with reduced O$_2$ affinity
  Carbon monoxide exposure

The actual content of arterial oxygen, CaO$_2$, is calculated as follows:

$$\text{CaO}_2 \text{ (ml O}_2/100 \text{ ml blood)} = \text{SaO}_2 \times 1.34 \times [\text{Hb}] \text{ (g/100 ml)}$$

This equation neglects the small amount of oxygen that is physically dissolved in the blood (0.003 ml O$_2$/100 ml per mm Hg PO$_2$). Given a normal hemoglobin concentration of 15 gm/100 ml and a PaO$_2$ of 100 mm Hg at sea level,

$$\text{CaO}_2 = 97.5 \times 1.34 \times 15 = 19.6 \text{ ml O}_2/100 \text{ ml blood.}$$

An additional 0.3 ml O$_2$ would be physically dissolved in the plasma giving a total CaO$_2$ of approximately 20 ml/100ml.

The laboratory determination of CaO$_2$ requires knowledge of hemoglobin concentration and SaO$_2$. SaO$_2$ may be directly obtained from spectrophotometric analysis of blood or derived indirectly from the oxyhemoglobin dissociation curve if PO$_2$, pH, and temperature are known. A convenient device for estimating SaO$_2$ during exercise is the ear or finger oximeter, which approximates SaO$_2$ from the capillary blood just beneath the skin. This is an important measurement in patients with chronic lung disease, where SaO$_2$ might significantly decrease during exercise.

It should be clear from the preceding discussion that there are a multitude of factors ranging from the PO$_2$ of inspired air to the hemoglobin concentration that can affect arterial oxygen content and potentially limit exercise. These are summarized in Figure 2.14 and Table 2.2. The workup for exercise intolerance should consider all these possibilities. Pulmonary function studies, blood gas analyses, and hematologic studies are all important aspects of the clinical evaluation for suspected exercise impairment and disability.

OXYGEN EXTRACTION BY SKELETAL MUSCLES.

The final determinant of $\dot{V}O_{2max}$ is the capacity of skeletal muscle to extract and utilize oxygen from the arterial blood. During exercise this is reflected by the arteriovenous O_2 content difference ($CaO_2 - C\bar{v}O_2$). Oxygen extraction by skeletal muscle depends on a number of factors, including the intensity of exercise, the capillary density (i.e., number of capillaries per unit of muscle tissue), the aerobic enzyme content within the muscle fiber mitochondria, and the number and size of the mitochondria. In healthy individuals at rest, approximately 25% of the arterial oxygen is extracted by the muscle fibers with resulting $CaO_2 - C\bar{v}O_2$ difference of 40 to 50 ml O_2/L; as exercise increases mixed venous O_2 content progressively falls, and the $CaO_2 - C\bar{v}O_2$ difference widens to 130 to 150 ml O_2/L (Fig. 2.13).

Although the maximal O_2 extraction capacity of skeletal muscle is, to a considerable extent, under genetic control, exercise training and deconditioning can significantly modify this capacity. Studies have shown that after several months of training, adaptations within the muscle fiber include increased density of capillaries and increased aerobic enzyme activity in the muscle mitochondria (31). These training-induced changes enable the muscle fibers to extract more oxygen per unit of blood flow. As much as 50% of the improvement in $\dot{V}O_{2max}$ with training is accounted for by peripheral adaptations in muscle (32). In cardiac patients, moreover, where central adaptations within the heart are often limited by myocardial damage and left ventricular dysfunction, the peripheral adaptations in skeletal muscle account for most, if not all, of the increased $\dot{V}O_{2max}$ with training (33). This has obvious implications for cardiac rehabilitation programs, because it implies that patients with major compromises in cardiac function can still benefit from a carefully designed exercise program.

In contrast, decreased physical activity, which occurs with deconditioning and prolonged periods of bed rest, results in a reduction in the oxidative metabolic capacity of skeletal muscles and accounts for much of the decline in $\dot{V}O_{2max}$ (31). It is not surprising, therefore, that individuals recovering from an illness involving several weeks or more of bed rest find that usual physical activities are associated with easy fatigability and weakness. It often takes several months to regain previous levels of conditioning as shown in the classic bed rest study of Saltin (34).

In addition to deconditioning there are diseases of skeletal muscle that interfere with oxygen extraction even when the supply is adequate. These diseases often have a profound effect on exercise tolerance. Primary muscle and neuromuscular diseases causing weakness and exercise intolerance include the muscular dystrophies (progressive muscle wasting of muscle fibers), glycogen storage diseases (enzymatic defects in glycogenolysis), periodic paralyses (intermittent attacks of muscle paralysis), and myasthenia gravis (failure at the neuromuscular junction). Decreased mitochondrial oxygen consumption is also a feature of hypothyroidism, a common endocrine abnormality. Finally, hypokalemia, a frequent side effect of diuretic therapy, may be associated with muscle weakness and reduced exercise tolerance.

ANAEROBIC PARAMETERS

Any discussion of anaerobic metabolism during dynamic, isotonic exercise is likely to be somewhat controversial because of the ongoing debate over the validity of the *ventilatory anaerobic threshold* ($\dot{V}_{at}$) (35, 36). Nevertheless, functional exercise testing often includes such measurements, and they have proven to be clinically useful in assessing functional impairment in CHF patients and in studying athletic performance (22, 37–40). Although the full debate over these issues is beyond the scope of this chapter, a brief discussion of anaerobic metabolism during exercise will be instructive.

Figure 2.17 illustrates the ventilatory and blood lactate responses to exercise as a function of $\dot{V}O_2$. During the initial (aerobic) phase of a progressive exercise activity, which lasts until 50 to 60% $\dot{V}O_{2max}$ is reached (in untrained subjects), expired ventilation ($\dot{V}_E$) increases linearly with $\dot{V}O_2$ and reflects aerobically produced CO_2 in the exercising muscles. Blood lactate levels are normal during this phase, as lactic acid production is minimal. During the latter half of exercise a significant increase in blood lactate occurs as a result of lactic acid production by the exercising muscles. Anaerobic metabolism occurs with lactate production

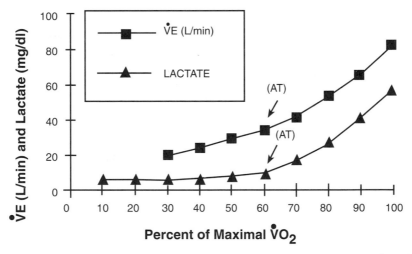

Figure 2.17. Ventilatory and blood lactate response to exercise as a function of oxygen uptake. The anaerobic threshold (*AT*) indicates the onset of significant anaerobic metabolism, which occurs at approximately 50 to 60% of $\dot{V}O_{2max}$. (Adapted from Yanowitz FG. CARDIO April 1993, pp. 56–64.)

when the O_2 supply can no longer keep up with the increasing metabolic requirements of the muscle fibers (14). The $\dot{V}O_2$ at the onset of blood lactate accumulation is often called the *anaerobic threshold or lactate threshold* ("AT" in Fig. 2.17). In the peripheral blood almost all of the lactic acid is buffered by sodium bicarbonate according to the following reactions:

$$\text{Lactic acid} + NaHCO_3 \rightarrow \text{Na lactate} + H_2CO_3$$

$$H_2CO_3 \rightarrow H_2O + CO_2$$

The excess CO_2 produced during this buffering process is added to the increasing amounts of CO_2 produced aerobically in the muscle fibers, causing the $\dot{V}_E$ to rise more steeply during later stages of exercise. Interestingly, it is during this phase that exercising subjects often experience dyspnea. Because the change in $\dot{V}_E$ at the onset of anaerobic metabolism is well defined theoretically, noninvasive methods have been developed to detect this transition (14, 22, 41). The $\dot{V}O_2$ at the onset of the ventilatory change is appropriately called the ventilatory threshold ($\dot{V}_{at}$). Specific techniques for estimating this threshold are discussed in Chapter 5. The controversy is over the validity of these noninvasive techniques and whether a true threshold exists (42).

MYOCARDIAL OXYGEN SUPPLY AND DEMAND

Unlike skeletal muscle, the heart depends almost entirely on aerobic metabolism (oxidative phosphorylation) for its energy requirements. Accordingly, coronary blood flow is exquisitely autoregulated to maintain a balance between myocardial oxygen supply and demand. Myocardial cells efficiently extract 60 to 70% of the oxygen delivered over a wide range of metabolic requirements. An increase in oxygen demand by the heart, therefore, can only be achieved by an increase in myocardial blood flow.

There are four major determinants of myocardial oxygen consumption ($M\dot{V}O_2$); (a) intramyocardial tension or stress (pressure × volume), (b) inotropic state (contractility), (c) heart rate, and (d) myocardial mass (2). Increases in one or more of these variables as occur during exercise, are normally matched by appropriate increases in coronary blood flow to maintain the oxygen supply-demand balance. Recent evidence suggests that autoregulation of coronary blood flow is mediated by the metabolite adenosine, a breakdown product of ATP and a potent vasodilator of the coronary vasculature (2).

According to the Laplace relationship myocardial wall tension (T) is directly proportional to intraventricular radius (r) and pressure (P) and inversely proportional to wall thickness (h) as in the following equation:

$$T = Pr/2h$$

Table 2.3. Acute and Chronic Adaptations to Exercise

	Acute Response to Exercise	Chronic Adaptation to Exercise Training	Effects of Deconditioning	Causes of Exercise Intolerance
$\dot{V}O_2$	Linear increase to $\dot{V}O_2$ max	Increase in $\dot{V}O_2$ max	Decrease in $\dot{V}O_2$ max	
HR	Linear increase to max HR (220 minus age)	No change or possible decrease in max HR; Decrease in resting HR and HR response to submaximal exercise	Increase HR response to submaximal workloads	Sinus node disease; AV node disease; Beta-blocking drugs
SV	Increase in early exercise to a plateau	Increase in max SV; Increase in resting SV and SV response to submaximal exercise	Decrease max SV and SV response to submaximal workloads	Valvular heart disease; Ischemic heart disease; Cardiomyopathy; Deconditioning
CaO_2	No change	No change	No change	High altitude ($\downarrow F_IO_2$); Hypoventilation ($\downarrow P_AO_2$); Ventilation/perfusion abnormalities ($\uparrow$ A-a$\bar{V}$); Hematologic abnormalities
$C\bar{v}O_2$	Progressive fall to minimal value	Decrease in min $C\bar{v}O_2$ with widening of CaO_2-$C\bar{v}O_2$ difference	Narrowing of CaO_2-$C\bar{v}O_2$ difference due to decreased oxidative enzyme activity in muscle fibers	Skeletal muscle disease; Neuromuscular disease; Systemic diseases affecting oxidative metabolism; Deconditioning

AV, Atrioventricular; *HR*, heart rate; *SV*, stroke volume.

Although wall tension cannot be measured directly, the determinants of tension are studied using various invasive and noninvasive cardiac techniques (see Chapter 3).

An indirect measure of $M\dot{V}O_2$ is the heart rate-systolic blood pressure product, commonly known as the *double product* or the *tension-time index* (2). Although this readily measured index of $M\dot{V}O_2$ does not take into consideration ventricular volume or myocardial contractility, studies during exercise have demonstrated that it correlates well with directly measured $M\dot{V}O_2$ in healthy subjects (2). Furthermore, the double product is a useful parameter to follow in patients with coronary artery disease. Calculating the double product at the onset of exercise-induced angina or ischemic ECG changes (see Chapter 5) provides an indirect index of the $M\dot{V}O_2$ threshold above which myocardial ischemia occurs. Changes in this threshold over time, resulting from various medical and/or surgical interventions or occurring naturally with progression of disease, correlate well with the patient's clinical status and coronary angiographic findings.

SUMMARY

This chapter has reviewed anatomic and physiologic concepts of the cardiovascular system at rest and during exercise. The sections provide a foundation for the subsequent chapters, which deal with more practical aspects of exercise testing, exercise training, and cardiac rehabilitation. The acute and long-term adaptations to exercise training were reviewed using the Fick principle to emphasize the close coupling of oxygen uptake, oxygen transport, and oxygen utilization. Table 2.3 summarizes these important adaptations from the perspective of the Fick variables. Finally, many of the causes of exercise intolerance that were discussed are reversible to some extent with exercise training, medical therapy, and surgical interventions.

REFERENCES

1. Schlant RC, Silverman ME, Roberts WC. Anatomy of the heart. In: Hurst JW, ed. The heart. 7th ed. New York: McGraw-Hill, 1990.
2. Schlant RC, Sonnenblick EH. Normal physiology of the cardiovascular system. In: Hurst JW, ed. The heart. 7th ed. New York: McGraw-Hill, 1990.
3. Ross R. The pathogenesis of atherosclerosis—an update. N Engl J Med 1986;314:488–500.
4. Guyton AC. Textbook of medical physiology. 6th ed. Philadelphia: WB Saunders, 1981.
5. Rushmer RF. Cardiovascular dynamics. 3rd ed. Philadelphia: WB Saunders, 1970.
6. DeSanctis RW, Ruskin JN. Disturbances of cardiac rhythm and conduction. In: Rubenstein E, ed. Scientific American medicine. New York: Scientific American, 1993.
7. Hutter AM. Ischemic heart disease: angina pectoris. In: Rubenstein E, ed. Scientific American medicine. New York: Scientific American, 1991.
8. American Heart Association. 1992 heart and stroke facts. AHA Publication 55-0386 (COM). National Centre, 7272 Greenville Avenue, Dallas, Tx 75231-4596.
9. Yanowitz FG, Charlton GA. Arguments for prevention. In: Yanowitz FG, ed. Coronary heart disease prevention. New York: Marcel Dekker, 1992.
10. Ross R, Glomset JA. The pathogenesis of atherosclerosis. N Engl J Med 1976;295:369–377.

11. Yanowitz FG. Atherosclerosis: processes versus origins. In: Yanowitz FG, ed. Coronary heart disease prevention. New York: Marcel Dekker, 1992.
12. Steinberg D, Parthasaratthy S, Carew TE et al. Beyond cholesterol. Modifications of low-density lipoprotein that increase its atherogenecity. N Engl J Med 1989;320:915–924.
13. Davies MJ, Thomas AC. Plaque fissuring—the cause of acute myocardial infarction, sudden ischemic death, and crescendo angina. Br Heart J 1985;53:363–373.
14. Wasserman K, Hansen JE, Sue DY, Whipp BF. Principles of exercise testing and interpretation. Philadelphia: Lea & Febiger, 1987.
15. Huxley HE. The contraction of muscle. Sci Am 1958;19:319–328.
16. Huxley HE. The mechanism of muscle contraction. Science 1969;164:1356–1360.
17. Huxley AF. Muscle contraction. J Physiol (Lond) 1974;243:1–17.
18. Astrand P, Rodahl K. Textbook of work physiology. 2nd ed. New York; McGraw-Hill, 1977.
19. Kirchberger MA. Excitation and contraction of skeletal muscle. In: West JB, ed. Best and Taylor's physiological basis of medical practice. 12th ed. Baltimore, Williams & Wilkins, 1991.
20. Carlson FD, Wilkie DR. Muscle physiology. Englewood Cliffs, NJ: Prentice-Hall, 1974.
21. Faulkner JA, White TP. Adaptations of skeletal muscle to physical activity. In: Bouchard C, Shephard RJ, Stephens T, Sutton JR, McPherson BD, eds. Exercise, fitness, and health. Champaign, IL: Human Kinetics Books, 1990.
22. Weber KT, Janicki JS. Cardiopulmonary exercise testing. Physiologic principles and clinical applications. Philadelphia: WB Saunders, 1986.
23. Mitchell JH, Blomqvist G. Maximal oxygen uptake. N Engl J Med 1971;284:1018–1023.
24. Yanowitz FG. Functional exercise testing in chronic congestive heart failure. CARDIO, April 1993; pp. 56–64.
25. Saltin B, Rowell LB. Functional adaptations to physical activity and inactivity. Fed Proc 1980; 39:1506–1513.
26. Mason DT, Zelis R, Longhurst J, Lee G. Cardiocirculatory responses to muscular exercise in congestive heart failure. Prog Cardiovasc Dis 1976;19:475–489.
27. Ellestad MH. Stress testing: Principles and practice. 2nd ed. Philadelphia: FA Davis, 1980.
28. West JB, ed. The cardiac pump. Best and Taylor's physiological basis of medical practice. 12th ed. Baltimore: Williams & Wilkins, 1991.
29. West JB, ed. Pulmonary gas exchange. Best and Taylor's physiological basis of medical practice. 12th ed. Baltimore: Williams & Wilkins, 1991.
30. Ranney HM, Rapaport SI. The red blood cell. In: West JB, ed. Best and Taylor's physiological basis of medical practice. 12th ed. Baltimore: Williams & Wilkins, 1991.
31. Saltin B, Rowell LB. Functional adaptations to physical activity and inactivity. Fed Proc 1980; 39:1506–1513.
32. Clausen JP. Effect of physical training on cardiovascular adjustments to exercise in man. Physiol Rev 1977;57:779–814.
33. Clausen JP. Circulatory adjustments to dynamic exercise and effects of physical training in normal subjects and patients with coronary artery disease. Prog Cardiovasc Dis 1976;18:459–495.
34. Saltin B, Blomqvist G, Mitchell JH et al. Response to exercise after bed rest and after training. Circulation 1968;38:1–78.
35. Brooks GA. Anaerobic threshold: review of the concept and directions for future research. Med Sci Sports Exerc 1985;17:22–31.
36. Davis JA. Anaerobic threshold: review of the concept and directions for future research. Med Sci Sports Exerc 1985;17:6–18.
37. Simonton CA, Higginbothan MB, Cobb FR. The ventilatory threshold: quantitative analysis of reproducibility and relation to arterial lactate concentrations in normal subjects and in patients in congestive heart failure. Am J Cardiol 1988;62:100–107.
38. Matsumura N, Nishijima H, et al. Determination of anaerobic threshold for assessment of functional state in patients with congestive heart failure. Circulation 1983;68:360–367.
39. Neuberg GW, Friedman SH, Weiss MB, Herman MV. Cardiopulmonary exercise testing. The clinical value of gas exchange data. Arch Intern Med 1988;148:2221–2226.
40. Wasserman K. The anaerobic threshold measurement to evaluate exercise performance. Am Rev Respir Dis 1984;129(Suppl):S35–S40.

41. Beaver WL, Wasserman K, Whipp BJ. A new method for detecting the anaerobic threshold by gas exchange. J Appl Physiol 1986;60:2020–2027.
42. Yeh MP, Gardner RM, Adams TD et al. "Anaerobic threshold": problems of determination and validation. J Appl Physiol 1983;55:1178–1186.

II.   EVALUATION AND EXERCISE PRESCRIPTION

3

Cardiovascular Assessment and Treatment

THE PRACTICE OF CARDIOVASCULAR medicine has undergone remarkable changes in recent years, primarily as a result of technologic advances in diagnostic and therapeutic procedures. There are both positive and negative consequences to this scientific explosion in medicine. On the positive side there is now an incredible array of sophisticated diagnostic techniques for quantitating cardiovascular abnormalities to a degree of accuracy never before imagined. In addition, new drugs and interventional procedures permit earlier and more effective treatments to be administered to increasing numbers of patients with cardiovascular disorders. Because of these important advances the decline in cardiovascular mortality that began in the 1970s has continued into the 1990s with no sign of leveling off (1).

On the negative side, however, the technologic advances have created a severe strain on our nation's health care budget. The American Heart Association estimated that in 1990 cardiovascular diseases cost our economy $95.5 billion, of which $60.7 billion was paid to hospitals and nursing homes, $13.6 billion for physician and nursing services, $4.7 billion for drugs, and $15.5 billion forfeited to the economy because of lost productivity (1). Almost 75% of these costs were

TABLE 3.1. Cardiovascular Assessment and Treatment

Introduction
Objectives of the cardiovascular examination
Methods of the cardiovascular examination
  Medical history
    Differential diagnosis of chest pain
    Other symptoms
  Cardiovascular physical examination
    Inspection
    Palpation
    Auscultation
  Electrocardiogram
  Chest x-ray
  Noninvasive cardiovascular techniques
    Echocardiography and Doppler studies
    Nuclear cardiology
  Invasive cardiovascular techniques
    Right and left heart catheterization
    Angiocardiography
Cardiovascular therapeutics
  Cardiovascular drugs
    Antianginal drugs
    Antihypertensive drugs
    Antiarrhythmic drugs
    Heart failure treatment drugs
  Invasive cardiovascular therapies
    Coronary artery bypass surgery
    Percutaneous transluminal coronary angioplasty
    New interventional procedures
Conclusions

spent on coronary heart disease, stroke, and hypertension, diseases that could have been prevented by risk factor modification and lifestyle changes.

A second negative consequence of modern scientific cardiology is the dehumanization that inevitably results when the medical focus is predominately on the quantitative and mechanical aspects of heart disease diagnosis and treatment. This increasing reliance on sophisticated technology has widened the emotional distance between physician and patient, causing a loss of some of the more humanistic skills that have traditionally characterized the physician-patient relationship.

This chapter reviews the process of cardiovascular diagnosis and treatment (Table 3.1). Although the focus is on technology, the major purpose is to illustrate logical and comprehensive strategies for managing patients with cardiovascular diseases. The discussion begins with a review of the objectives of the cardiovascular evaluation. What information is needed to successfully manage a patient with suspected or known cardiovascular disease? The next section considers specific methods of the cardiovascular assessment, beginning with the low-cost medical history and physical examination and progressing to more sophisticated and expensive technologies that may be needed in select situations. The chapter concludes with a review of current cardiovascular therapeutics. Throughout, an attempt is made to present a humanistic and cost-effective approach to the workup and treatment of cardiac patients. Specific examples are considered that are most appropriate for students and health professionals working in cardiac rehabilitation and other preventive programs.

OBJECTIVES OF THE CARDIOVASCULAR EXAMINATION

The evaluation of a patient with known or suspected cardiovascular disease must be tailored to the specific needs of the patient. Table 3.2 lists the questions that might form the basis for a cardiovascular evaluation. These questions fall into two different categories: (a) questions concerned with the diagnosis of cardiovascular disease, and (b) questions related to patient management. The design of an optimal management strategy depends, in part, on the specific diagnoses, but is also influenced by prognostic and quality-of-life considerations.

A comprehensive classification system for cardiovascular diagnoses has been described by the New York Heart Association in their publication *Nomenclature and Criteria for the Diagnosis of Diseases of the Heart and Great Vessels* (2). Although the specific criteria for various diagnoses may have changed since the last edition of this book in 1988, the nomenclature and categories of diagnoses are quite

TABLE 3.2. Questions for the Cardiovascular Examination

1.	Is cardiovascular disease present?
2.	What is its cause? (i.e., etiologic diagnosis)
3.	What are the structural abnormalities? (i.e., anatomic diagnoses)
4.	Are there abnormalities in cardiac function or myocardial contractility?
5.	Are there abnormalities in cardiac rhythm or conduction?
6.	Is myocardial ischemia present?
7.	Is treatment needed?
8.	What are the most appropriate therapies?
9.	What is the prognosis?
10.	How does the cardiovascular disease affect the patient's quality of life?

TABLE 3.3. Elements of the Cardiovascular Diagnosis[a]

1. The etiologic diagnosis
2. The anatomic diagnosis
3. The physiologic diagnosis
4. Cardiac status
5. Prognosis

[a] From the Criteria Committee of the New York Heart Association. Nomenclature and criteria for diagnoses of diseases of the heart and great vessels. 8th ed. Boston: Little, Brown, 1979.

TABLE 3.4. Examples of Etiologic Cardiovascular Diagnoses

1. Atherosclerotic cardiovascular disease
2. Congenital heart disease
3. Rheumatic heart disease
4. Hypertensive heart disease
5. Pulmonary heart disease
6. Infectious heart disease
7. Idiopathic heart disease (unknown etiology)

relevant to current practices in cardiovascular medicine. The classification scheme subdivides the cardiovascular "diagnoses" into the five categories listed in Table 3.3.

The *etiologic* diagnoses refer to the causes of heart and blood vessel diseases. Often this is not known for a particular patient, and the term *idiopathic* is sometimes used to express an unknown etiology. Most of the time, however, a careful evaluation of the patient's clinical data will enable an etiologic diagnosis to be made with a reasonable degree of certainty. Examples of etiologic diagnoses are listed in Table 3.4. By far the most common diagnosis in this country and one that provides the large majority of patients for cardiac rehabilitation and other preventive programs is *atherosclerotic* cardiovascular disease. Patients may have more than one etiologic diagnosis (e.g., the combination of atherosclerotic and hypertensive heart disease). Also an etiologic diagnosis does not necessarily imply a complete understanding of the cause. In atherosclerosis, for example, the causes in any one individual are often multiple and include host factors (e.g., genetic predisposition), lifestyle factors (e.g., smoking), and environmental factors (e.g., social isolation). Another patient with the same degree and distribution of atherosclerotic lesions may have an entirely different set of etiologic factors.

The *anatomic* diagnoses are usually more easily determined by the various diagnostic tools discussed in this chapter. Structural abnormalities may involve the chambers of the heart (hypertrophy, enlargement, infarction, etc.), the

TABLE 3.5. Cardiac Status and Prognosis[a]

Cardiac Status	Prognosis
Uncompromised	Good
Slightly compromised	Good, with therapy
Moderately compromised	Fair, with therapy
Severely compromised	Guarded, despite therapy

[a] From the Criteria Committee of the New York Heart Association. Nomenclature and criteria for diagnoses of diseases of the heart and great vessels. 8th ed. Boston: Little, Brown, 1979.

cardiac valves (stenosis, insufficiency), the arteries (atheroma, aneurysms), and the veins. Anatomic diagnoses also include specific tumors of the heart, pathologic diagnoses obtained from biopsy specimens, and abnormalities of the pericardium.

Physiologic diagnoses refer to abnormalities of cardiovascular function (systolic and diastolic dysfunction, abnormalities of myocardial contractility, etc.), electrical disturbances of cardiac rhythm and conduction, and hypertension in the systemic or pulmonary circulation. These abnormalities are detected by an assortment of simple and sophisticated diagnostic tools described in this chapter.

Cardiac status and *prognosis* are determined after establishing the etiologic, anatomic, and physiologic diagnoses and after deciding on the most appropriate therapy (Table 3.5). Clinical judgment and experience, knowledge of the natural history and therapy of cardiovascular diseases, and careful evaluation of the patient's limiting symptoms are all important in making this assessment.

One of the challenges in modern cardiovascular practice is knowing how far to go in a particular patient's workup and management. Given the sophistication of diagnostic and therapeutic technologies available today, along with the economic incentives for those physicians and hospitals providing the services, there is an increasing tendency to include costly and possibly unnecessary procedures in the workup of patients with cardiovascular symptoms and findings. Less reliance is given to information obtained during the history and physical examination in favor of the more quantitative data provided by expensive noninvasive and invasive procedures. Practice guidelines developed by consensus panels of experts are beginning to appear in the medical literature in an effort to better define the indications for various cardiovascular diagnostic and treatment procedures (3–8). It is too early, however, to evaluate the impact of these guidelines on the practice of cardiovascular medicine.

An important and relevant concept to this discussion is the distinction between *disease* and *illness*. Disease refers to the specific pathologic processes taking place within the cells, tissues, and organ systems of the body that may or may not be causing symptoms. The disease process is defined by etiologic, anatomic, and physiologic characteristics that are determined from the history, physical examination, and other diagnostic tests. An illness, on the other hand, is characterized by a constellation of symptoms and findings related to the patient's clinical state of well-being. The complaints experienced by the patient are often heavily influenced by cultural and psychosocial determinants that are best evaluated during interaction of patient and health professional. This aspect of the cardiovascular evaluation is frequently neglected while too much emphasis is given to the "hard data" derived from invasive and noninvasive tests. Ideally, the cardiovascular workup and subsequent therapeutic interventions should be tailored to both the underlying disease and the resulting illness, if any. This distinction between disease and illness is especially pertinent to cardiac rehabilitation where the primary goals are initially directed towards managing the illness resulting from an acute cardiac event rather than the basic disease process.

The methods of the cardiovascular examination are reviewed in the next section. The basic database of history, physical examination, electrocardiogram (ECG), and chest radiograph are considered first. This is followed by a brief description of the invasive and noninvasive procedures that are the "bread-and-butter" techniques of cardiovascular specialists.

METHODS OF THE CARDIOVASCULAR EXAMINATION

Medical History

The most humanistic and cost-effective diagnostic procedure is the medical history. Occasionally, a complete diagnosis and management plan can be determined from the patient history alone. More often, the history provides important clues to the etiologic, anatomic, and physiologic diagnoses, which are then confirmed by other diagnostic procedures. As already discussed, the history may be the only means of evaluating possible psychosocial variables that contribute to the patient's illness. Also, the actual process of obtaining the medical history may have a therapeutic benefit because of the nature of the relationship that develops between patient and physician during the interaction. Although much of the medical history can be obtained from self-administered questionnaires or a computer terminal, the physician-administered history is a necessary element in the medical care process. In some circumstances such as a cardiac rehabilitation or wellness program, the history may be obtained by a health professional such as a nurse practitioner or exercise specialist.

Table 3.6 lists the components of the medical history that are important in the cardiovascular workup. The actual sequence of data collection will depend on the particular circumstances of the physician-patient encounter. Often the patient is seeking medical attention because of a specific complaint or an illness

TABLE 3.6. The Cardiovascular History

History of the present illness (if any)

Review of cardiovascular symptoms
- Chest pain or discomfort
- Dyspnea
- Palpitations
- Syncope
- Edema
- Fatigue

Past cardiovascular history
- Rheumatic fever
- Myocardial infarction (MI)
- Cardiovascular surgery
- Congestive heart failure
- Pulmonary embolism
- Bacterial endocarditis
- Cardiovascular drugs and procedures

Cardiovascular risk factors
- Cigarette smoking
- Hypertension
- Hyperlipidemia
- Diabetes mellitus
- Family history of premature coronary disease
- Lifestyle assessment
    Exercise history
    Diet history
    Stress and personality factors

that is worrisome. In this situation the history should begin with a detailed description of the present illness and particular symptomatology. At other times an individual may be undergoing a routine checkup in the absence of any illness. In these situations the history might begin with a review of previous cardiovascular problems, followed by the symptoms review and risk factor assessment. It is important to emphasize that patients who do not *complain* of cardiovascular symptoms may still be experiencing symptoms although perhaps not appreciating their significance.

Differential Diagnosis of Chest Pain

One of the most frequent diagnostic challenges encountered by physicians is chest pain and/or discomfort. The evaluation of chest symptoms is also of

TABLE 3.7. Causes of Chest Discomfort

Noncardiovascular conditions
    Chest wall abnormalities
    Esophageal disorders
    Pleural disease
    Gastrointestinal disturbances
    Pulmonary disease
    Psychogenic
Cardiovascular diseases
    Coronary heart disease (CHD)
        Stable angina pectoris
        Unstable angina pectoris
        Variant angina
        Acute myocardial infarction
        Postmyocardial infarction syndrome (Dressler's)
    Other cardiovascular disorders
        Aortic valve disease
        Hypertrophic cardiomyopathy
        Mitral valve prolapse
        Pericarditis
        Pulmonary hypertension
        Pulmonary infarction
        Dissecting aortic aneurysm

considerable importance to those working in cardiac rehabilitation, adult fitness, and exercise testing laboratories. The medical history is the primary diagnostic procedure for this assessment, although additional tests might be needed to confirm a particular diagnosis. In obtaining the history it is important to assess descriptors of pain quality, location and duration of discomfort, precipitating and relieving factors, and associated symptoms. Questions dealing with discomfort in the neck, jaw, arms, epigastrium, as well as terms such as burning, numbness, pressure, and difficulty breathing should be included in the history. Table 3.7 lists the possible causes of chest discomfort that need to be considered in the differential diagnosis. Most of these conditions can be diagnosed by a detailed history and physical examination. Occasionally more expensive diagnostic procedures are required to resolve atypical symptoms and physical findings. The use of exercise testing in the evaluation of chest pain is discussed in Chapter 5.

The distinction between *typical angina pectoris, atypical angina*, and *nonanginal chest pain* is an important consideration in the evaluation of patients with suspected coronary artery disease. The clinical characteristics of typical angina are listed in Table 3.8. This classic syndrome is almost always caused by

TABLE 3.8. The "Pain" of Typical Angina Pectoris

Quality	Tightness, aching, squeezing, burning, pressing
Location	Substernal, but may also involve left chest, arms, neck, or jaw
Duration	3 to 5 minutes, up to 15 minutes
Precipitating factors	During exertion, emotional upset, cold weather, exertion after meals
Relieving factors	Within 3 to 5 minutes after rest or sublingual nitroglycerin

TABLE 3.9. Probability of Coronary Heart Disease by Symptoms[a]

Age	Nonanginal Discomfort	Atypical Angina	Typical Angina
Males			
35-44	0.11	0.45	0.81
45-54	0.21	0.60	0.91
55-64	0.28	0.69	0.94
65-74	0.28	0.70	0.94
Females			
35-44	0.03	0.16	0.45
45-54	0.07	0.32	0.68
55-64	0.13	0.47	0.84
65-74	0.17	0.54	0.95

[a] From Diamond GA, Forrester JS. N Engl J Med 1979; 300:1350–1359.

fixed coronary atherosclerotic lesions and occurs predictably whenever myocardial oxygen demands exceed the available coronary blood supply. Because this is usually a threshold phenomenon, the precipitating factors of exercise and emotional excitement can bring on an attack in a rather reproducible manner. Typical angina is also called *secondary angina* because the ischemic symptoms are secondary to factors increasing myocardial oxygen demand.

In contrast, atypical angina is defined as a clinical syndrome that is somewhat suggestive of angina pectoris but lacking in one or two of the typical features listed in Table 3.8. Atypical anginal symptoms are associated with an increased likelihood of coronary artery disease but to a lesser degree of certainty than typical angina. One frequent setting where these symptoms occur is during coronary artery spasm superimposed on a fixed obstructive atherosclerotic lesion (*mixed angina*). Another form of atypical angina is caused by coronary artery spasm without underlying atherosclerosis (*primary angina*). Angina caused by spasm usually occurs at rest and is often associated with transient ST segment elevation. This anginal syndrome is sometimes called *Prinzmetal's angina* or *variant angina* (9, 10).

Finally, nonanginal chest pain refers to symptoms lacking three or more of the classic features described in Table 3.8 and is very unlikely to be caused by ischemic heart disease. Other causes of chest pain listed in Table 3.7 need to be considered and the appropriate workup carried out.

Diamond and Forrester (11) have published data for men and women of various ages estimating the probability of underlying coronary disease for patients presenting with typical angina, atypical angina, and nonanginal chest pain. These probabilities based on symptoms are listed in Table 3.9 and can be used as pretest probabilities for various noninvasive diagnostic procedures such as exercise ECG testing (Chapter 5).

In patients with typical or atypical angina, it is important to further classify the symptoms as *stable* or *unstable*. Stable angina pectoris implies that the symptoms have been present and stable for at least 1 month. Unstable angina includes recent onset angina (within 1 month), progressive or accelerating angina, and angina-at-rest (12). Patients with unstable symptoms are usually not candidates for exercise testing, but are in need of further workup and management. Often this requires hospitalization and bed rest.

Other Symptoms

The other symptoms listed in Table 3.6 may or may not be related to cardiovascular disorders. Dyspnea on effort, for example, may be secondary to cardiac or respiratory disorders, or it may simply be a manifestation of deconditioning. Cardiac dyspnea, a manifestation of left ventricular failure and pulmonary congestion, is usually exertional; although if difficulty breathing occurs at night when the patient is lying flat, it is called *orthopnea*. Orthopnea is often accompanied by *paroxysmal nocturnal dyspnea*, sudden shortness of breath that awakens the patient at night and feels like suffocation.

Palpitations refer to the subjective awareness of the heartbeat and may be the result of disturbances in heart rate or rhythm. Syncope or sudden loss of consciousness is frequently secondary to heart disease, although many other causes, including the common faint and adverse drug reactions (postural hypotension), need to be included in the differential diagnosis. Subcutaneous edema has many different causes, including diseases of the heart, peripheral veins, liver, and kidneys. Finally, fatigue is almost a universal symptom in patients with a variety of disease and nondisease conditions.

Cardiovascular Physical Examination

The physical examination of the cardiovascular system is often the first opportunity to appreciate significant structural or functional abnormalities that may be responsible for limiting symptoms or impairment. There are three components to this examination: *inspection, palpation*, and *auscultation*. Each of these modalities requires considerable skill and clinical experience. Unfortunately, there is a tendency today to rely less and less on physical findings in favor of more quantitative information derived from expensive, noninvasive, imaging techniques. Although these procedures are sometimes needed to confirm a particular diagnostic impression, many abnormalities of the cardiovascular system can be detected and managed successfully using simple clinical skills at the bedside.

Inspection

Inspection begins with a general overview of the patient at rest and, if possible, during activity looking for abnormalities of body habitus, facial appearance, and gait. Occasionally the detection of specific skeletal abnormalities will suggest the presence of underlying congenital heart defects.

There are a number of clinical signs of hyperlipidemia that can be detected during inspection, which suggest the possibility of underlying atherosclerosis. Examination of the skin may reveal yellow, waxy plaques of *xanthelasma* around the soft periorbital tissues. These lesions may or may not be associated with ringlike deposits of phospholipids and cholesterol in the cornea called *arcus cornealis*. Although a normal phenomenon with aging (*arcus senilis*), when these lesions are seen in patients under the age of 50 years, they suggest hyperlipidemia. Tendon xanthomata, more specific findings of familial hypercholesterolemia, are lumpy, nodular swellings of cholesterol deposits over the extensor surfaces of knee, elbow, and finger joints as well as in the Achilles tendons. If one or more of these lesions are detected during physical examination, a fasting blood lipid evaluation should be done.

Inspection of the jugular venous pulse in the neck often provides important clues to the functional status of the right heart chambers and valves. The right internal jugular pressure and waveform are most suitable for this examination. The patient should be positioned for optimal visualization of venous pulsations just beneath the sternocleidomastoid muscle (~30° trunk elevation for normal subjects). In right heart failure or tricuspid valve disease, the jugular venous pressure increases abnormally as a reflection of elevated pressures in the right heart; greater trunk elevation up to the sitting position may be necessary to see the top of the oscillating venous column. The central venous pressure is estimated by taking the vertical distance from the top of the venous column to the sternal angle of Lewis and adding 5 cm for the distance to the center of the right atrium below the sternal angle. Normal pressure is ≤8 cm of water.

The jugular venous waveform normally consists of two positive waves and two negative waves (Fig. 3.1A). The *A wave* is a positive presystolic event that occurs during atrial contraction and peaks just before the first heart sound (S_1).

A. Normal

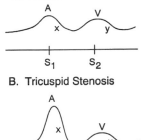

B. Tricuspid Stenosis

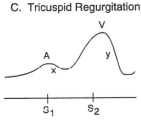

C. Tricuspid Regurgitation

FIGURE 3.1. Jugular venous pulse (JVP) tracings relative to the timing of the 1st and 2nd heart sounds. **A.** The normal JVP with "A" and "V" waves, and the x- and y-descents (see text). **B.** JVP in tricuspid valve stenosis. **C.** JVP in tricuspid valve regurgitation.

The *V wave* is a positive late systolic wave that reflects atrial filling against a closed tricuspid valve. The V wave peaks near the second heart sound (S_2). Between the A and V waves is the negative *x-descent*, which is caused by atrial relaxation and systolic collapse. The x-descent is often the most easily observed motion of the jugular venous waveform. The *y-descent* occurs after the V wave and represents early ventricular filling immediately after opening of the tricuspid valve. Prominent A waves occur in right ventricular hypertrophy, pulmonary hypertension, and tricuspid stenosis (Fig. 3.1*B*). Giant A waves, also called Cannon A waves, are caused by simultaneous contraction of the atrium and ventricle, usually the result of an arrhythmia such as a PVC or ventricular tachycardia with atrioventricular dissociation. In tricuspid regurgitation the V wave becomes especially prominent with decrease or obliteration of the x-descent and fusion with the A wave (Fig. 3.1*C*). Often a clue to underlying cardiac structural and functional abnormalities can be obtained by careful inspection of the jugular venous waveform.

Palpation

During the cardiovascular examination all major arterial pulses, including carotid, brachial, radial, femoral, posterior tibial, and pedal pulses, should be palpated for patency and waveform characteristics. Pulse intensity should be graded from 0 to 3+, where 0 refers to complete absence of pulsation, 1+ is diminished pulsation, 2+ is normal pulsation, and 3+ is bounding or large pulsation. Auscultation over the major arteries, including the abdominal aorta and its branches, should be carried out to detect audible bruits caused by turbulence of blood flow resulting from partial occlusion usually from atherosclerosis.

The carotid pulse examination is especially important, since occlusive vascular disease may lead to catastrophic cerebrovascular accidents (CVA) and neurologic impairment. The auscultation of a bruit over the carotid arteries is often followed up with ultrasound studies to quantitate the degree of obstruction and determine if surgical intervention is needed. The contour of the carotid artery pulsation often provides clues to particular cardiac abnormalities (Fig. 3.2). The

FIGURE 3.2. Carotid artery pulse tracings relative to the timing of the 1st and 2nd heart sounds. **A.** Normal carotid artery pulse with the dicrotic notch identified. **B.** Carotid artery pulse in aortic valve stenosis. **C.** Carotid artery pulse in hypertrophic subaortic stenosis.

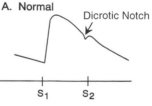

A. Normal

Dicrotic Notch

S_1 S_2

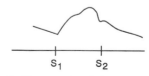

B. Aortic Stenosis

S_1 S_2

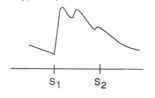

C. Hypertrophic Subaortic Stenosis

S_1 S_2

carotid upstroke begins just after the first heart sound (S_1). The *dicrotic notch* (not palpable) occurs in timing with the second heart sound (S_2). A low-volume, slowly rising, carotid artery waveform (pulsus parvus et tardus) is often the best physical finding for assessing the severity of aortic valve stenosis (Fig. 3.2B). In contrast, a *bisferiens* pulse has a dynamic, rapid upstroke with two peaks during systole (Fig. 3.2C). This abnormal pulse contour is sometimes seen in combined aortic regurgitation and stenosis, as well as in idiopathic hypertrophic subaortic stenosis (IHSS).

Palpation of the precordium is an important means of assessing the characteristics of right and left ventricular contractions. Left ventricular size is best appreciated by palpating the apex impulse while the patient is sitting up, leaning forward in held expiration. The center of the point of maximal impulse (PMI) correlates reasonably well with the left heart border. Normally, the PMI is in the fifth intercostal space, midclavicular line. In left ventricular enlargement the PMI is displaced to the left and downward. A sustained, lifting impulse indicates left ventricular hypertrophy usually secondary to aortic stenosis, hypertensive heart disease, or cardiomyopathy. In a patient recovering from a large anterior wall myocardial infarction, an abnormal systolic impulse medial to the apex in the third or fourth intercostal space suggests a ventricular aneurysm. Right ventricular hypertrophy is often the cause of a sustained left parasternal lift, best appreciated with the palm of the hand placed over the left parasternal region. Heart sounds and murmurs may also be detected during palpation, although their definitive characteristics are better determined with auscultation.

Auscultation

The stethoscope was introduced by Laennec in 1826 and quickly became the most important examination tool of the cardiovascular physician. Although in today's fast-moving, high-technology medicine the stethoscope has lost much of

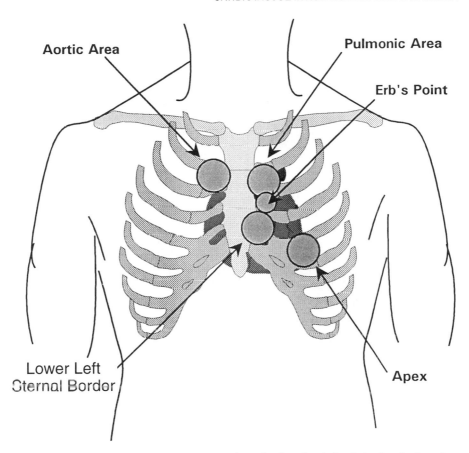

FIGURE 3.3. Standard auscultatory regions in the chest for listening to heart sounds and heart murmurs.

its glamour, skillful auscultation of the heart remains one of the most rewarding diagnostic techniques in medicine.

A systematic approach to cardiac auscultation is necessary to avoid missing significant findings. Table 3.10 summarizes the important aspects of auscultation that are considered in this section. Initially, the patient should be resting comfortably with approximately 30° trunk elevation in a quiet room. There are approximately four important auscultatory regions of the chest with variable overlap (Fig. 3.3). The aortic area is located in the right second intercostal space near the sternum. Aortic sounds and murmurs are also heard in the left third intercostal space near the sternum (Erb's point) and at the apex. The murmur of valvular aortic stenosis may be loudest in any one of these areas. The pulmonic area is primarily confined to the upper left sternal border, while the tricuspid area involves the lower left sternal border. The mitral area is at the cardiac apex and may extend into the left axilla.

69

TABLE 3.10. Auscultation of the Heart

Regions of auscultatory interest:

 Aortic areas: right 2nd intercostal space, left 3rd intercostal space, and apex
 Pulmonic area: upper left parasternal region
 Tricuspid area: lower left parasternal region
 Mitral area: cardiac apex and axilla

Heart sounds:

 S_1: mitral and tricuspid valve closure
 S_2: pulmonic and aortic valve closure
 S_3: ventricular filling sounds
 S_4: atrial systole (when there is decreased ventricular compliance)
 Ejection click: aortic or pulmonic valve opening
 Midsystolic click: mitral valve prolapse
 Opening snap: opening of mitral valve in mitral stenosis

Heart murmurs:

 Systolic ejection murmurs:
  Functional or innocent flow murmurs
  Aortic stenosis
  Pulmonic stenosis
  Idiopathic hypertrophic subaortic stenosis
  Atypical mitral regurgitation
 Pansystolic or holosystolic murmurs:
  Mitral regurgitation
  Tricuspid regurgitation
  Ventricular septal defect
 Late systolic murmurs:
  Mitral valve prolapse
 Immediate diastolic decrescendo murmurs:
  Aortic regurgitation
  Pulmonic regurgitation
 Delayed diastolic murmurs:
  Mitral stenosis
  Tricuspid stenosis
 Continuous murmurs (systole and diastole):
  Patent ductus arteriosus
  Arteriovenous fistula

Auscultation should proceed from one area to the next, using both the bell and diaphragm of the stethoscope. The diaphragm, when pressed firmly to the chest wall, selects high-frequency sounds and murmurs. The bell, when held lightly on the chest is best for low-frequency murmurs and gallop sounds. Examination of the cardiac apex in the left lateral decubitus position with the bell is optimal for detecting mitral stenosis murmurs and left ventricular gallop sounds. Early diastolic murmurs of aortic and pulmonary regurgitation are best detected with the diaphragm over the right and left parasternal regions while the patient is sitting up, leaning forward in held expiration.

First Heart Sound (S_1). The first heart sound initiates ventricular systole and has several components, the loudest of which is mitral valve closure (Fig. 3.4).

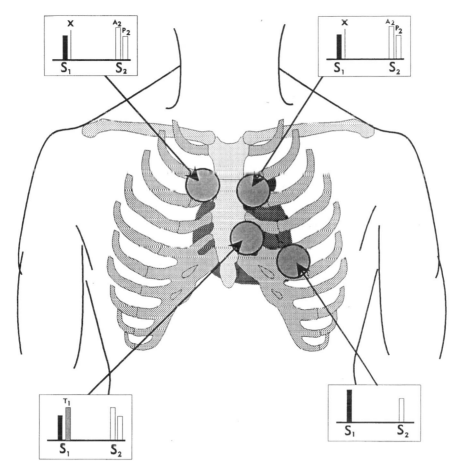

FIGURE 3.4. Diagram of heart sounds as heard in the four auscultatory regions. S_1, 1st heart sound(s); S_2, 2nd heart sound(s); T_1, tricuspid component of 1st heart sound along lower left sternal border; x, ejection click; A_2, aortic component of 2nd heart sound; P_2, pulmonic component of 2nd heart sound.

71

HEART SOUNDS AND GALLOPS

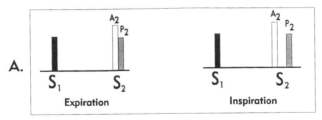

Normal Physiologic Splitting of S2

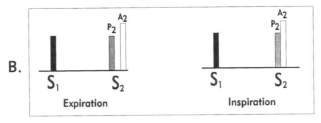

Paradoxical Splitting of S2

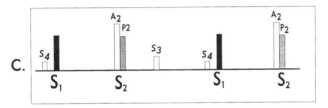

S3 and S4 Gallop Sounds at the Apex

FIGURE 3.5. Heart sounds and gallops. **A.** Normal physiologic splitting of S_2. **B.** Paradoxical splitting of S_2 in left bundle branch block. **C.** S_3 and S_4 gallop sounds recorded at the apex.

Splitting of S_1 in the tricuspid area is usually caused by tricuspid valve closure, which closely follows mitral closure. At the base of the heart, however, the second component of a split S_1 may be an ejection sound from the aortic or pulmonary valves. S_1 is usually loudest at the apex. The loudness or intensity of S_1 at the apex is affected by several factors, including the position of the mitral valve leaflets at the onset of ventricular systole. Increased intensity occurs in patients with mitral stenosis, high-output states, and short PR intervals. Soft S_1 sounds are heard in mitral regurgitation, low-output states, and prolonged PR intervals (1°AV block). Variable intensity of S_1 is usually caused by cardiac arrhythmias such as atrial fibrillation or ventricular tachycardia.

Second Heart Sound (S_2). In normal subjects the second heart sound splits physiologically in the pulmonic area (Fig. 3.5A). The initial louder component (A_2) is caused by aortic valve closure; the second and softer component (P_2) is caused by pulmonic valve closure. With inspiration A_2 moves inward (closer to S_1), P_2 moves outward, and the split widens; during expiration the split narrows until a single sound is heard. Normally P_2 is only heard in the pulmonic area. In pulmonary hypertension P_2 gets louder and can be heard at the apex. Very loud P_2 sounds may actually be palpable in the pulmonic area. Fixed splitting with respiration is found in atrial septal defects. Increased physiologic splitting is found in conditions that prolong or delay right ventricular ejection (right bundle branch block, pulmonic stenosis). In paradoxical splitting A_2 is delayed and follows P_2 during expiration (Fig. 3.5B). With inspiration the split paradoxically narrows and often becomes a single sound. This is seen in conditions that delay or prolong left ventricular ejection (left bundle branch block, aortic stenosis, left ventricular failure).

Gallop Sounds (S_3, S_4). Gallop sounds are abnormal heart sounds that reflect abnormalities in ventricular structure or function. They may originate in either ventricle, although they are more common in the left ventricle. These low frequency sounds in the left ventricle are best heard with the bell of the stethoscope at the apex with the patient lying in the left lateral decubitus position. Figure 3.5C illustrates the timing of gallop sounds relative to the first and second heart sounds. In a patient with a dilated, failing left ventricle, an S_3 gallop occurs in early diastole in timing with the peak of rapid ventricular filling. A similar sound, called a physiologic S_3, is often heard in young healthy individuals. An S_4 is always an abnormal finding and indicates decreased compliance of the ventricle; it occurs late in diastole just before S_1 during atrial systole. In coronary artery disease an S_4 gallop is often heard during ischemic episodes and in acute myocardial infarction. It may also be detected immediately after exercise testing in a patient with ischemic ECG abnormalities.

Midsystolic Clicks. These are sounds heard in mid-to-late systole caused by prolapse of the mitral valve leaflets into the left atrium. A late systolic murmur following the click is indicative of mitral regurgitation, which occurs while the leaflets are prolapsed into the left atrium (Fig. 3.6A). This is a very common and usually benign developmental abnormality, found especially in young women. The clinical importance of this auscultatory finding is related to the resting and exercise ST-T wave changes that may mimic ischemic heart disease.

Systolic Ejection Murmurs. These systolic murmurs begin after S_1, end before S_2, and have a diamond-shaped configuration (Fig. 3.6B). They are harsh, medium-pitched murmurs that are usually caused by turbulent blood flow across the aortic or pulmonic valves. The most common ejection murmur is the benign functional or innocent murmur, best heard along the left sternal border in young healthy individuals. These murmurs are generally soft, rather brief in duration, and not associated with any cardiac pathology. Murmurs of aortic or pulmonic valve stenosis are usually harsher in quality and occupy most of systole. In aortic stenosis the murmur radiates into the carotid arteries, although the intensity may be loudest at the mitral area or Erb's point (Fig. 3.5). The murmur of mitral regurgitation caused by ischemia- or infarction-related papillary muscle dysfunction is often confused with aortic stenosis. Other diagnostic techniques (e.g., echocardiography) may be needed to differentiate these two valve lesions.

Pansystolic Murmurs. These murmurs begin with S_1 and usually end with S_2 (Fig. 3.6*C*). They are usually caused by mitral or tricuspid valve regurgitation and have a high-pitched blowing quality. The murmur of mitral regurgitation is best heard at the apex and radiates into the axilla and back. Tricuspid regurgitation is best heard along the lower left sternal border and intensifies with inspiration. It is also associated with giant V waves in the jugular venous pulse (Fig. 3.1*C*). The murmur of ventricular septal defect is loudest along the left sternal border, but is more medium pitched and often associated with a palpable "thrill." This lesion may be the result of a congenital malformation or secondary to myocardial infarction with ruptured septum.

Diastolic Murmurs. Murmurs in diastole are of two types. The immediate, high-pitched decrescendo murmurs of aortic and pulmonic regurgitation are best heard along the right and left sternal borders with the diaphragm of the stethoscope and with the patient sitting up, leaning forward, breath held at end expiration (Fig. 3.6*D*). The murmur of mitral stenosis is a delayed (i.e., beginning after S_2), low-pitched, rumbling diastolic murmur at the apex, best heard with the bell of the stethoscope with the patient in the left lateral decubitus position (Fig. 3.6*E*). This murmur often begins with an "opening snap" sound caused by the opening of the fibrotic mitral valve leaflets. Mild mitral stenosis may only result in a late diastolic murmur with presystolic accentuation (Fig. 3.6*F*). Tricuspid stenosis is an uncommon abnormality that causes a similar murmur but one that is heard best along the lower left sternal border.

An accurate description of a heart murmur includes the intensity (grades 1 to 6), location (on chest) and radiation, timing (systolic, diastolic, early, or late), configuration, pitch, and duration. In addition, certain maneuvers may be helpful in the differential diagnosis. These include respiratory variations, Valsalva maneuver, exercise, postural changes, pharmacologic agents (e.g., amyl nitrite), and postpremature beat intensity changes. Although a careful physical examination will often lead to the correct diagnosis, the definitive diagnosis is usually made with an echocardiographic study.

Electrocardiogram (ECG)

This section considers the clinical applications of the ECG in evaluating suspected anatomic, physiologic, and functional cardiac abnormalities. Because of its low cost, simplicity, and extensive usage over the years, the ECG continues to be one of the most effective clinical tools in all of medicine. It is especially important to workers in cardiac rehabilitation and exercise testing laboratories.

Heart Murmurs

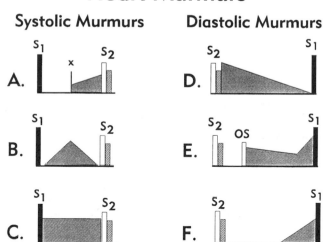

Systolic Murmurs   **Diastolic Murmurs**

FIGURE 3.6. Systolic and diastolic heart murmurs. **A.** Midsystolic click *(x)* and late systolic murmur of mitral valve prolapse heard at the apex. **B.** Systolic ejection murmur of aortic valve stenosis heard in the aortic area. **C.** Pansystolic or holosystolic murmur of rheumatic mitral valve regurgitation heard at the apex. **D.** Immediate decrescendo murmur of aortic regurgitation heard along the left sternal border. **E.** Delayed diastolic murmur with presystolic accentuation of mitral stenosis beginning with the mitral opening snap *(OS)* and heard at the apex. **F.** Late diastolic or presystolic murmur of mild mitral stenosis.

In addition to the resting ECG, which has become an essential diagnostic study in the cardiac workup, there are several advanced ECG applications that have clinical utility in certain situations. *Ambulatory electrocardiography* involves the continuous recording of one or more ECG leads for a prolonged period (usually 24 to 48 hours) while the patient carries out usual daily activities. This is used in the evaluation of suspected or known cardiac arrhythmias and conduction abnormalities and in the study of episodic ischemia, silent or symptomatic (13, 14). The *signal-averaged electrocardiogram* is a new method for studying high-frequency components in the ECG, particularly at the end of the QRS complex (15, 16). These so-called *late potentials* are a marker for increased likelihood of malignant ventricular arrhythmias and sudden death. They occur most often in the post-MI patient population. Finally, the *exercise electrocardiogram* is a useful method for the study of suspected myocardial ischemia and other exercise-related symptoms. Because of its importance to cardiac rehabilitation and adult fitness, exercise testing is discussed in considerable detail in Chapter 5.

The standard recording system for the resting ECG is the 12-lead ECG, which requires 10 electrodes (Fig. 3.7). Four electrodes are placed distally on

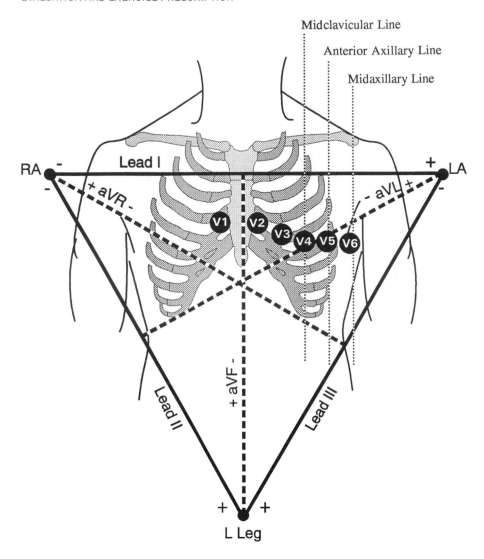

FIGURE 3.7. Standard electrode placement and orientation of the 12-lead ECG. The arm and leg electrodes are placed distally near the hands and feet *(see text).*

each limb, from which the six frontal plane leads are derived (the right leg electrode is the ground). Six precordial lead electrodes make up the horizontal plane and are placed as follows: V_1, parasternal right fourth intercostal space; V_2, parasternal left fourth intercostal space; V_3, halfway between V_2 and V_4; V_4, left 5th intercostal space, midclavicular line; V_5, anterior axillary line horizontal to V_4; V_6, midaxillary line horizontal to V_5. The 12-lead electrocardiogram provides cardiac electrical information in three orthogonal directions: (a) right-to-left

TABLE 3.11. The Standard 12-Lead ECG Orientation

(Note: It is important to think of the 12-lead ECG as providing electrical information in three orthogonal directions: right-left orientation, superior-inferior orientation, and anterior-posterior orientation. Each of the 12 leads has a particular direction of orientation.)

A. **Bipolar Limb Leads**
   Lead I: RA (-) to LA(+): (right-to-left orientation, "lateral")
   Lead II: RA (-) to LL(+): (superior-to-inferior orientation)
   Lead III: LA (-) to LL(+): (superior-to-inferior orientation)

B. **Augmented Unipolar Limb leads**
   Lead aVR: RA(+) to [LA & LL](-): (right superior orientation)
   Lead aVL: LA(+) to [RA & LL](-): (left superior orientation, "lateral")
   Lead aVF: LL(+) to [RA & LA](-): (superior-to-inferior orientation)

C. **Unipolar Chest (Precordial) Leads** (each lead is +)
   Leads V_1–V_4: (posterior-to-anterior orientation, "anterior")
   Leads V_5–V_6: (right-to-left orientation, "lateral")

RA, Right arm; *LA*, left arm; *LL*, left leg; "+" = electrical forces moving toward electrode (positive deflection on ECG); "-" = electrical forces moving away from electrode (negative deflection on ECG).

orientation, (b) superior-to-inferior orientation, and (c) anterior-to-posterior orientation. Table 3.11 describes the orientation of the 12 leads and indicates the positive and negative poles for each lead. The negative pole for the "unipolar" precordial leads is called the *central terminal* and is derived from the combination of right arm (RA), left arm (LA), and left leg (LL) electrodes. By convention, electrical activity moving towards the (+) pole of a lead during depolarization is seen as a positive deflection on that lead; electrical activity moving away from the positive pole and toward the negative pole is seen as a negative deflection.

Method of Interpretation

The complete interpretation of the 12-lead resting electrocardiogram requires a systematic approach to avoid missing important findings. Table 3.12 describes the recommended sequence of steps for ECG analysis. The terminology and format for ECG data presentation are illustrated in Figure 3.8, assuming the standard paper speed of 25 mm/sec. A normal 12-lead ECG is shown in Figure 3.9. The sections to follow review briefly each of the steps of ECG analysis.

Heart Rate. Usually there is a one-to-one relationship between atrial and ventricular events, and a single heart rate is measured. If the rhythm is reasonably regular, the ventricular rate is determined by dividing the RR interval

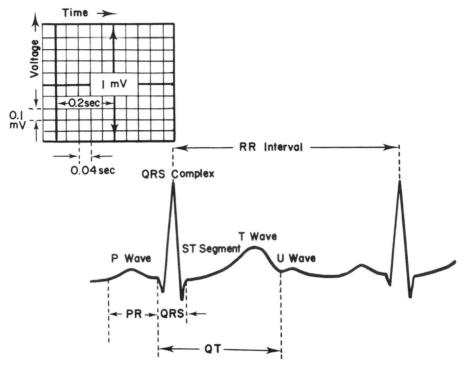

FIGURE 3.8. Standard ECG format and terminology. The paper speed is 25 mm/sec and the 1-mV calibration equals 10 mm.

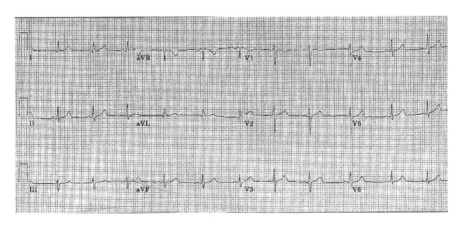

FIGURE 3.9. Normal 12-lead ECG.

TABLE 3.12. A "Method" of ECG Interpretation

(Note: This "method" is the recommended approach to reading all 12 lead ECGs. It is desirable to follow a standardized method so that subtle abnormalities—some of which have important clinical implications—are not overlooked. The six major sections in the "method" should be followed in the order presented below.)

A. Measurements (Usually made in the frontal plane leads)
  1. Heart rate (atrial and ventricular, if different)
       Normal range: 50–90 bpm
  2. PR interval (onset of P to onset of QRS complex)
       Normal range: 0.12–0.20 sec (120–200 ms)
  3. QRS duration (width of QRS complex)
       Normal range: 0.06–0.10 sec (60–100 ms)
  4. QT interval (onset of QRS to end of T wave)
       Normal range: depends on heart rate
  5. Frontal plane QRS axis (i.e., the average direction of forces during QRS)
       Normal range for adult: +90 degrees to -30 degrees

B. Rhythm Analysis
  1. Normal: Normal sinus rhythm (NSR)
  2. Normal variants:
       a. Sinus tachycardia (HR >90 bpm)
       b. Sinus bradycardia (HR <50 bpm)
  3. Abnormal rhythms: consider all rhythm abnormalities originating in the atria, AV junction, and ventricles)

C. Conduction Analysis
  1. Normal: normal SA, AV, and IV conduction
  2. Abnormalities: Consider the following conduction abnormalities:
       a. SA block: 2nd degree (type I or II)
       b. AV block: 1st, 2nd (type I or II), and 3rd degree
       c. IV block: BBBs, fascicular blocks, and nonspecific IVCD
       d. Exit block: block just distal to pacemaker (e.g., junctional rhythm with exit block; also applies to SA block)

TABLE 3.12. Cont.

D. Waveform Description
    1. P waves (consider atrial enlargement)
    2. QRS complexes (consider infarction, ventricular hypertrophy)
    3. ST segment (elevation or depression?)
    4. T waves (flattened or inverted?)
    5. U waves (prominent or inverted?)

E. ECG Interpretation
    This is the conclusion of the above analyses. The ECG should be interpreted as "Normal," "Borderline Abnormal," or "Abnormal," and the abnormalities should be listed as in the following examples:
    1. Inferior MI, probably acute
    2. Old anteroseptal MI
    3. Left anterior fascicular block
    4. Left ventricular hypertrophy
    5. Nonspecific ST-T-wave changes
    6. ST-T- and U-wave abnormalities suggestive of hypokalemia, etc. . . .

F. Comparison With Previous ECG (*if one is available*)

HR, Heart rate; *bpm*, beats per minute; *SA*, sinoatrial; *AV*, atrioventricular; *IV*, intraventricular; *IVCD*, intraventricular conduction disorder; *BBB*, bundle branch block.

(measured in sec) into 60 to get beats per minute (bpm). For example, if the RR interval (Fig. 3.8) is 0.6 sec, the corresponding heart rate is 60/0.6 or 100 bpm. If the paper speed is 25 mm/sec, it is convenient to remember that atrial or ventricular events (i.e., P waves or QRS complexes) occurring one large box apart on the ECG paper (0.2 sec) have a rate of 300 bpm; two boxes (0.4 sec), 150 bpm; three boxes, 100 bpm; four boxes, 75 bpm; five boxes, 60 bpm; and six boxes, 50 bpm. This is an easy way to quickly establish the heart rate at a glance. The traditional and generally accepted resting heart rate limits for *normal sinus rhythm* are 60 to 100 beats/min. A more clinically relevant range, from 50 to 90 bpm, based on actual data, has been reported by Spodick et al. (17). Heart rates <50 bpm are called *sinus bradycardia*, and heart rates >90 bpm are called *sinus tachycardia*. Slight beat-to-beat variation in heart rate with normal respiration is called *sinus arrhythmia*.

PR Interval. The PR interval is measured from the beginning of the P wave to the onset of the QRS complex, usually in the frontal plane leads (Fig. 3.8). This measurement represents the conduction time from the onset of atrial electrical activation (i.e., depolarization) to the beginning of ventricular muscle activation and includes conduction through the AV node, bundle of His, and bundle branches. The normal PR interval range is 0.12 to 0.20 sec. PR intervals <0.12 sec are found in ventricular preexcitation (e.g., the Wolff-Parkinson-White syndrome). In AV junctional rhythms the PR interval may also be <0.12 sec, but the morphology of the P wave suggests a *retrograde* origin (i.e., inverted P waves in leads II, III, and aVF). PR intervals >0.20 sec imply conduction delay between the atria and the ventricles, usually in the AV node (i.e., first-degree AV block).

QRS Duration. This measurement represents the ventricular muscle activation time (Fig. 3.8), and normally ranges from 0.06 to 0.10 sec. These narrow QRS durations reflect the simultaneous activation of the right and left ventricles. In bundle branch block, however, the ventricles are activated sequentially and the QRS duration is prolonged (≥0.12 sec). Other nonspecific intraventricular conduction disorders (IVCD) also prolong the QRS duration beyond 0.10 sec. Rhythms originating in the ventricles (e.g., ventricular tachycardia) will almost always have wide QRS durations.

QT Interval. This important measurement (Fig. 3.8) is from the QRS onset to the end of the T wave and roughly corresponds to the duration of ventricular systole. The normal range is heart rate or cycle length dependent; slower heart rates have longer QT intervals. As an approximate guide, the QT interval should be ≤0.40 sec at 70 bpm. For every 10 beat/min increase in the heart rate, the upper limit of QT interval decreases by 0.02 sec; for every 10 beat/min decrease in heart rate, the upper limit increases by 0.02 sec (e.g., if heart rate is 50 bpm, the QT should be ≤0.44 sec; for a heart rate of 90 bpm, the QT should be ≤0.36 sec). These are only approximate upper limits; more accurate tables of normal limits based on heart rate or RR intervals are provided in many textbooks of electrocardiography.

Prolonged QT intervals are found in many clinical conditions, including CHD, drug therapies (e.g., quinidine, procainamide, tricyclic antidepressants), electrolyte abnormalities (e.g., hypokalemia), central nervous system diseases (e.g., stroke), and hereditary disorders (18). In all of these conditions there is an increased vulnerability to serious, often life-threatening, ventricular arrhythmias and sudden death.

Frontal Plane QRS Axis. The QRS axis in the frontal plane reflects the average direction of ventricular activation in that plane. The measurement is based on the assumption that the six frontal plane leads can be represented by an equilateral triangle as illustrated in Figure 3.10. The axis is determined by vector summation of the individual components of the QRS complexes from any two frontal plane leads, using the reference system shown in Figure 3.10. The normal range in adults is from −30° to +90°. An axis to the left (i.e., more negative) of −30° is called *left axis deviation* and one to the right (i.e., more positive) of +90° is called *right axis deviation.* Axis deviation is seen in several different

FIGURE 3.10. Frontal plane lead diagram for axis determination. The normal range for the QRS axis is shaded.

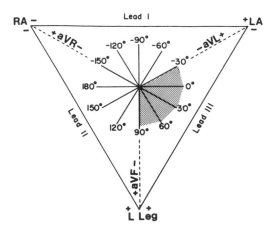

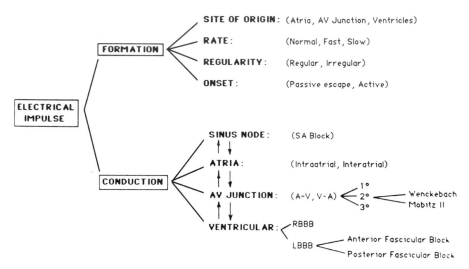

FIGURE 3.11. Approach to the classification of rate, rhythm, and conduction disturbances. (Courtesy of Alan E. Lindsay, M.D.)

conditions, including ventricular hypertrophy and fascicular blocks involving the left bundle branch.

Rhythm and Conduction Analysis. Figure 3.11 offers a useful approach for conceptualizing arrhythmias and conduction disturbances. Abnormalities of impulse formation may be considered in the following sequence: (a) site of origin (atria, AV junction, ventricles); (b) rate of occurrence (normal, slow, fast); (c) regular or irregular response; and (d) active (premature) or passive (escape) onset.

In a similar manner, conduction delays or block may be approached in terms of (a) site of delay (sinoatrial, intraatrial, atrioventricular, intraventricular); (b) direction of block (antegrade, retrograde); and (c) degree of block (1°, 2°, 3°). In 1° block conduction through the tissues in question always succeeds, but the conduction time is prolonged (e.g., the prolonged PR interval in 1° AV block). In 2° block there is intermittent failure of conduction. Some impulses get through the tissues in question; some do not. Also 2° block, especially in the AV junction, can be further divided into type I (Wenckebach), which is a progressive form of block, and type II (Mobitz), which is an all-or-none form of block. Finally, in 3° block, none of the impulses are able to get through the tissues in question.

Figure 3.12 presents an abbreviated atlas of common arrhythmias and conduction disturbances, along with a brief description of pertinent findings of each abnormality. A more thorough discussion of these disorders can be found in many excellent textbooks (19–22).

Waveform Description. Analysis of the individual components of the ECG waveform often provides clues to specific structural abnormalities within the heart. Beginning with the P wave, evidence for right or left atrial enlargement should be sought (Fig. 3.13). Right atrial enlargement (RAE) is manifest by tall, peaked P waves in leads II, III, and aVF. Left atrial enlargement (LAE) causes widening and notching of the P waves in the frontal plane leads and an increase in the terminal negative component of the P wave in lead V_1.

Abnormalities of the QRS complex may show evidence for ventricular hypertrophy. Right ventricular hypertrophy (RVH) causes one or more of the following: (a) rightward shift in the frontal plane QRS axis (usually beyond +90°), (b) increased R-wave forces in V_{1-2}, and (c) increased S-wave forces in V_{5-6}. Left ventricular hypertrophy (LVH) causes increased R-wave voltage in leads V_{5-6}, increased S-wave voltage in V_{1-2}, a leftward shift of the QRS axis, and is often associated with evidence of left atrial enlargement. Both RVH and LVH are often accompanied by secondary ST-T-wave changes deflected in the opposite direction of the major QRS forces. Unfortunately, the ECG is quite insensitive for these anatomic abnormalities. The echocardiogram is a much better diagnostic tool for evaluating chamber size and wall thickness.

The ECG diagnosis of myocardial infarction requires careful analysis of the QRS complex, as well as the ST-T wave. In acute myocardial infarction the most characteristic sequence of ECG changes begins with (a) increasing T-wave amplitude and width in leads corresponding to the anatomical location of infarction. This is shortly followed by (b) ST-segment elevation and later by (c) "pathologic" Q waves in the same set of leads. An abnormal Q wave is defined as one that is wide (0.04 sec), and/or deep (~$\frac{1}{3}$ QRS amplitude). As the infarct evolves, (d) the ST-segment elevation becomes less and the terminal portion of the T wave inverts. With healing and with time, the ECG often returns toward normal, although in large infarcts the abnormalities in QRS and ST-T waves can persist indefinitely. These changes are illustrated in Figure 3.14. Some acute

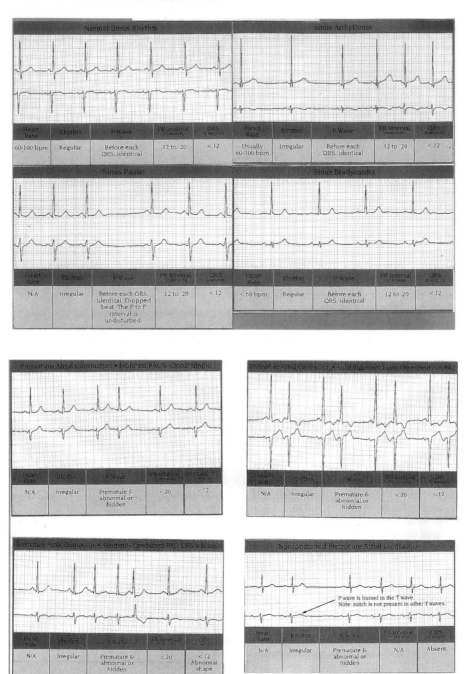

FIGURE 3.12. Brief atlas of common arrhythmias and conduction defects. (Courtesy of Marquette Electronics, Inc.)

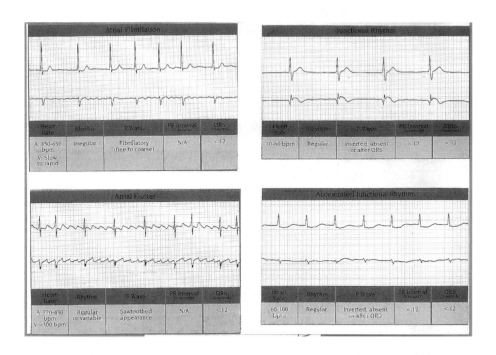

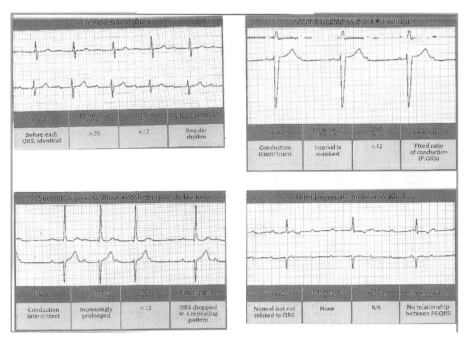

FIGURE 3.12. Cont.

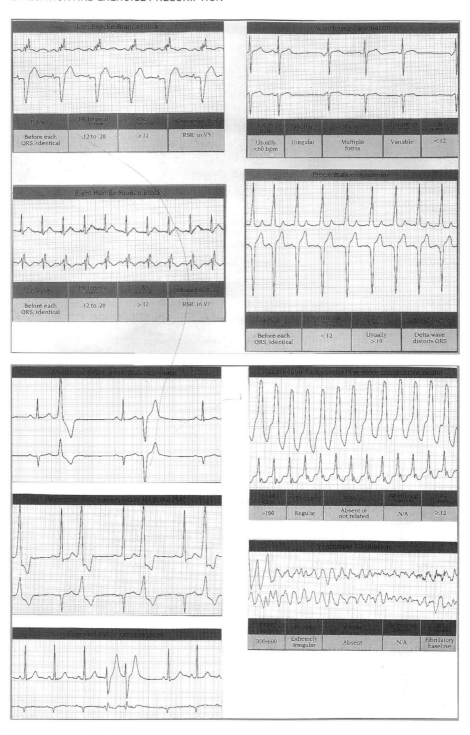

FIGURE 3.12. Cont.

86

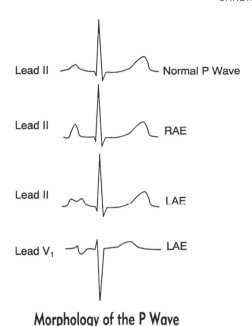

FIGURE 3.13. Morphology of the P wave. *RAE*, Right atrial enlargement; *LAE*, Left atrial enlargement.

Lead II — Normal P Wave

Lead II — RAE

Lead II — LAE

Lead V₁ — LAE

Morphology of the P Wave

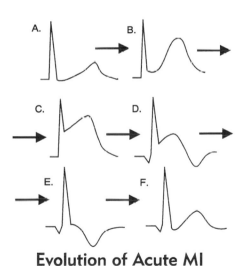

A.

B.

C.

D.

E.

F.

FIGURE 3.14. Typical sequence of ECG changes in inferior myocardial infarction. **A.** Normal lead II ECG waveform before acute MI. **B.** Hyperacute T-wave changes of acute MI. **C.** Acute ST-segment elevation with hyperacute T-wave changes. **D.** Pathologic Q wave, decreasing ST-segment elevation, terminal T-wave inversion (fully evolved acute MI). **E.** Late T-wave inversion of healed MI. **F.** Normalization of T-wave changes in old MI.

Evolution of Acute MI

MIs do not evolve Q-wave abnormalities and are called "non-Q wave MIs." Pathologically, these infarcts have nonhomogeneous necrosis, and they are often associated with subtotaled coronary occlusions. Older textbooks called these non-Q MIs "nontransmural," but this is incorrect.

Table 3.13 classifies infarct locations based on the ECG leads showing the typical changes illustrated in Figure 3.14. Since there are no ECG leads directly

87

TABLE 3.13. ECG Localization of Myocardial Infarctions

(Note: These ECG-defined locations of MIs have only an approximate correlation with actual anatomic locations of myocardial infarctions.)

I. *Inferior* family of infarctions (right coronary or dominant left circumflex lesions):
   A. *Inferior MI*:
      1. Pathologic Q waves and evolving ST-T changes in II, III, aVF
      2. Q waves largest in III, next largest in aVF, smallest in II
   B. *True posterior MI*
      1. Increasing R-wave amplitude in V_1 and/or V_2
      2. R/S ratio in V_1 or $V_2 \geq 1.0$ (prominent anterior forces)
      3. Acute ST-T changes: ST depression, T inversion in V_1 or V_2
      4. Late normalization of ST-T waves in V_{1-2} with upright T waves
   C. *Inferoposterior MI*:
      1. Changes of inferior and posterior MI
   D. *Inferolateral MI*:
      1. Changes of inferior MI
      2. Q waves and/or loss of R waves in V_{4-6}
      3. Evolving ST-T wave changes in V_{4-6}
   E. *Inferoposterolateral MI*:
      1. Changes of inferior, posterior, and lateral MI
   F. *Right ventricular MI*:
      1. ST elevation in right chest leads (V_3R and V_4R)

II. *Anterior* family of infarctions (left anterior descending or left main coronary lesions):
   A. *Anteroseptal MI*:
      1. Q or QS in V_{1-3} with typical ST-T changes
   B. *Anterior MI*:
      1. Q or QS in V_{2-4} with typical ST-T changes
   C. *Anterolateral MI*:
      1. Q or QS in V_{4-6} with typical ST-T changes
      2. May or may not see similar changes in I and/or aVL
   D. *High lateral MI*:
      1. Q or QS in I and aVL with typical ST-T changes
   E. *Extensive anterior MI*:
      1. Q or QS in most precordial leads

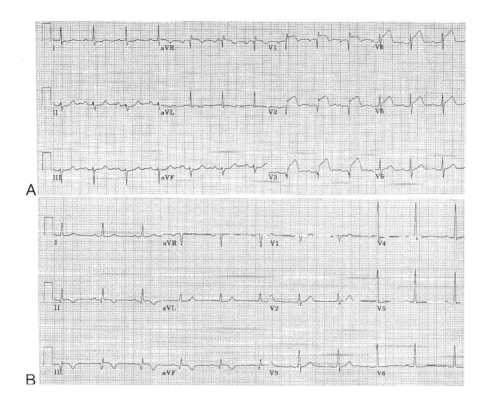

FIGURE 3.15. **A.** Recent anterior wall MI. **B.** Recent inferior wall MI.

over the posterior surface of the heart, the *true posterior* MI is recognized in the anterior leads (V_{1-2}) by changes that are 180° reciprocal to the usual changes; i.e., tall, wide R waves, ST-segment depression, and terminal T waves directed in the positive direction. Two ECG examples of MI are illustrated in Figure 3.15. The ECG recognition of myocardial ischemia is discussed in Chapter 5.

There are many subtle ECG abnormalities that can only be understood when the ECG data are analyzed within the clinical context of the particular patient being evaluated. This is especially true when interpreting the significance of ST-T-wave changes. ST-segment depression and T-wave inversion have many causes, including electrolyte abnormalities, drugs, myocardial ischemia or infarction, ventricular hypertrophy, and central nervous system diseases. The interpretation of a particular ST-T-wave change is dependent on knowing the patient's clinical status at the time the ECG was obtained. The term "*nonspecific*

89

ST-T-*wave changes*" is used when clinical information is not available or when the specific abnormalities are unclear.

If available, it is important to compare the patient's most recent ECG with any previous ECGs. Subtle changes from one ECG to the next may be the only clues to the presence of a new pathologic process.

Chest X-ray

The chest radiograph completes the four essential tools used in the workup of patients with known or suspected heart disease. Along with the history, physical examination, and resting ECG, the chest x-ray provides important information regarding the heart, great vessels, and pulmonary vasculature. The standard roentgenographic assessment of the heart consists of four views: posteroanterior, lateral, and right and left anterior obliques. A barium swallow is often included to outline the posterior cardiac structures, which are adjacent to the barium-filled esophagus. Unfortunately, the more expensive echocardiographic study has replaced the chest x-ray in many clinical situations where the x-ray had previously been used.

As was discussed for the ECG, a systematic approach to "reading" the chest film is necessary to avoid missing subtle abnormalities. In addition, it is important to correlate the abnormal radiographic findings with other clinical information and laboratory data obtained from the patient. The following sequential approach is recommended for complete radiographic analysis: (a) soft tissues and bones of the thorax; (b) pulmonary vasculature and lungs; (c) size and contour of the heart and individual chambers; (d) great vessels and mediastinal structures; (e) abnormal densities and lucencies; and (f) pleura and diaphragms. There are several excellent texts and review articles discussing various aspects of cardiovascular radiology (23–25).

Noninvasive Cardiovascular Techniques

Noninvasive diagnostic procedures have revolutionized the study of patients with cardiovascular diseases by providing quantitative and qualitative analyses of anatomic and physiologic disease processes to a degree of clarity never before imagined. These procedures generally require expensive, highly sophisticated electronic instrumentation, and they demand considerable expertise of the cardiovascular specialist. Many of these tests have become so routine in the practice of cardiovascular medicine that they are often performed without considering their cost-effectiveness relative to a more simple, clinical, bedside examination. Table 3.14 lists the questions that should be addressed in considering the indications for specialized noninvasive testing (26).

The following noninvasive tests are briefly considered: (a) echocardiography and Doppler studies; (b) nuclear imaging techniques; (c) magnetic resonance imaging (MRI) techniques.

TABLE 3.14. Questions To Be Considered Before Doing Specialized Cardiovascular Diagnostic Tests[a]

1. What is *pretest* probability of the disease based on initial clinical findings?
2. What is the overall management objective?
3. What specific questions still need to be answered?
4. How well does the proposed test answer these questions?
5. How will a negative or positive test result be interpreted?
6. What treatments will be recommended based on test results?
7. Is the specific test worth the cost, risk, and inconvenience?

[a] From Patterson RE, Horowitz SF. J Am Coll Cardiol 1989; 13:653–662.

Echocardiography and Doppler Studies

Echocardiography, or cardiac ultrasound, involves the transmission of ultrahigh-frequency sound waves into the body to detect and image stationary and moving structures. Short bursts of ultrasound are emitted from a transducer held on the body surface and directed in different directions and tomographic planes. The depth and position of the reflected echoes returning from various anatomic structures are detected by the transducer and electronically amplified to produce either time-motion strip-chart recordings (M-mode) or two-dimensional (2-D) images in a video format. Computer processing of the data is done to enhance the images and to provide quantitative analyses of chamber size, ventricular function, wall motion, and valve areas.

The echocardiographic examination is performed while the patient is supine or in the left lateral decubitus position. Various acoustic windows are chosen for both M-mode and 2-D imaging to obtain multiple views of the cardiovascular structures. The M-mode images represent an "ice pick" or one-dimensional time-motion analysis of moving and stationary cardiac structures. By scanning the M-mode beam in an arc, as illustrated in Figure 3.16, the different cardiac structures from apex to base can be imaged. The simultaneously recorded ECG signal permits accurate timing of events. The major disadvantage of M-mode echocardiography is the limited spatial views available with this technique. As a result, M-mode images today are only obtained in conjunction with 2-D echocardiography.

Two-dimensional, or tomographic, imaging is the primary echocardiographic technique used today in clinical medicine. Various tomographic cuts of the heart along its long and short axes are obtained by varying the transducer location on the body surface and the ultrasound beam plane (Fig. 3.17). The images are recorded on videotape for subsequent playback and analysis. Imaging quality is occasionally limited by interference from other anatomic structures in the echo

91

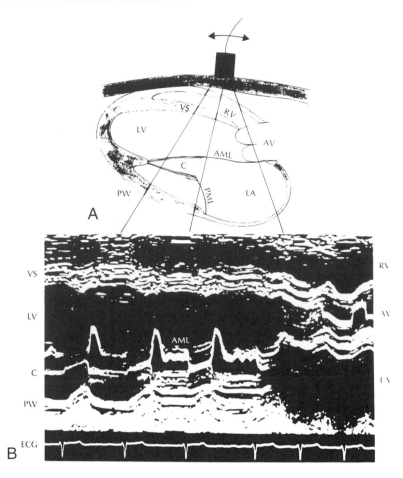

FIGURE 3.16. M-mode echocardiography. **A.** M-mode scan (*diagram*). **B.** M-mode scan data. (Reproduced by permission from Nanda NC, Gramiak R. Clinical echocardiography. St Louis: CV Mosby, 1978.)

beam, including subcutaneous fat, ribs, lung tissue, and other chest-wall abnormalities. A recent advance in 2-D imaging is the transesophageal echocardiographic (TEE) technique, which has opened up several new and unique anatomic windows to cardiac anatomy (27). In this technique the transducer is passed endoscopically into the esophagus and positioned at various locations behind the heart to obtain the different views. Patients are usually premedicated for the TEE study to minimize gagging, retching, and laryngospasm. This technique is especially useful in diagnosing aortic dissection, vegetations from endocarditis, and prosthetic valve malfunction.

Echocardiography has many important clinical applications, which are listed in Table 3.15 (28). In recognizing chamber enlargement, hypertrophy, and myo-

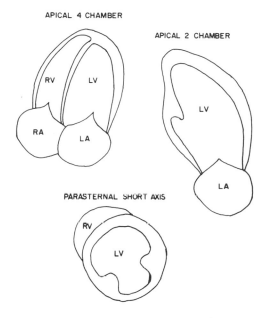

APICAL 4 CHAMBER

APICAL 2 CHAMBER

PARASTERNAL SHORT AXIS

FIGURE 3.17. Two-dimensional echocardiographic views. (Reproduced by permission from Selzer A. Principles and practice of clinical cardiology. 2nd ed. Philadelphia: WB Saunders, 1983.)

TABLE 3.15. Applications of Echocardiography

I. Evaluation of *valvular heart disease*
    A. Differential diagnosis and evaluation of heart murmurs
        1. Functional murmur versus organic valvular abnormality
        2. Specific etiology of mitral regurgitation murmurs
        3. Aortic valve stenosis versus hypertrophic cardiomyopathy
        4. Quantitation of valve areas
    B. Prosthetic valve abnormalities
    C. Detection of valvular vegetations (e.g., endocarditis)
    D. Evaluation of ventricular function in valvular heart disease

II. Evaluation of known or suspected *coronary heart disease*
    A. Global and segmental wall motion abnormalities
    B. Detection of ventricular aneurysm
    C. Detection of mural thrombus
    D. Assessment of left ventricular ejection fraction
    E. Detection of right ventricular infarction
    F. Differential diagnosis of chest pain in emergency room

III. Diagnosis of *congenital heart disease*

IV. Diagnosis of *pericardial disease*

V. Evaluation of *cardiomyopathy*

VI. Diagnosis of *cardiac tumors*

cardial infarction location and size, the echo examination has surpassed the ECG. The ECHO is also a very important adjunct to the physical examination in the differential diagnosis of heart murmurs. In addition to identifying the origin of a heart murmur, the ECHO provides quantitative information regarding the severity of valve lesions, the etiology, and the functional consequences to the myocardium. Quantitation of valve areas, chamber size, wall thickness, and ventricular function are all necessary prerequisites to determining the need for corrective surgery. The ECHO is also the procedure of choice for recognizing pericardial effusion, tamponade, and atrial myxomas.

Echocardiography has many applications in coronary heart disease (29). Beginning in the emergency room, the ECHO is now being used to help diagnose acute myocardial infarction in patients with atypical presentations (30). Once admitted to the coronary care unit the ECHO can assess ventricular function and ejection fraction for risk stratification. The detection of mural thrombi and ventricular aneurysms in patients recovering from acute MI facilitates the decision to administer anticoagulant and other specific therapies. In the post-MI period exercise and pharmacologic stress echocardiographic studies are now being carried out to detect myocardial ischemia, especially in patients whose abnormal resting ECGs preclude adequate ischemia recognition (see Chapter 5).

The Doppler imaging technique is now a routine part of the ultrasound examination of the cardiovascular system (31). This method quantitates blood flow velocity, direction, and timing in the heart and blood vessels. This information complements the anatomic data from echocardiography and improves the quantitation of valve stenosis and regurgitation. In some patients being evaluated for valve surgery, a good ECHO-Doppler study obviates the need for invasive cardiac catheterization.

Four modalities of Doppler imaging are used to assess cardiovascular diagnoses and function (32). *Pulsed-wave Doppler* (PWD) uses a probe that alternates as a transmitter and receiver of ultrasound signals. The ultrasound beam is focused on selected sites in the heart to detect blood flow velocity and turbulence in the various chambers and vessels. The localization of heart murmurs and the severity of valve lesions can be determined with this technique. *Continuous-wave Doppler* (CWD) transmits and receives ultrasound continuously using two groups of piezoelectric crystals in the probe. This technique permits an accurate assessment of blood flow velocity in the heart and great vessels similar to an electromagnetic flowmeter. The CWD technique, however, does not give information regarding the origin of the reflected signals. *High–pulse repetition frequency* (HPRF) *Doppler* combines the advantages of PWD with those of CWD and permits recording of high flow velocities and sites of origin in the cardiovascular system. This technique is useful in distinguishing several high-velocity jets in close proximity to each other such as is found in combined aortic stenosis and mitral regurgitation. The most recent Doppler technique to be introduced is *Doppler flow imaging* (DFI), which provides two-dimensional images of blood flow in color. The technique is also called *color-flow imaging*. Different colors are used to distinguish flows moving in various directions relative to the transducer. Color-shading is used to characterize flow velocities. This technique is used in conjunction with 2-D echocardiography to analyze flow patterns in the various chambers of the heart during systole and diastole.

Nuclear Cardiology

The rapid development of radioactive isotope techniques in the 1970s coincided with the need to improve the recognition of myocardial ischemia and the quantitation of ventricular function as more definitive therapies became available for patients with CHD. Numerous reports in the literature have documented the improved sensitivity and specificity of these techniques for diagnosis of CHD (33). Recent applications of nuclear cardiology have focused more on the functional and prognostic assessment of patients with known cardiovascular disease rather than on diagnostic issues. Additional applications of these techniques include detection of right-to-left shunts, assessment of right ventricular function, and quantitation of valvular regurgitation.

The two major nuclear imaging methods in clinical use today are (a) myocardial perfusion imaging, and (b) radionuclide blood pool ventriculography. The radiographic images are obtained using a high-sensitivity, high-resolution gamma-ray scintillation camera (33). The images are visually analyzed, as well as computer processed for more quantitative analyses. The techniques may be carried out at rest, during and after exercise, or following pharmacologic stress. Exercise and pharmacologic stress imaging are discussed in Chapter 5.

Myocardial Perfusion Imaging. Thallium-201 (^{201}Tl) is a radioactive isotope that is an analog of potassium. It is distributed in the myocardium in proportion to blood flow distribution and cellular viability. When injected intravenously in a patient with normal coronary blood flow and myocardial perfusion, there is a rapid accumulation of the radioisotope in an even distribution throughout the myocardium. Ischemic myocardium is initially underperfused and therefore appears as a defect or "cold-spot" surrounded by normally perfused myocardium. If the ischemic abnormality is only transient, as seen during exercise or coronary spasm, there will be a delayed uptake (usually after several hours) into the previously ischemic zone with disappearance of the defect. In MI, however, the defect is permanent, since the infarcted or scarred myocardium remains underperfused indefinitely. Most laboratories utilize quantitative and tomographic ^{201}Tl imaging techniques to enhance contrast and provide information about the extent and localization of disease. The specific applications of ^{201}Tl perfusion imaging to exercise testing are discussed in Chapter 5.

Radionuclide Ventriculography. This nuclear imaging technique uses radioactive technetium (^{99m}Tc) bound either to albumin in the blood or to the patient's own red blood cells. The test is comparable to contrast ventriculography performed during invasive cardiac catheterization. It is done to assess heart chamber size, segmental and global wall motion abnormalities, contractile function, ejection fraction, and intracardiac shunts at rest and during exercise. In patients with CHD the functional consequences of myocardial ischemia or infarction can be evaluated from the perspective of wall motion abnormalities and ejection fraction measurements. The test is also valuable in assessing the severity of congestive heart failure for the purpose of making therapeutic decisions and identifying prognostic indices.

Two techniques are available for assessing cardiovascular performance (33). The *first-pass radionuclide angiocardiography* technique involves the rapid bolus injection of radiotracer intravenously, and only the initial pass through the central circulation is analyzed using a gamma scintillation camera. Computer image processing is used to compute end-systolic volumes, end-diastolic volumes, and ejection fractions. The *multiple-gated equilibrium cardiac blood-pool imaging* (MUGA) technique uses the ECG signal to control the temporal sequences of images throughout the cardiac cycle. Data are acquired over several hundred cardiac cycles until a sufficient count density is achieved to create a well-defined sequence of images spanning the entire cardiac cycle. Unlike the first-pass technique, the MUGA allows for sequential studies and studies in multiple positions at rest and during exercise from a single radioisotope injection.

Magnetic Resonance Imaging (MRI) Techniques

The newest and most expensive addition to the noninvasive imaging armamentarium is the MRI technique (34). Anatomic images result from the interaction of hydrogen nuclei of biologic tissues with strong magnetic fields introduced from the MRI device. Regions of weakly magnetized tissue can then be localized within the magnetic field to form an image of the particular structures being investigated. High-contrast tomographic sections can be obtained in different planes using ECG-gated acquisition of data to analyze cardiac structure and function throughout the cardiac cycle. Cardiovascular applications of this technique are growing and include assessment of complex congenital heart abnormalities, diagnosis of cardiac tumors, diagnosis of pericardial disease, evaluating global and segmental ventricular function, and characterization of specific tissue abnormalities within heart muscle. Many of these applications overlap with those of echocardiography and radionuclide imaging, and the exact role for the more expensive MRI techniques is evolving.

Invasive Cardiovascular Diagnostic Procedures

The invasive techniques that are used in the evaluation of patients with cardiovascular disease are listed in Table 3.16. Without a doubt, these procedures have

TABLE 3.16. Invasive Cardiovascular Diagnostic Procedures

1. Right and left heart catheterization
2. Contrast angiography
3. Cardiac function evaluation
4. Electrophysiologic studies
5. Myocardial biopsy

resulted in major advances in diagnostic and therapeutic cardiology over the past 35 years. They have become indispensable prerequisites to making many therapeutic decisions. Invasive procedures, however, are associated with increased risk, considerable cost, and some discomfort to the patient. At a time when the health care reform process is encouraging more cost-saving strategies in medicine, it is imperative that the indications for invasive procedures be carefully defined based on cost-benefit analyses of outcomes.

Right and Left Heart Catheterization

Patients undergoing elective cardiac catheterization studies are usually admitted to the hospital the day of the procedure after undergoing a preliminary workup in the physician's office. The specific catheterization protocol will depend on the particular questions raised during the preliminary workup.

The right heart catheterization procedure usually uses a percutaneous femoral vein approach, although other venous entry sites are possible. Information obtained includes (a) pressure measurements in the right atrium, right ventricle, pulmonary arteries, and pulmonary capillary "wedge" position (an indirect reflection of left atrial pressures); (b) pressure gradients across tricuspid and pulmonic valves; (c) cardiac output measurements by thermodilution; and (d) oxygen contents of blood in the right heart chambers and pulmonary circulation (used to calculate left-to-right shunts).

Left heart catheterization usually involves a percutaneous femoral artery approach, although other sites are also used. Hemodynamic data include (a) pressures in the aorta and left ventricle, (b) pressure gradients across the aortic valve to assess the severity of aortic stenosis, and (c) oxygen contents of blood in the left ventricle and aorta (used to calculate right-to-left shunts). When the right heart catheter is in the pulmonary "wedge" position and the left heart catheter is in the left ventricle, the pressure gradient across the mitral valve can be measured to determine the severity of mitral stenosis. The pressure gradients and flow measurements in systole and diastole permit calculating aortic and mitral valve areas, respectively, using appropriate formulas and assuming no valve regurgitation (35). This is rarely done, however, because valve areas are better assessed with the echocardiographic technique.

In addition to measuring pressures and blood flow during routine cardiac catheterization, two special invasive procedures have recently been introduced to address difficult diagnostic and management questions: (a) intracardiac electrophysiologic studies, and (b) endomyocardial biopsy. Electrophysiologic studies are performed to evaluate and treat complex cardiac arrhythmias and conduction abnormalities (36). The myocardial biopsy procedure is used to obtain heart tissue for pathologic studies (37).

One of the earliest applications of intracardiac electrophysiology in the 1970s was direct recordings from the AV node and bundle of His to identify the site of slowed conduction or heart block in patients with AV conduction disorders. The information was useful in determining the need for permanent pacemaker therapy. More recently, these techniques have increasingly been performed to evaluate and treat complex ventricular arrhythmias that are associated with an increased risk for syncope and sudden death. The extrastimulus pacing technique is used to induce ventricular tachycardia by delivering one or more premature stimuli to various ventricular sites. If the ECG morphology of the induced arrhythmia is similar to the patient's spontaneous arrhythmia, the patient is then placed on antiarrhythmic drug therapy and the procedure repeated. If a drug can be found that prevents the pacing-induced ventricular tachycardia, then it is likely that the drug will be effective in preventing the patient's spontaneous arrhythmia. Intracardiac electrophysiologic studies are also being done to identify and ablate the anatomic substrate for reentrant supraventricular arrhythmias. A full discussion of these techniques is beyond the scope of this chapter.

Endomyocardial biopsy was initially developed to study the rejection phenomenon in patients who have had cardiac transplants (37). The technique involves the use of a specially designed biopsy catheter with a forceps handle to manipulate the cutting jaws at the catheter tip. Samples of right and left ventricular endocardium can be obtained for microscopic examination. It is usual for heart transplant patients to have frequent biopsy procedures during the first year after surgery. As investigators gained skill and experience with this procedure, the clinical indications for biopsy increased to include patients with idiopathic cardiomyopathy and suspected myocarditis. In addition, the technique has been found to be a useful method of monitoring the cardiotoxic effects of chemotherapeutic agents. The pathologic diagnosis made from the biopsy samples often permits more specific therapies to be administered to patients with severely compromised cardiac function.

Angiocardiography

Angiographic procedures are often performed during right and left heart catheterization studies. The procedure involves the selective injection of radiopaque dye into cardiac chambers and blood vessels to visualize various segments of the cardiovascular system. X-ray images are analyzed using cineangiographic techniques or cut-film angiography. Right heart studies are done to detect certain congenital abnormalities and to evaluate the pulmonary circulation. Abnormalities of the right ventricular outflow tract and pulmonic valve are easily visualized by this technique. Left ventricular angiography is performed to quantitate the degree of mitral regurgitation and evaluate left ventricular function. Global and segmental abnormalities of left ventricular wall motion can be assessed by this technique. Aortic root angiography is done to evaluate abnormalities of the aortic valve and ascending aorta.

The coronary angiogram is the definitive test for diagnosing and quantitating the severity of coronary atherosclerosis. The purpose of coronary angiography, according to a recent joint task force of the American Heart Association (AHA) and American College of Cardiology (ACC) (4) is "to define the anatomy of the coronary arteries when such information is needed for patient management." Furthermore, "this anatomic definition includes assessment of the presence, extent and severity of obstructive atherosclerotic coronary artery disease, coronary artery size, coronary collateral flow, thrombus formation, dynamic obstructions (coronary spasm) or congenital coronary artery anomalies" (4).

In this technique arterial catheters are introduced into the right and left coronary arteries to selectively visualize different segments of the coronary circulation (35). Multiple cineangiographic views of each major coronary artery are obtained using hand injections of radiopaque dye. In patients who have had coronary artery bypass surgery, the saphenous vein grafts can also be visualized. Left ventricular angiograms are routinely done in conjunction with coronary artery studies to evaluate left ventricular function.

Coronary angiography is the "bread-and-butter" technique of the practicing invasive cardiologist. Most often this procedure is performed to detect surgically correctable lesions or to identify lesions that can be dilated by catheter angioplasty techniques. Occasionally an angiogram is done to evaluate asymptomatic individuals who have abnormal resting or exercise ECGs. In addition, patients being evaluated for heart valve surgery often undergo coronary angiographic studies to identify those needing coronary artery bypass surgery at the time of valve surgery. The joint AHA/ACC task force has carefully defined and published guidelines for coronary angiography based on the consensus of experts in the field (4).

The interpretation of coronary angiography requires a systematic evaluation of each coronary artery. A significant lesion is usually defined as one that occludes at least 70 to 75% of the luminal diameter. The extent of disease is determined by the number of vessels with significant lesions; e.g., single-, double-, or triple-vessel disease. A lesion of 50% or greater of the left main coronary artery is considered to be the equivalent to double-vessel disease. In addition to the degree of obstruction, the length of the narrowing is also an important determinant of coronary blood flow beyond the lesion. Finally, the

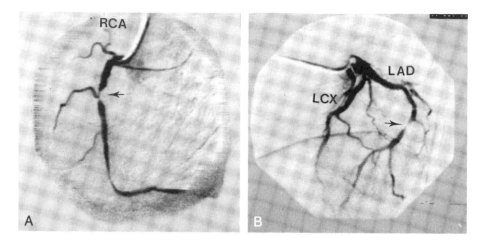

FIGURE 3.18. Coronary angiograms. **A.** High-grade lesion of the proximal right coronary artery *(arrow)*. **B.** High-grade lesion of the middle segment of the left anterior descending *(LAD)* coronary artery *(arrow)*. The left circumflex *(LCX)* artery is also shown.

location of the lesion in the diseased artery may be an important consideration in determining optimal therapy. Proximal lesions that are not totally obstructing may be relieved by angioplasty procedures. Two examples of significant lesions on angiography are illustrated in Figure 3.18.

CARDIOVASCULAR THERAPEUTICS

The following is a brief discussion of treatment strategies in cardiovascular medicine. These treatments can be classified as *specific therapies* directed against particular diseases or manifestations of disease and as *nonspecific therapies* designed to improve the patient's overall state of well-being. Cardiac rehabilitation and adult fitness, the principal subjects of this book, are primarily nonspecific therapies, although there may be some direct effect in reversing or ameliorating the atherosclerotic process. Therapies can also be categorized as *remedial* (i.e., directed against an actual disease manifestation) or *prophylactic* (i.e., aimed at preventing a disease or recurrence of an existing disease). To some extent, exercise therapy is both remedial and prophylactic for patients with CHD, although the major benefits are related to improvements in functional capacity. Finally, therapies may be *nonpharmacologic*, *pharmacologic*, or *invasive*. Nonpharmacologic therapies are directed toward changes in behaviors and lifestyles. These are extremely important in the long-term management of patients with cardiovascular disease and will be discussed in Chapter 11. Pharmacologic therapies are directed against specific manifestations and symptoms of disease. Invasive therapies include surgical procedures, angioplasty, and other invasive manipulations of the body. The comprehensive management of cardiovascular diseases often involves many different therapeutic approaches.

A primary consideration in selecting a particular treatment is the cost-benefit ratio. The therapeutic benefits to the patient should clearly outweigh the potential risks, discomforts, and financial obligations. In addition, the objectives of each therapy should be carefully defined and discussed with the patient prior to its initiation. Periodic follow-up should be done to evaluate the therapeutic effects. Decisions to modify or discontinue a particular therapy are usually based on cost-benefit issues, which vary from patient to patient.

Cardiovascular Drugs

In the natural history of most diseases drug therapy frequently becomes necessary to relieve symptoms or other disease manifestations. The various clinical indications for initiating drug therapy are listed in Table 3.17. For each of these indications there are several different classes of drugs that may be effective, and within each class there are many choices. The factors that lead to the selection of a specific drug for a given patient are many and involve both the science and the art of medicine. Included in the decision-making process are physician experience, desired therapeutic response, ease of administration, side effects, cost, and potential interactions with other drugs. In addition, the pharmaceutical industry may have subtle and not so subtle influences in the selection of specific drugs through the use of clever advertisements, convincing salesmen, exhibits at scientific meetings, and enticing gifts to health care professionals.

Antianginal Drugs

Drugs that relieve symptoms of angina pectoris and episodes of silent ischemia are effective because they restore the balance between coronary blood flow (i.e., oxygen supply) and myocardial oxygen demands. Three classes of drugs are most applicable to the management of ischemic manifestations: (a) nitrates, (b) beta-adrenergic blocking drugs, and (c) calcium-channel blocking drugs. Each of these classes is briefly considered.

TABLE 3.17. Common Indications for Cardiovascular Drug Therapy

- Relief of angina pectoris
- Treatment of heart failure
- Control of cardiac arrhythmias
- Management of hypertension
- Antiplatelet, anticoagulant, and thrombolytic therapy
- Management of hyperlipidemia

Nitrates. The organic nitrates are the oldest and most commonly prescribed drugs for the treatment of symptomatic and silent ischemia (38). They are also prescribed in congestive heart failure and frequently used in the treatment of acute myocardial infarction. Although potent coronary vasodilators, the nitrates also work primarily by dilating the systemic and pulmonary venous circulations. As a result, the venous return to the right heart is reduced, pulmonary venous return to the left heart is reduced, left ventricular filling pressures are reduced, and myocardial oxygen demands are lowered. Coronary vasodilation may improve the supply of oxygenated blood to the myocardium, especially in the setting of coronary artery spasm. Finally, nitrates cause systemic arteriolar vasodilation and lower blood pressure.

The two most common forms of nitrate therapy are nitroglycerin and isosorbide dinitrate. Both drugs are available as short-acting (sublingual spray, tablets, and chewable forms), intermediate-acting (oral and topical ointments), and long-acting (oral and transdermal patches) preparations. Short-acting drugs take effect within minutes and may be effective for 15 minutes to several hours. Intermediate-acting preparations are effective for 3 to 6 hours; the long-acting drugs may have an effect for 8 to 12 hours or longer. Intravenous nitrates are used in acute care settings in the management of unstable angina and myocardial infarction. The newest long-acting oral preparation, isosorbide mononitrate, has kinetics favorable for the elderly population who may have liver or kidney impairment.

Headaches and postural light-headedness are the most common side effects of the nitrates. For most patients the headaches diminish after several weeks of therapy, although in some the headaches are so severe that continued therapy becomes impossible. Postural hypotension may be severe enough to cause syncope. When initiating nitrate therapy, patients should be instructed to be sitting or supine when first taking the short-acting preparations. In patients taking long-acting preparations the development of tolerance to the desired hemodynamic effects often occurs unless there is a daily nitrate-free interval of 8 to 12 hours' duration (39). Usually this is recommended during the nighttime hours when the myocardial oxygen demands are lowest.

β-Adrenergic Blockers. The β-blocking agents have been used for over 20 years in the treatment of angina pectoris, hypertension, and arrhythmias. In recent years many new agents in this class have been introduced with a variety of desirable and undesirable effects (40). These drugs are competitive inhibitors of catecholamine binding at β-adrenergic receptor sites. In the heart this results in decreased myocardial contractility and slowing of the heart rate, both of which reduce myocardial oxygen requirements. In patients with angina these effects are associated with fewer anginal attacks and increased exercise tolerance.

The available β-blockers differ in their pharmacologic properties. Cardioselective agents (e.g., metoprolol, atenolol) have advantages over nonselective

102

drugs (e.g., propranolol, timolol, nadolol) because they minimize undesirable β-blocking effects on other tissues such as the pulmonary airways (i.e., broncho-constriction). This is particularly dangerous in patients with reactive airways disease (asthma, chronic bronchitis) since these unwanted effects may produce bronchospasm. Beta-blockers also differ in their lipid solubility. Lipid-soluble drugs (e.g., propranolol, metoprolol, timolol) have a relatively short half-life and must be administered 2 to 4 times daily. In contrast, water-soluble agents (e.g., atenolol, nadolol) have a long half-life and can be administered once daily. Recently, sustained-release lipid-soluble preparations (e.g., metoprolol succinate) that permit once-a-day dosing have become available.

The major side effects of these drugs are related to their basic mechanisms of action (i.e., bradycardia and depressed myocardial function). In patients with preexisting left ventricular failure, β-blockers are relatively contraindicated, and therefore they should be used with caution. As already mentioned, β-blockers can exacerbate bronchospasm in individuals with reactive airways disease (asthma, chronic bronchitis). In insulin requiring diabetes mellitus, β-blockers can mask the symptoms of hypoglycemia. Other common side effects include fatigue, weakness, depression, decreased libido, and gastrointestinal disturbances.

Calcium Channel Blockers. The newest class of antianginal drugs are the calcium channel blocking agents, also known as calcium antagonists (41). By blocking the entry of ionic calcium into vascular smooth muscle cells these drugs relax the muscle cells and produce vasodilation. Although initially approved for the relief of coronary artery spasm, the calcium blockers are also effective for treating anginal symptoms caused by coronary atherosclerosis. They are also commonly prescribed for the treatment of hypertension, cardiac arrhythmias, and hypertrophic cardiomyopathies.

The first generation calcium antagonists (nifedipine, diltiazem, and verapamil) have been used for over 20 years. Newer agents are appearing on the market all the time. These drugs are all reasonably effective in relieving symptoms of myocardial ischemia, although they have differing properties on myocardial contractility and cardiac conduction (41). Verapamil and diltiazem depress myocardial contractility, decrease heart rate, and slow conduction in the AV node. This last property makes them useful in the treatment of paroxysmal supraventricular tachycardias and atrial fibrillation. Nifedipine, on the other hand, has more peripheral vasodilating effects and often results in reflex acceleration in heart rate and AV conduction. In the treatment of angina, all three calcium channel blockers work well as single agents or in combination with nitrates and/or β-blockers. Each drug has short- and long-acting formulations. In general, the calcium antagonists are better tolerated than nitrates or β-blockers.

Antihypertensive Drugs

Hypertension is mostly a silent disease. The major objective in treating hypertension therefore is to reduce the cardiovascular, renal, and central nervous system morbidity and mortality associated with long-standing elevations in blood pressure. It is now well established that antihypertensive drugs are effective in controlling high blood pressure and prolonging life (42). Nonpharmacologic management of hypertension is discussed in Chapter 11.

A major stimulus to the management of hypertension has been the publications of the *Joint National Committee on Detection, Evaluation, and Treatment of High Blood Pressure*. The *Fifth Report* (JNC-V) of this influential body sponsored by the National Institutes of Health was published in January 1993 (42). Table 3.18 illustrates the new classification scheme of adult blood pressure and the recommendations for follow-up based on the initial blood pressure measurements. The JNC-V and ongoing education programs strongly recommend treatment goals of systolic blood pressures <140 mm Hg and diastolic blood pressures <90 mm Hg. Further reduction to 130/85 mm Hg is encouraged for

TABLE 3.18. Classification of Blood Pressure and Recommended Follow-Up[a]

Range (mm HG)	Classification[b]	Recommended Follow-Up
Diastolic		
<85	Normal blood pressure	Recheck in 2 years
85–89	High normal blood pressure	Recheck in 1 year
90–99	Stage 1 (mild)	Confirm within 2 months
100–109	Stage 2 (moderate)	Evaluate or refer within 1 month
110–119	Stage 3 (severe)	Evaluate or refer within 1 week
≥120	Stage 4 (very severe)	Evaluate or refer immediately
Systolic		
<130	Normal blood pressure	Recheck within 2 years
130–139	High normal	Recheck in 1 year
140–159	Stage 1 (mild)	Confirm within 2 months
160–179	Stage 2 (moderate)	Evaluate or refer within 1 month
180–209	Stage 3 (severe)	Evaluate or refer within 1 week
≥210	Stage 4 (very severe)	Evaluate or refer immediately

[a]Adapted from the report of the Joint National Committee on Detection, Evaluation, and Treatment of High Blood Pressure (JNC-V). Arch Intern Med 1993;153:154–183.
[b]Not on antihypertensive drugs or acutely ill. When systolic and diastolic BP fall into different categories, the *higher* category should be selected to classify the BP status and dictate follow-up strategy. For example, 160/92 should be stage 2, and 180/120 should be stage 4. Isolated systolic hypertension (ISH) is defined as SBP ≥140 mm Hg and DBP <90 mm Hg, and staged appropriately.

select individuals with some caution in older persons. As in previous reports, a "stepped-care" approach is preferred, beginning with lifestyle modifications as the first and often the most important step (Chapter 11). Figure 3.19 illustrates the JNC-V treatment algorithm which includes the recommended choices of drugs.

Because of costs and proven efficacy in reducing cardiovascular morbidity and mortality, diuretics and β-blockers are the preferred first-line drugs for

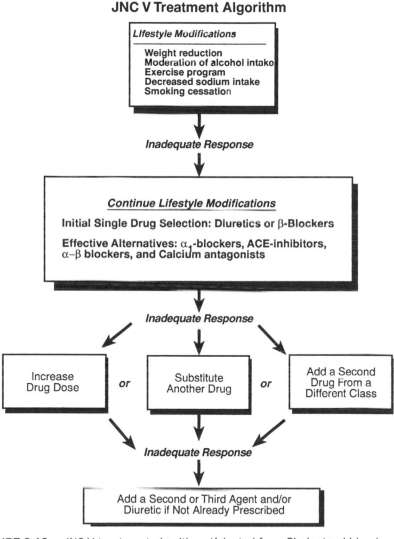

FIGURE 3.19. JNC-V treatment algorithm. (Adapted from Cholesterol blood pressure update. Vol 5. [Bethesda, MD:] Citizens For Public Action on Blood Pressure and Cholesterol, January 1993.)

treating newly diagnosed hypertension. Beta-blockers were previously discussed for the treatment of ischemic syndromes. Their role in treating hypertension is based on their ability to decrease cardiac output and lower plasma renin activity. Diuretics, which are predominately of the thiazide type, act initially by decreasing plasma and extracellular fluid volume and cardiac output, followed later by reducing total peripheral resistance and normalization of cardiac output. They should be initiated at the lowest effective dose, usually the equivalent of 12.5 to 25 mg per day of hydrochlorothiazide. The majority of patients with stage 1 and 2 hypertension (Table 3.18) will respond to these first-line drug therapies, especially if nonpharmacologic self-management is also practiced.

There are several alternative drug classes that are equally effective initial treatment choices. The α_1-receptor blockers (e.g., doxazosin, prazosin) block postsynaptic α_1-receptors of the sympathetic nervous system and cause vasodilation. The α-β blockers (e.g., labetalol) have both beta-blocking properties and α_1-receptor blocking properties. They are possibly more effective in hypertensive blacks than other β-blockers. Angiotensin-converting-enzyme (ACE) inhibitors (e.g., captopril, enalapril, lisinopril) are especially attractive new agents because of their low side-effect profile and convenient dosing, although they are considerably more expensive than the diuretics and β-blockers. They work by blocking the formation of the potent vasoconstrictor, angiotensin II, causing vasodilation and decreased circulating aldosterone. Finally, the calcium antagonists (e.g., diltiazem, verapamil, nifedipine), discussed above for the treatment of ischemic syndromes, are effective antihypertensive agents because of their ability to cause smooth muscle relaxation. Unlike the diuretics and β-blockers, however, these alternative drug classes have not been shown to lower cardiovascular morbidity and mortality in controlled clinical trials (42).

If adequate blood pressure control is not achieved with single drug therapy, then the algorithm illustrated in Figure 3.19 should be followed. The choices include increasing the drug dose, substituting another drug, or adding a second agent from another class. Continued emphasis on lifestyle restructuring should be reinforced. Adding a third agent is rarely necessary in the management of severe, refractory hypertension. Occasionally a detailed workup for secondary causes of hypertension (e.g., endocrine tumor, renal artery stenosis) is indicated in cases of hypertension unresponsive to conventional drug therapies or the sudden onset of severe hypertension in older individuals (43).

Isolated systolic hypertension (ISH), defined as systolic blood pressures >140 mm Hg and diastolic blood pressures <90 mm Hg, is increasingly being recognized as an important cause of cardiovascular morbidity and mortality in the elderly (42). Whereas in the past ISH was considered a benign condition associated with "aging" and hardening of the arteries, it is now clear that this is a widely prevalent and dangerous cardiovascular risk factor, even more so than diastolic hypertension. In a recently completed, randomized, placebo-controlled trial, the Systolic Hypertension in the Elderly Program (SHEP) concluded that low-dose thiazide diuretics, supplemented if necessary by a β-blocker, significantly reduced the morbidity and mortality from stroke and myocardial infarction compared to the placebo (44). Since cardiovascular diseases are the leading causes of death for men and women over age 65 years, it is important to detect and successfully manage this form of hypertension.

Antiarrhythmic Drugs

Cardiac arrhythmias of various types are found in normal healthy individuals, as well as in patients with a variety of cardiac and other diseases. In the absence of organic heart disease, drug therapy is usually not indicated unless the cardiac rhythm disturbance is so severe that it is associated with disabling or uncomfortable symptoms. Preventing sudden hemodynamic collapse and sudden death are the most serious indications for the treatment of cardiac arrhythmias. These catastrophic complications, however, are most likely to occur in patients with established heart disease, often with severely compromised ventricular function. Unfortunately, in this group of patients antiarrhythmics are least likely to be effective.

Once an arrhythmia has been detected by resting, exercise, or ambulatory ECG monitoring, the initial treatment consideration in the hemodynamically stable patient is to identify and remove any precipitating or contributing factors. These might include ischemia, hypoxia, electrolyte abnormalities, or adverse drug effects. More urgent therapy is indicated in the hemodynamically unstable patient and might include intravenous antiarrhythmic medications, cardioversion, or defibrillation. The decision to initiate oral antiarrhythmic therapy should be made only after careful consideration of the risk:benefit ratio. Studies published in the last decade have indicated that antiarrhythmic treatment of certain arrhythmias such as PVCs in patients with coronary heart disease might be associated with a higher mortality than no treatment or placebo (45). This is because of the *proarrhythmic* side-effect profile of many antiarrhythmic drugs (46). In these situations the treatment of a condition is worse than the condition itself, even when the treatment appears to be working!

There are four classes of antiarrhythmic drugs based on electrophysiologic properties (Table 3.19) (47). Class I agents are further subclassified into three categories. All three subclasses are sodium-channel blockers and work by slowing electrical conduction through cardiac muscle as a result of the slowed depolarization of action potentials. They differ, however, in their effects on repolarization. Class IA agents are the oldest drugs in this class and include quinidine, procainamide, and disopyramide. Although moderately effective in controlling ventricular arrhythmias, these drugs have considerable side effects

107

TABLE 3.19. Classification of Antiarrhythmic Agents

Class I (sodium channel blocking agents)

    Class IA: quinidine, procainamide, disopyramide
    Class IB: lidocaine, mexiletine, phenytoin
    Class IC: flecainide, encainide, propafenone

Class II (β-adrenergic blocking agents)

    Examples: propranolol, metoprolol, atenolol, timolol

Class III (potassium channel-blocking agents)

    Examples: amiodarone, sotolol, bretylium

Class IV (calcium channel-blocking agents)

    Examples: diltiazem, verapamil

---

and proarrhythmic potential. Class IB agents include lidocaine, which is only available as an intravenous preparation, and mexiletine. Lidocaine is very effective in managing ventricular arrhythmias in the intensive care units, but should not be used prophylactically to prevent arrhythmias in all acute myocardial infarction patients. Mexiletine has a favorable side-effect profile, but unfortunately is not as effective as other class I agents in treating arrhythmias. The most effective class I agents are the IC agents, flecainide and propafenone. These drugs, however, have a significant proarrhythmic profile in patients with coronary artery disease.

The class II antiarrhythmics are the beta-adrenergic blockers. These drugs are particularly effective in managing arrhythmias caused by myocardial ischemia or circulating catecholamines. They also effectively slow the heart rate in atrial fibrillation by increasing AV conduction time. In clinical trials these drugs have been shown to increase survival during the first year post-MI presumably by reducing the incidence of sudden death (48). Because of their low proarrhythmic potential and generally favorable side-effect profile, the beta-blockers are often agents of first choice for treating ventricular arrhythmias in patients with coronary and other forms of heart disease.

Class III antiarrhythmics are also known as potassium-channel blockers and work by slowing the repolarization phase of the cardiac action potential. These are the only antiarrhythmics that raise the threshold for ventricular fibrillation. Included in this class of drugs are bretylium, which is only available as an intravenous preparation; amiodarone, a complex drug with many adverse side-effects; and sotolol, a very effective new drug that has beta-blocking properties, as well as class III properties (49).

Finally, class IV drugs are the calcium antagonists, verapamil and diltiazem. These drugs are primarily used for the acute treatment of paroxysmal supraventricular tachycardia and for slowing the heart rate in atrial fibrillation. They may also have a role in the management of some patients with exercise-induced ventricular tachycardia.

Two other drugs that have antiarrhythmic properties but are not part of the classification system just described are digoxin and adenosine. Digoxin is the only digitalis preparation in common use today. Its antiarrhythmic properties are caused by vagotonic effects, which slow AV nodal conduction. As a result digoxin is useful in the long-term management of atrial tachyarrhythmias, including atrial fibrillation, atrial flutter, and other supraventricular arrhythmias. Adenosine, on the other hand, is a new intravenous drug that is very effective in the acute management of paroxysmal supraventricular tachycardia, including those seen in the Wolff-Parkinson-White syndrome (50).

Heart Failure Treatment Drugs

Congestive heart failure is a common end-stage consequence of many cardiovascular diseases. Treatment considerations range from the simple (e.g., dietary salt restriction) to the very complex (e.g., cardiac transplantation, ventricular assist devices). There are three pharmacologic approaches to managing patients with heart failure: (a) inotropic agents to increase myocardial contractility; (b) diuretics to treat fluid overload and reduce ventricular filling (preload); and (c) peripheral vasodilators to reduce the impedance to left ventricular ejection (afterload). Inotropic agents increase myocardial work and oxygen requirements; the afterload and preload reducing agents, on the other hand, reduce myocardial work and oxygen requirements. Often these drugs are used in combination.

Digitalis preparations, most commonly digoxin, are the oldest and most familiar of the inotropic agents, having been used for over 200 years (51). The primary mechanism of action is to increase the availability of calcium ions to the contractile proteins within cardiac muscle cells through inhibition of the enzyme, sodium-potassium adenosine-triphosphatase (Na-K ATPase) in the cell membrane (52). Inhibition of this enzyme enhances sodium-calcium exchange across the cell membrane, thus increasing intracelluar calcium. The resultant increased force of myocardial contraction is modest but often effective in improving symptomatology from congestive heart failure (53).

Two intravenous beta-sympathetic agonists, dopamine and dobutamine, are inotropic agents often used in the intensive care setting to treat acute heart failure and cardiogenic shock (54). Dopamine, in low doses, has a unique action in dilating renal blood vessels, which promotes diuresis. In high doses, however, there may be alpha-adrenergic-induced peripheral vasoconstriction that may adversely affect cardiac function. Dobutamine primarily acts by stimulating cardiac beta-adrenergic receptors to increase stroke volume and cardiac output.

A new class of heart failure treatment agents, the phosphodiesterase inhibitors, has both positive inotropic and vasodilating properties (54). Inhibition of the cyclic-AMP–specific phosphodiesterase enzyme increases the "second" messenger, cyclic-AMP, in the cell and improves contractility. These agents, which include amrinone, milrinone, and enoximone, are primarily used in the treatment of acute congestive heart failure.

Diuretics have a long and successful role in the management of acute and chronic congestive heart failure (55). They work by promoting salt and water excretion by the kidneys, thereby relieving the preload burden of the already overloaded heart. In patients with advanced heart failure there is often a delicate balance between volume overload and diuretic-induced volume depletion. Overdiuresis with these agents can result in excessive intravascular volume loss, low-output states, orthostatic hypotension, and increased fatigue. The popular "loop" diuretics, furosemide and bumetanide, are the most rapidly acting of all diuretics and act by inhibiting the reabsorption of salt in the ascending limb of the kidney's loop of Henle. Given intravenously, these agents act within minutes; taken orally, they usually have an effect within several hours. Potassium depletion is a common side effect and is treated by oral potassium chloride supplements. Thiazide diuretics such as hydrochlorothiazide reduce salt reabsorption in the distal tubule and have a slower onset and longer duration of action.

Vasodilators represent the most significant pharmacologic advance in the treatment of heart failure (55, 56). Several subclasses of vasodilators exist that have differential effects on the arterial and venous circulations. Drugs that act primarily on the venous system (e.g., nitrates) work by reducing the preload and are more useful in acute heart failure conditions. More important in long-term management, however, are the direct and indirect acting arterial vasodilators that have afterload-reducing properties. Direct-acting vasodilators include hydralazine, minoxidil, and the calcium-channel blockers. The ACE-inhibitors, however, are the most popular and effective of the vasodilators, and they work by blocking the formation of the potent vasoconstrictor, angiotensin II. As a result of afterload reduction, left ventricular function and cardiac output improve significantly. ACE-inhibitors not only improve symptomatology and exercise tolerance in patients with chronic heart failure, they also irrefutably improve survival (57).

Invasive Cardiovascular Therapies

The most advanced and expensive therapies for cardiovascular diseases are the invasive therapies, which include surgical procedures, catheterization procedures, and implantable devices to control cardiac rate and rhythm. By necessity, these techniques require considerable training and technical expertise of surgeons, cardiologists, and their support personnel. The clinical indications for these complex procedures have been defined to varying degrees in the medical literature, although in many situations much controversy exists over their real value. Unlike new drugs, which undergo extensive testing and clinical trials before FDA approval and widespread use, new invasive therapies often become "standards-of-care" long before they are scientifically proven to be of value. In fact, many of the invasive therapies of the past have eventually been shown to be of no value. The following sections briefly review several invasive procedures that are frequently encountered by health care providers working in cardiac rehabilitation, exercise testing laboratories, and adult fitness programs.

Coronary Artery Bypass Graft (CABG) Surgery

Surgical attempts to revascularize ischemic myocardium were totally unsuccessful until direct coronary bypass surgery was introduced in the late 1960s. Within a few years CABG became the most frequently performed cardiac operation in the world.

The techniques for CABG involve using the patient's greater saphenous vein as a bypass graft between the proximal aorta and the diseased coronary artery distal to an atherosclerotic lesion (58). Alternatively, the internal mammary artery may be used as an artery-to-artery graft, provided the diameter of the artery is large enough for adequate blood flow. Internal mammary grafts are technically more complicated and can only be grafted to the left anterior descending coronary artery and its diagonal branches. In spite of technical difficulties, however, most authorities feel that internal mammary grafts have superior patency and better clinical outcomes than saphenous vein grafts.

The indications for CABG surgery are continuously evolving as data from prospective randomized trials comparing surgery to other management strategies are published. Studies comparing surgery to medical management have generally shown that surgery improved survival in patients with three-vessel and left-main coronary artery disease, especially those with left ventricular dysfunction or inducible ischemia during stress testing (59). Surgery has also been associated with a better quality of life in terms of symptomatic improvement and increased exercise tolerance than has medical treatment. Operative mortality in experienced centers should be close to 1%, but may be higher depending on age, number of bypassed vessels, and left ventricular function. Five-year survival rates are also excellent, ranging from 90 to 95%. Occlusion of vein grafts eventually occurs over time in 20 to 30% of grafts and may be associated with recurrent angina, myocardial infarction, and rarely, sudden death (59). Progression of coronary atherosclerosis also accounts for return of symptoms and other adverse clinical outcomes.

Percutaneous Transluminal Coronary Angioplasty (PTCA)

The field of "interventional cardiology" suddenly emerged in 1977 when Gruntzig and coworkers introduced the PTCA procedure. Since that time there has been a virtual revolution in cardiovascular therapeutics directed at unplugging diseased blood vessels. In the PTCA technique the narrowed coronary artery is dilated by a balloon-tip catheter introduced through a peripheral artery (60). After the catheter tip is positioned within the lumen of the narrowed artery, inflation of the balloon compresses the lesion. Successful dilation is documented by observing smaller pressure gradient across the lesion, reduced obstruction, and improved coronary blood flow.

The National Heart, Lung, and Blood Institute (NHLBI) established a PTCA registry in 1979 to evaluate this technique. Initial guidelines for PTCA were limited to proximal, single-vessel lesions in patients with stable angina pectoris. As new catheters were introduced and techniques improved, the indications for this procedure broadened to include multivessel disease, more distal lesions, unstable angina, and even acute myocardial infarction (5). The immediate success rate for PTCA is now approximately 90%, although there is a 30 to 50% restenosis rate within 6 months of the procedure that varies with the number of vessels dilated (61). There has been an enormous effort by various investigators to lower the restenosis rate by using various drugs, including aspirin, dipyridamole, warfarin, calcium antagonists, and fish-oil supplements. None of these interventions have been shown to have reproducible benefits in carefully controlled clinical trials (61). And so, the search goes on. Direct studies comparing PTCA with CABG in comparable patients are now under way to see which procedure is more cost-effective.

New Interventional Procedures

Beginning with the introduction of balloon catheters in the late 1970s and the subsequent emergence of interventional cardiologists, there has been widespread interest in the development of new catheter techniques for opening up diseased coronary arteries. The options were best stated in an article published in the *Journal of the American College of Cardiology* entitled, "Crackers, Breakers, Stretchers, Drillers, Scrapers, Shavers, Burners, Welders, and Melters—The Future Treatment of Atherosclerotic Coronary Artery Disease?" (62). Three techniques are undergoing considerable investigation at the present time: (a) atherectomy, (b) intracoronary stents, and (c) lasers.

Atherectomy. This procedure involves the actual removal of atherosclerotic plaque using a special catheter system with a side window positioned alongside the plaque (63). The catheter is held in place by an inflatable balloon. A motor-driven rotating cutter within the catheter shaves the plaque tissue, which is then stored in the distal housing of the cutter capsule in the catheter. Rotation of the catheter enables radial excision of the lesion. Although this represents an attractive alternative to the PTCA technique, studies to date have shown that long-term restenosis rates are comparable for both procedures (63).

Intracoronary Stents. Because of frequent problems of acute dissection, abrupt closure, and late restenosis with the PTCA technique, stents were developed as a strategy to prevent these adverse outcomes (63). The stent is a 15 to 23 mm woven wire mesh that fits snugly over the end of a catheter delivery system and can be placed in an appropriate location by positioning the catheter. These devices are used after PTCA if evidence of acute dissection, abrupt closure, or unsuccessful dilatation of the primary lesion occurs. After the stent has been positioned in the desired location, it is released and self-expands radially within the lumen of the vessel. Once released, the catheter is withdrawn and the stent cannot be retrieved. Early angiographic studies after this procedure have shown reduced lesion size as a result of the radial expansion of the stent. Unfortunately, restenosis rate has remained high and comparable to that following PTCA without stents. Also, acute closure following the stent procedure sometimes occurs as a result of intracoronary thrombosis secondary to the reaction of blood constituents with the stent material. Continued improvements in the design of stents is an ongoing process.

Lasers. The most futuristic of the advanced catheter techniques is the use of lasers to vaporize the atherosclerotic plaque (63). Laser applications, however, have been slow to develop because of complex technologic problems and the worry of inducing heat damage to normal segments of the coronary arteries. Laser angioplasty has worked better in peripheral vasculature where the vessels are straighter and more easily approached. Nevertheless, several laser-based methods are being investigated in the coronary circulation, and it is anticipated that the technical problems will eventually be overcome.

CONCLUSIONS

Although the practice of cardiovascular medicine is rapidly evolving as new diagnostic technologies and treatments become available, it is unlikely that the basic strategy of the cardiovascular workup will change in the years to come. Diagnostic procedures should begin with the simple, inexpensive, and qualitative methods of the history, physical examination, and resting electrocardiogram. Additional tests should be undertaken only if the more expensive and quantitative data are necessary for making management decisions that will significantly improve clinical outcomes. Considerable skill is needed by the practicing physician in deciding just how far to go in the workup of a particular patient. Organizations such as the American Heart Association, the American College of Cardiology, and the American College of Sports Medicine are providing valuable guidelines for making cost-effective clinical decisions concerning particular tests and treatments. It is also likely that the health care reform process of the 1990s will significantly impact the practice of medicine in terms of availability and justification of various expensive diagnostic and treatment procedures.

REFERENCES

1. American Heart Association. 1992 heart and stroke facts. American Heart Association National Center, 7272 Greenville Avenue, Dallas, Tx 75231–4596, 55–0386 (COM).
2. The Criteria Committee of the New York Heart Association. Nomenclature and criteria for diagnoses of diseases of the heart and great vessels. 8th ed. Boston: Little, Brown & Co. 1979.
3. Subcommittee on Exercise Testing. Guidelines for exercise testing. A report of the American College of Cardiology/American Heart Association Task Force on Assessment of Cardiovascular Procedures. J Am Coll Cardiol 1986;8:725–738.
4. Subcommittee on Coronary Angiography. Guidelines for coronary angiography. A report of the American College of Cardiology/American Heart Association Task Force on Assessment of Diagnostic and Therapeutic Cardiovascular Procedures. J Am Coll Cardiol 1987;10:935–950.
5. Subcommittee on Percutaneous Transluminal Coronary Angioplasty. Guidelines for percutaneous transluminal coronary angioplasty. A report of the American College of Cardiology/American Heart Association Task Force on Assessment of Diagnostic and Therapeutic Cardiovascular Procedures. Circulation 1988;78:486–502.
6. Woolf SH. Practice guidelines: a new reality in medicine. I Recent developments. Arch Intern Med 1990;150:1811–1818.
7. Woolf SH. Practice guidelines: a new reality in medicine. II Methods of developing guidelines. Arch Intern Med 1992;152:946–952.
8. Woolf SH. Practice guidelines: a new reality in medicine. III Impact on patient care. Arch Intern Med 1993;153:2646–2655.
9. Prinzmetal M, Kennamer R, Merliss R, et al. Angina pectoris I. A variant form of angina pectoris: preliminary report. Am J Med 1959;27:375–388.
10. Maseri A, Davies G, Hackett D, et al. Coronary artery spasm and vasoconstriction. The case for a distinction. Circulation 1990;81:1983–1990.
11. Diamond GA, Forrester JS. Analysis of probability as an aid in clinical diagnosis of coronary artery disease. N Engl J Med 1979;300:1350–1359.
12. Braunwald E. Unstable angina. A classification. Circulation 1989;80:410–414.
13. Subcommittee on Ambulatory Electrocardiography. Guidelines for ambulatory electrocardiography. A report of the American College of Cardiology/American Heart Association Task Force on Assessment of Diagnostic and Therapeutic Cardiovascular Procedures. J Am Coll Cardiol 1989;13:249–258.
14. DiMarco JP, Philbrick JT. Use of ambulatory electrocardiographic (Holter) monitoring. Ann Intern Med 1990;113:53–68.
15. Berbari EJ, Lazzara R. An introduction to high-resolution ECG recordings of cardiac late potentials. Arch Intern Med 1988;148:1859–1863.
16. Hall PAX, Atwood JE, Myers J, et al. The signal averaged surface electrocardiogram and the identification of late potentials. Prog Cardiovasc Dis 1989;31:295–317.
17. Spodick DH, Raju P, Bishop RL, et al. Operational definition of normal sinus heart rate. Am J Cardiol 1992;69:1245–1246.
18. Jackman WM, Friday KJ, Anderson JL, et al. The long QT syndromes: a critical review, new clinical observations and a unifying hypothesis. Prog Cardiovasc Dis 1988;31:115–172.
19. Marriott HJL, Conover MH. Advanced concepts in arrhythmias. St Louis: CV Mosby, 1983.
20. Goldschlager N, Goldman MJ. Principles of clinical electrocardiography. Norwalk, CN: Appleton & Lange, 1989.
21. Conover MH. Understanding electrocardiography. Arrhythmias and the 12–lead ECG. St Louis: Mosby-Year Book, 1992.
22. Goldberger AL, Goldberger E. Clinical electrocardiography. A simplified approach. St Louis: Mosby-Year Book, 1990.
23. Chen JTT. Essentials of cardiac roentgenology. Boston: Little, Brown and Co, 1987.
24. Cooley RN. Radiology of the heart and great vessels. 3rd ed. Baltimore: Williams & Wilkins, 1979.
25. Shuford WH. Detection of cardiac chamber enlargement with the chest roentgenogram. Heart Dis Stroke 1992;1:341–347.

26. Patterson RE, Horowitz SF. Importance of epidemiology and biostatistics in deciding clinical strategies for using diagnostic tests: a simplified approach using examples from coronary artery disease. J Am Coll Cardiol 1989;13:653–662.

27. Currie PJ. Transesophageal echocardiography. New window to the heart. Circulation 1989; 80:215–217.

28. Sahn D, Kisslo J. Report of the Council on Scientific Affairs. Ultrasonic imaging of the heart: report of the ultrasonography task force. Arch Intern Med 1991;151:1288–1294.

29. Kloner RA, Parisi AF. Acute myocardial infarction: diagnostic and prognostic applications of two-dimensional echocardiography. Circulation 1987;75:521–530.

30. Sasaki H, Charuzi Y, Beeder C, et al. Utility of echocardiography for the early assessment of patients with nondiagnostic chest pain. Am Heart J 1986;112:494–497.

31. Nishimura RA, Miller FA, Callahan JM, et al. Doppler echocardiography: theory, instrumentation, technique, and application. Mayo Clin Proc 1985;60:321–343.

32. Pearlman AS. The use of Doppler in the evaluation of cardiac disorders and function. In: Hurst JW, ed. The heart. 7th ed. New York: McGraw-Hill, 1990.

33. Zaret BL, Berger HJ. Nuclear cardiology. In: Hurst JW, ed. The heart. 7th ed. New York: McGraw-Hill, 1990.

34. Pettigrew RI. Magnetic resonance imaging of the heart and great vessels. In: Hurst JW, ed. The heart. 7th ed. New York: McGraw-Hill, 1990.

35. Franch RH, King SB, Douglas JS. Techniques of cardiac catheterization including coronary angiography. In: Hurst JW, ed. The heart. 7th ed. New York: McGraw-Hill, 1990.

36. Walter PF. Technique of electrophysiological testing. In: Hurst JW, ed. The heart. 7th ed. New York: McGraw-Hill, 1990.

37. Lutz JF. Technique of endomyocardial biopsy. In: Hurst JW, ed. The heart. 7th ed. New York: McGraw-Hill, 1990.

38. Abrams J. Nitroglycerin and long-acting nitrates in clinical practice. Am J Med 1983;76(Suppl 6A):85–94.

39. Abrams J. Interval therapy to avoid nitrate tolerance: paradise regained? Am J Cardiol 1989; 64:923–924.

40. Frishman WH. Clinical differences between beta-adrenergic blocking agents: implications for therapeutic substitution. Am Heart J 1987;113:1190–1198.

41. McCall D, Walsh RA, Frohlich ED, et al. Calcium entry blocking drugs: mechanisms of action, experimental studies and clinical uses. Curr Probl Cardiol 1985;10(8):1–80.

42. Joint National Committee on Detection, Evaluation, and Treatment of High Blood Pressure. The fifth report of the Joint National Committee on Detection, Evaluation, and Treatment of High Blood Pressure (JNC -V). Arch Intern Med 1993;153:154–183.

43. Kaplan N. Management of hypertension. Dis Mon, November 1992.

44. SHEP Cooperative Research Group. Prevention of stroke by antihypertensive drug treatment in older persons with isolated systolic hypertension. JAMA 1991;265:3255–3264.

45. Epstein AE, Hallstrom AP, Rogers WJ, et al. Mortality following ventricular arrhythmia suppression by encainide, flecainide, and moricizine after myocardial infarction. JAMA 1993; 270:2451–2455.

46. Brugada P, Wellens HJJ. Arrhythmogenesis of antiarrhythmic drugs. Am J Cardiol 1988;61:1108–1113.

47. Woosley RL. Antiarrhythmic agents. In: Hurst JW, ed. The heart. 7th ed. New York: McGraw-Hill, 1990.

48. Teo KK, Yusuf S, Furberg CD. Effects of prophylactic antiarrhythmic drug therapy in acute myocardial infarction. An overview of results from randomized controlled trials. JAMA 1993; 270:1589–1595.

49. Anderson JL. Effectiveness of sotalol for therapy of complex ventricular arrhythmias and comparisons with placebo and class I antiarrhythmic drugs. Am J Cardiol 1990;65:37A-42A.

50. Camm AJ, Garratt CJ. Adenosine and supraventricular tachycardia. N Engl J Med 1991;325: 1621–1629.

51. Fisch C. William Withering: An account of the foxglove and some of its medical uses 1785–1985. J Am Coll Cardiol 1985;5:1A–2A.
52. Fozzard HA, Sheets MF. Cellular mechanism of action of cardiac glycosides. J Am Coll Cardiol 1985;5:10A-15A.
53. Kulick DL, Rahimtoola SH. Current role of digitalis therapy in patients with congestive heart failure. JAMA 1991;265:2995–2997.
54. Om A, Hess HL. Intropic therapy of the failing myocardium. Clin Cardiol 1992;16:5–14.
55. Arai AE, Greenberg BH. Medical management of congestive heart failure. West J Med 1990; 153:406–414.
56. Deedwania PC. Angiotension-converting enzyme inhibitors in congestive heart failure. Arch Intern Med 1990; 150:1798–1805.
57. Weintraub NL, Chaitman BR. Newer concepts in the medical management of patients with congestive heart failure. Clin Cardiol 1993;16:380–390.
58. Jones EL, Hatcher CR. Techniques for the surgical treatment of atherosclerotic coronary artery disease and its complications. In: Hurst JW, ed. The Heart. 7th ed. New York: McGraw-Hill, 1990.
59. Nwasaokwa ON, Koss JH, Friedman GH, et al. Bypass surgery for chronic stable angina: predictors of survival benefit and strategy for patient selection. Ann Intern Med 1991;114:1035–1049.
60. Douglas JS, King SB, Roubin GS. Technique of percutaneous transluminal angioplasty of the coronary, renal, mesenteric, and peripheral arteries. In: Hurst JW, ed. The heart. 7th ed. New York: McGraw-Hill, 1990.
61. Klein LW, Rosenblum J. Restenosis after successful percutaneous transluminal coronary angioplasty. Prog Cardiovasc Dis 1990;32:365–382.
62. Waller BF. "Crackers, breakers, stretchers, drillers, scrapers, shavers, burners, welders, and melters"—the future treatment of atherosclerotic coronary artery disease? A clinical-morphologic assessment. J Am Coll Cardiol 1989;13:969–987.
63. Holmes DR, Vlietstra RE, Reiter SJ, et al. Advances in interventional cardiology. Mayo Clin Proc 1990;65:565–583.

4

SCREENING FOR EXERCISE PROGRAMS

THIS CHAPTER DESCRIBES assessment techniques that are recommended before initiating an exercise program. Many of these tests are available in physicians' offices, hospitals, and health clubs. It is likely that the number of facilities and the scope of the evaluation procedures will expand to accommodate the growing public interest in healthy lifestyles.

Patients with known cardiovascular, pulmonary, or metabolic diseases should undergo a careful medical examination, including exercise electrocardiogram

(ECG) testing before starting an aerobic exercise program. Additional tests are recommended for these populations, as well as for apparently healthy individuals. Indentifying persons at risk for exercise-related cardiovascular complications is the primary concern among health professionals working in this area. A second purpose of the screening evaluation is to identify adverse lifestyles or behaviors that should be altered during the exercise training program. Many of these behaviors increase the risk for developing cardiovascular disease. Third, the assessment should include some degree of orthopedic screening to detect existing or potential musculoskeletal problems that might be aggravated by certain modes of exercise or require special training considerations. Fourth, the evaluation establishes a baseline for those parameters likely to change with training and provides a more objective means for quantifying the degree of improvement. Finally, information from screening is used for developing individualized exercise and lifestyle intervention.

This chapter considers the use of questionnaires and simple assessment techniques that can be administered easily by allied health personnel. Discussions of exercise ECG testing and other physician-administered procedures are found in Chapters 3 and 5.

HEALTH HISTORY AND LIFESTYLE QUESTIONNAIRES

Self-administered questionnaires have a number of advantages over interview techniques for obtaining medical history and lifestyle information. They can be completed prior to the individual's fitness evaluation, thereby saving valuable professional time during the assessment. The database obtained is generally more comprehensive than that obtained by an interviewer. Much of the data can be standardized and collected in a computer-usable format that will facilitate data management and provide an important database for performing follow-up studies and for gaining a better understanding of the individual to help with intervention design. Table 4.1 lists the categories of data that are of interest in screening individuals for exercise and other health-enhancing programs. The completed questionnaires should be reviewed by a health professional and, if necessary, further details obtained by interviewing the client. An example of a comprehensive questionnaire developed for cardiovascular risk assessment is shown in Figure 4.1.

PHYSICAL ASSESSMENT TECHNIQUES

In evaluating candidates for adult fitness and cardiac rehabilitation programs, there are several important physical measurements that should be obtained. These include (a) weight and height, (b) body composition, (c) blood pressure, (d) muscle strength, flexibility, and endurance, (e) exercise testing (maximal or

TABLE 4.1. Questionnaire Data for Fitness Evaluations

Medical history
  Past history of:
    Cardiovascular disease
    Cardiovascular disease risk factors
    Pulmonary disease
    Neuromuscular problems
    Orthopedic problems
    Surgery
  Current symptoms
  Current medications
  Family history
Lifestyle information
  Smoking history
  Nutrition and weight history
  Exercise habits
  Substance abuse
Psychosocial information
  Personality classification (type A/B)
  Analysis of life stressors

submaximal), and (f) pulmonary function screening tests. Although these procedures are rather easily administered, they must be performed carefully by experienced personnel. Often the simplest techniques are carried out most carelessly.

Weight and Height

Accurate weight and height measurements are desirable for utilizing the height-weight charts developed by the Metropolitan Life Insurance Company (see Tables 4.2 and 4.3) (1). The Metropolitan tables have been revised on several occasions, most recently in 1983, although most professionals prefer to use the earlier more conservative values (1). Although these optimal weights have several limitations—for example, in subjects with high lean body mass such as athletes with considerable skeletal muscle tissue (2), they provide useful guidelines for the average person. If possible the same scale should be used each time the subject is weighed. The zero position should be checked before each weighing, and the scale should be recalibrated periodically. Subjects should be weighed without shoes and with minimal clothing, and weight should be recorded to the nearest $1/4$ lb or 0.1 kg. For height measurements the subject should stand without shoes with the back to the measuring device, feet

119

1. GENERAL INFORMATION

A. PERSONAL

Name _____
(Last)   (First)   (Middle)

Sex: _____

Date of Birth _____
(Month)   (Day)   (Year)

Age: _____

Address: _____

Phone _____
(Home)   (Work)

Marital Status:

☐ Single ☐ Married ☐ Divorced ☐ Widowed ☐ Separated

Total Number of Children: (including adopted) _____

Race:

☐ Caucasian ☐ Black ☐ Asian ☐ Hispanic ☐ Other

Education: (Check highest level attained)

☐ Grade School ☐ Jr. High ☐ High School ☐ College ☐ Graduate School

Occupation: _____

Blood Type: _____   What is your Rh Type: _____

B. MEDICAL COVERAGE

Carrier(s) or Provider(s) including Medicare:

_____
_____

Policy or Identification Number(s):

_____
_____

Name of Policy Holder:

_____
_____

Employer and Address:

_____
_____

(Note: When visiting your doctor, please take insurance/Medicare forms with you.)

C. DOCTORS

Primary Care: _____
Address: _____ Phone: _____
Specialist: _____
Address: _____ Phone: _____
Specialist: _____
Address: _____ Phone: _____

Eye: _____
Address: _____ Phone: _____
Dentist: _____
Address: _____ Phone: _____
Dentist: _____
Address: _____ Phone: _____

2. MEDICAL HISTORY

A. MEDICAL ILLNESS

Have you ever been told BY A DOCTOR that you suffer from any of the following health problems?	AGE AT 1st DIAGNOSIS.	Have you taken prescription medication for this health problem?	Have you ever been hospitalized for this health problem?	Have you ever had any special tests performed for this health problem?
	Yes No	Age	Yes No	Yes No	Yes No
1. Heart Attack (Myocardial Infarction [MI], Coronary Thrombosis)	☐ ☐	____	☐ ☐	☐ ☐	☐ ☐
2. Angina Pectoris	☐ ☐	____	☐ ☐	☐ ☐	☐ ☐
3. Rheumatic or other Heart Disease Please list: _____	☐ ☐	____	☐ ☐	☐ ☐	☐ ☐
4. Stroke	☐ ☐	____	☐ ☐	☐ ☐	☐ ☐
5. High Blood Pressure	☐ ☐	____	☐ ☐	☐ ☐	☐ ☐
6. High Blood Pressure during Pregnancy only	☐ ☐	____	☐ ☐	☐ ☐	☐ ☐
7. High Blood Cholesterol or Triglycerides, and/or Low HDL	☐ ☐	____	☐ ☐	☐ ☐	☐ ☐
8. Diabetes	☐ ☐	____	☐ ☐	☐ ☐	☐ ☐
9. Cancer	☐ ☐	____	☐ ☐	☐ ☐	☐ ☐

Do you currently have or have you ever had any of the following: (please indicate the year)

10. ____ anemia	15. ____ malaria	20 ____ mumps	25 ____ varicose veins or phlebitis
11. ____ asthma	16. ____ jaundice or hepatitis	21. ____ polio	26. ____ venereal disease
12. ____ chickenpox	17. ____ measles	22. ____ scarlet fever	27. Other:
13. ____ hemorrhoids	18. ____ liver disease	23. ____ thyroid disease	_____
14 ____ hives	19 ____ mononucleosis	24. ____ typhoid	

FIGURE 4.1. Health assessment and medical history questionnaire.

HEART DISEASE

28. If you answered "Yes" to Number 1 (**Heart Attack**), circle any of the following that apply:

    a. Hospitalized for _____ days.
    b. Was placed in a Coronary or Intensive Care Unit.
    c. Experienced chest pain for one hour or more.

    Please circle any of the following terms used by your doctor to describe your situation:

    1 - Coronary thrombosis
    2 - Myocardial infarction (MI)
    3 - Congestive heart failure
    4 - Unstable angina
    5 - Other: _____

29. If you had **other heart problems**, circle any of the following that apply:

    a. Congestive heart failure
    b. Rheumatic heart disease
    c. Congenital heart disease
    d. Atrial fibrilation
    e. Paroxysmal atrial tachycardia (PAT)
    f. Premature ventricular contractions (PVC)
    g. Other heart rhythm problems
    h. Cardiomyopathy (diseased heart muscle)
    i. Pulmonary heart disease
    j. Any heart murmurs
    k. Any heart valve problems (stenosis, regurgitation, etc.)
    l. Other: _____

STROKE

30. If you answered "Yes" to Number 4 (**Stroke**), circle any of the following that apply:

    a. My muscles suddenly became weak or paralyzed on one side of my body.
    b. I suddenly had difficulty talking.
    c. I suddenly had partial or complete loss of vision in one eye.
    d. Fainted or passed out (usually not due to a stroke).
    e. I was hospitalized for _____ days.
    f. Some of the above problems were still present to some degree several months after the stroke.
    g. Other: _____

HIGH BLOOD PRESSURE

31. If you answered "Yes" to Number 5 or 6 (**High Blood Pressure**) circle any of the following that apply:

    a. Currently take prescription medication for high blood pressure.
    b. Previously took prescription medication for high blood pressure, but stopped taking it on my own.
    c. Previously took prescription medication for high blood pressure, but my doctor told me to stop.
    d. Only had high blood pressure when I was pregnant.
    e. Do not take prescription medication, but the doctor follows my high blood pressure (see doctor regularly to check blood pressure).

HIGH BLOOD CHOLESTEROL

32. If you answered "Yes" to Number 7 (**High Blood Cholesterol**, etc.), circle any of the following that apply:

    a. Has your blood cholesterol ever been measured ? Yes ☐ No ☐
    b. My highest blood cholesterol level was: _____ Date: _____.
    c. My current cholesterol level is: _____ Date: _____.
    d. My highest triglyceride level was: _____ Date: _____.
    e. My current triglyceride level is: _____ Date: _____.
    f. My lowest HDL level was : _____ Date: _____.
    g. My current HDL level is: _____ Date: _____.
    h. Medication has been prescribed by my doctor for my high blood lipids.

DIABETES

33. If you answered "Yes" to Number 8 (**Diabetes**), circle any of the following that apply:

    a. Insulin injections have been prescribed by my doctor for control of my blood sugar.
    b. Medication (pills or tablets) have been prescribed for control of my blood sugar.
    c. I monitor my urine and/or blood sugar at home as directed by my doctor.
    d. A special diet for control of my blood sugar has been prescribed by my doctor.

CANCER

34. If you answered "Yes" to Number 9 (**Cancer**) please answer the following questions:

    a. The type of cancer your doctor said you had: _____
    b. Did you undergo any surgical therapy for this cancer? _____ yes _____ no
    c. Did you have chemotherapy? _____ yes _____ no
    d. Did you have radiation therapy? _____ yes _____ no

B. MEDICAL PROCEDURES

Tests
(indicate previous tests and year performed:)

Operations and Hospitalizations
(Please list past hospitalization and operations/major procedures)

Was the test normal ?

		Year	Yes	No		
☐	upper GI X-ray	_____	☐	☐	_____	Year:
☐	lower GI X-ray	_____	☐	☐	_____	Year:
☐	gallbladder X-ray	_____	☐	☐	_____	Year:
☐	proctoscopic exam	_____	☐	☐	_____	Year:
☐	chest X-ray	_____	☐	☐	_____	Year:
☐	TB skin test	_____	☐	☐	_____	Year:
☐	tetanus shot	_____	☐	☐	_____	Year:
☐	allergy tests	_____	☐	☐	_____	Year:
☐	complete physical examination	_____	☐	☐	_____	Year:
☐	electrocardiogram (resting EKG)	_____	☐	☐	_____	Year:
☐	exercise electrocardiogram (stress test)	_____	☐	☐	_____	Year:
☐	mammogram	_____	☐	☐	_____	Year:
☐	pap smear	_____	☐	☐		
☐	colonoscopy	_____	☐	☐		

☐ Other X-rays

Year   Kind of X-ray

_____   _____

_____   _____

FIGURE 4.1. Cont.

C. MEDICATIONS, DRUG REACTION(S) and ALLERGIES

1. MEDICATIONS

(Please list the medications, vitamins and dietary supplements you take, prescription and non-prescription, even ones taken on an occasional basis.)

Name	When did you start this medication?	How often do you take this medication?	Dose

2. DRUG REACTIONS

(Please list any drug reaction you have had and the year you had this reaction.)

Date _____

Drug:
Side Effect:

Drug:
Side Effect:

Drug:
Side Effect:

Drug:
Side Effect:

Drug:
Side Effect:

3. ALLERGIES

(Please list the things you are allergic to and any reactions you have had.)

Date _____

Allergic to:
Side Effect:

Allergic to:
Side Effect:

Allergic to:
Side Effect:

Allergic to:
Side Effect:

Allergic to:
Side Effect:

Allergic to:
Side Effect:

3. REVIEW OF SYSTEMS

A. GENERAL REVIEW

(Check the appropriate boxes:)

☐ Do you have an intolerance to heat?

☐ Do you have an intolerance to cold?

☐ Do you often notice excessive fatigue or exhaustion?

☐ Do you have difficulty getting to sleep or staying asleep?

☐ Have you noticed any unusual thirst?

☐ Are you always hungry?

☐ Has your appetite disappeared or decreased?

☐ Have you noticed any lymph node swelling?

☐ Have you ever been exposed to radiation of head or neck? (other than dental or other diagnostic X-rays)

☐ Do you ever feel faint?

☐ Do you lose feeling in any part of your body?

☐ Have you noticed shaking or trembling?

☐ Have you ever had convulsions?

☐ Have you had excessive bleeding from a cut?

☐ Are you prone to bruise easily?

☐ Are you bothered with any skin abnormalities?

☐ Do you have any physical handicaps?

B. DIGESTIVE SYSTEM

☐ Do you notice any discomfort or pain in your upper abdomen or stomach?

☐ Do you have much abdominal gas?

☐ If you notice pain or discomfort in your abdomen, is it made worse by eating?

Is it made better by eating? ☐ Yes ☐ No

Is it improved with antacids? ☐ Yes ☐ No

☐ Are you bothered with heartburn, belching or do you have trouble swallowing? (underline which)

☐ Are you constipated more than once weekly?

☐ Do you have loose bowels for more than one or two days?

☐ Have you had any black or bloody stools in the last five years?

☐ Have you had any rectal bleeding in the last five years?

☐ Are your bowel movements painful?

☐ Do you have rectal pain?

☐ Do you have a hernia?

☐ Do you have hemorrhoids?

☐ Have you been told you have diverticulitis?

FIGURE 4.1. Cont.

C. GENITO-URINARY SYSTEM

☐ Do you notice pain or burning when urinating?

☐ Do you have trouble starting to urinate?

☐ Does your urination seem too slow?

How many times per night do you generally urinate? _____

How many times per day do you generally urinate? _____

☐ Do you have frequent urinary tract infections?

☐ Have you had past kidney trouble?

D. MEN

☐ Has the force of urine stream markedly decreased?

☐ Do you notice any dribbling after stopping urination?

☐ Have you noticed any discharge from the penis?

☐ Have you been told you have prostate trouble?

☐ Do your testicles become tender and swollen?

E. WOMEN

☐ Have you noticed any breast lumps?

☐ Have you noticed any discharge from your breasts?

☐ Are your periods regular with normal flow?

☐ Do you ever bleed between periods?

☐ Do you have vaginal itching or discharge?

☐ Have you ever taken birth control pills?

☐ Have you ever taken any hormone (estrogen or progesterone)replacement therapy?

☐ Have you ever been pregnant? If yes, how may pregnancies? _____

F. EYES, EARS, NOSE, THROAT and MOUTH

☐ Do you wear corrective lenses?

☐ Do you ever notice blurred or double vision?

☐ Are you bothered with eye pains or itching?

☐ Do you have excessive eye watering?

☐ Do you have difficulty hearing?

☐ Do you have ringing in your ears?

☐ Do you often have headaches?

☐ Have you had pain or swelling in your neck?

☐ Do you have sore areas on your gums?

☐ Is your tongue or the inside of your mouth sore?

☐ Do you have frequent stuffiness and drainage from your nose?

☐ Do you frequently notice drainage in the back of your throat?

☐ Are you bothered with nosebleeds?

☐ Is your throat sore or hoarse when you don't have a cold?

G. RESPIRATORY SYSTEM

☐ Do you ever have periods of wheezing?

☐ Do you have a regular cough?

☐ Do you often cough up anything?

☐ Have you ever coughed up blood?

☐ Do you need more than one pillow to sleep?

☐ Do you have or have you had the following?

☐ Bronchitis
☐ Emphysema
☐ Pneumonia

4. LIFESTYLE HISTORY (Personal Habits)

A. CIGARETTE SMOKING

1 Please circle the one that applies:

  a. **Smoker:** Have smoked daily for one year or more.

  b. **Ex-smoker:** Have not smoked for at least one year after having smoked daily for at least one year.

  c. **Non-smoker:** Have never smoked daily for at least one year.

2. If **smoker** or **ex-smoker**, circle **average** amount and indicate number of years smoked. Choose one only.

  a. Less than one pack a day for _____ years.

  b. About one pack a day for _____ years.

  c. One-two packs a day for _____ years.

  d. Two or more packs a day for _____ years.

3. List the last year in which you smoked _____

4. Do you smoke cigars? _____ yes _____ no cigars per day? _____

5. Do you smoke a pipe? _____ yes _____ no bowls per day? _____

6. Would you like to quit smoking? _____ yes _____ no

7. Do you use smokeless tobacco? _____ yes _____ no

8. On the average, how many hours per day are you exposed to other people's cigarette smoke?

  _____ 0 hours   _____ 5-8 hours

  _____ 1-2 hours   _____ more than 8 hours

  _____ 3-4 hours

B. ALCOHOL CONSUMPTION

1. Do you drink alcoholic beverages (beer, wine, or liquors)? Please circle the one that applies:

  a No.

  b Less than once a month.

  c. Once a month or more with an average of:

    1 _____ 12-16 oz. cans of beer per week.

    2 _____ 4-6 oz. glasses of wine per week.

    3 _____ shots, jiggers or mixed drinks per week.

C. DIETARY INFORMATION

1. How would you describe your tendency to lose weight? (If in doubt circle #3.)

  1) Lose weight easily by cutting food intake slightly.

  2) Lose weight with difficulty, even if I cut my food intake greatly.

  3) Average - neither tendency above noticed.

2. What is your current weight? _____ lbs. What is the most you have ever weighed (excluding pregnancy)? _____ lbs.

3. If you feel you need to lose weight, how much weight would you like to lose? _____ lbs.

4. How do you feel about your current weight?

  1) very satisfied
  2) satisfied
  3) not concerned
  4) dissatisfied
  5) very dissatisfied

5. Do you follow any special diet most of the time?

  1) No
  2) Yes, low calorie
  3) Yes, low fat or low cholesterol
  4) Yes, diabetic
  5) Yes, low salt
  6) Yes, other _____

6. In a typical week, how many meals or snacks do you eat away from home?

  1) _____ Breakfast (where) _____
  2) _____ Morning Snack (where) _____
  3) _____ Lunch (where) _____
  4) _____ Afternoon Snack (where) _____
  5) _____ Dinner (where) _____
  6) _____ Evening Snack (where) _____

FIGURE 4.1. Cont.

List of Salty Foods:

Bacon or Ham	Salted Crackers
Hot Dogs	Seasoning Salts
Sausage	(celery, garlic, onion)
Bologna and Luncheon	Pickles
Meats	Sauerkraut
Chipped or Corned Beef	Bouillon
Smoked or Salted Meats	Catsup
Herring, Sardines	Canned Soups
Potato Chips	Dried Soups
Pretzels	Chili Sauce
French Fries	Mustard
Salted Snacks	Olives
(popcorn, nuts, etc.)	Relishes
Sauces (soy, steak, etc.)	Meat Tenderizers

7. How often do you salt your food from a shaker at the dinner table or eat salty foods such as potato chips, bacon, or other foods listed above?

   1) 2 or more times a day
   2) Once a day
   3) 2-5 times a week
   4) Once a week
   5) Less than once a week
   6) Almost never (I'm on a special low salt diet)

8. When was the last time you used a salt shaker on your food or ate one of the salty foods listed above?

   1) Within the last three meals
   2) A day ago
   3) 2-5 days ago
   4) A week ago
   5) Over a week ago
   6) Over a year ago

9. Do you place specific emphasis of high fiber in your diet? _____ yes _____ no

10. How many cups of coffee containing caffeine do you drink in an average day? ☐☐

11. How many cups of tea containing caffeine do you drink in an average day? ☐☐

12. If you drink coffee or tea, how do you normally drink it?

    1) black, no cream or sugar
    2) cream, no sugar
    3) cream, one spoon of sugar
    4) cream, two spoons of sugar
    5) cream, three or more spoons of sugar
    6) no cream, one spoon of sugar
    7) no cream, two spoons of sugar
    8) no cream, three or more spoons of sugar

13. During the last week, how many days did you experience difficulty in limiting candy eating?
    1 2 3 4 5 6 7 Zero

14. During the past week, how many days did you experience difficulty in limiting your eating of fatty foods?
    1 2 3 4 5 6 7 Zero

15. During the past week, how many days did you plan what you would eat at the start of the day?
    1 2 3 4 5 6 7 Zero

16. During the past week, how many days did you eat your meals at set times?
    1 2 3 4 5 6 7 Zero

17. During the past week, on how many days did you decide not to eat a snack that you wanted, even though the food was available?
    1 2 3 4 5 6 7 Zero

18. How many carbonated soft drinks do you have in a week? ☐☐

19. How many are diet drinks? ☐☐

20. How many of the drinks you consume contain caffeine? (Drinks like Coca Cola, Pepsi, Dr. Pepper, Mountain Dew, contain caffine.)

21. How many cups of hot chocolate do you drink each day? ☐☐

22. How many cups of water do you drink each day? ☐☐

List of foods high in Cholesterol or Saturated Fat

Bacon	Sweet Rolls
Hot Dogs	Butter
Sausage	Shortening
Marbled and Fatty Meats	Coconut Oil
(beef, pork, lamb)	French Fries
Spare Ribs	Potato Chips
Fish fried in shortening	Other Fried Foods
Liver or other organ meats	Lard
Hamburger	Cream and Ice Cream
Luncheon Meats	Cheese
Egg Yolks	Butter Rolls
Cakes and Pies	Donuts
Whole Milk	Egg Noodles

23. When was the last time you ate eggs, whole milk, meat or other high cholesterol foods from the above list?

    1) Within the last three meals
    2) A day ago
    3) 2-5 days ago
    4) A week ago
    5) Over a week ago
    6) Over a year ago

24. How often do you eat any of the foods listed above?

    1) 2 or more times a day
    2) Once a day
    3) 2-5 times a week
    4) Once a week
    5) Less than once a week
    6) Almost never

25. In an average month, how may times do you skip:

    1) Breakfast? ☐☐
    2) Lunch? ☐☐
    3) Dinner? ☐☐

D. PHYSICAL ACTIVITY INFORMATION

1. Are you currently participating in a physical activity program? _____ yes _____ no
2. Please list the type, the frequency and the duration with which you participate in physical activity, that either includes brisk walking, jogging, swimming, gardening, aerobics, stationary cycling, country cycling, carpentry, calisthentics, etc. (please include only the time you are physically active).

Type of physical activity	Number of times per week	Time Spent in each activity session hours	minutes	Number of weeks per year (approximately)

3. If you walk briskly on a regular basis, how many miles do you walk each session? _____ How long does it take you to walk one mile? _____ (minutes).

4. On a usual weekday and a weekend day, how much time do you spend on the following activities

	Usual weekday hours/day	Usual weekend day hours/day
a. Vigorous activity (digging in the garden, strenuous sports, jogging, chopping wood, sustained swimming, brisk walking, heavy carpentry, bicycling on hills, etc.)		
b. Moderate activity (housework, light sports, regular walking, golf, yard work, lawn mowing, painting, repairing, light carpentry, dancing, bicycling on level ground, etc.)		
c. Light activity (office work, driving a car, strolling, personal care, standing with little motion, etc.)		
d. Sitting activity (eating, reading, desk work, watching TV, listening to radio, etc.)		
e. Sleeping or reclining		

FIGURE 4.1. Cont.

124

E. PSYCHOLOGICAL INFORMATION

Circle the number, from 0 (never) to 4 (frequently), that represents the degree to which the following thoughts, feelings, and behaviors have bothered you during the past month.

THOUGHTS — BOTHERED: Never / Rarely / Sometimes / Often / Frequently

THOUGHTS	Never	Rarely	Sometimes	Often	Frequently
1. Awfulizing (taking things to their worst possible outcome)	0	1	2	3	4
2. Blaming myself	0	1	2	3	4
3. Blaming others	0	1	2	3	4
4. Difficulty concentrating	0	1	2	3	4
5. Holding grudges	0	1	2	3	4
6. Thinking and rethinking the same situation	0	1	2	3	4
7. Wishing I could "turn my mind off"	0	1	2	3	4
8. Constantly criticizing other people or situations	0	1	2	3	4
9. Worrying	0	1	2	3	4
10. Thinking something is wrong with my mind	0	1	2	3	4
11. Needing to be right	0	1	2	3	4
12. Feeling out of control	0	1	2	3	4

BEHAVIORS	Never	Rarely	Sometimes	Often	Frequently
1. Nail or cuticle biting	0	1	2	3	4
2. Using tobacco in any form	0	1	2	3	4
3. Taking tranquilizers or "street" drugs to change mood	0	1	2	3	4
4. Drinking alcoholic beverages	0	1	2	3	4
5. Chewing gum or sucking candies	0	1	2	3	4
6. Talking a lot	0	1	2	3	4
7. Crying a lot	0	1	2	3	4
8. Sleeping problems (too much or too little)	0	1	2	3	4
9. Eating problems (too much or too little)	0	1	2	3	4
10. Trouble communicating	0	1	2	3	4
11. Avoiding responsibilities	0	1	2	3	4
12. Too much caffeine	0	1	2	3	4

EMOTIONS	Never	Rarely	Sometimes	Often	Frequently
1. Afraid of specific places or circumstances	0	1	2	3	4
2. Feeling like a victim	0	1	2	3	4
3. Anxious	0	1	2	3	4
4. Blue	0	1	2	3	4
5. Lonely	0	1	2	3	4
6. Irritable	0	1	2	3	4
7. Wanting to throw things or hit people	0	1	2	3	4
8. Guilty	0	1	2	3	4
9. Feeling unfriendly	0	1	2	3	4
10. Uptight	0	1	2	3	4
11. Hopeless about the future	0	1	2	3	4
12. Wanting to "pull the covers over my head"	0	1	2	3	4
13. Feeling that other people don't like me	0	1	2	3	4
14. Upset over criticism	0	1	2	3	4

F. SEAT BELT USAGE

1. Do you wear seat belts when riding in or driving motor vehicles?

_____no _____sometimes _____usually _____always

G. SLEEP

1. How many hours of sleep do you usually get a night? _____ hours

2. How would you best describe your night's sleep?

_____restful _____ difficult to get to sleep

_____wake at night and can't get back to sleep

3. Do you take naps during the day on a regular basis?

_____yes _____no

If yes, how long is your nap? _____minutes

5. GENETIC HISTORY

Please use the guide above to enter the information below:

(Start with [1. You] above and enter your health information in the number (1) slot below. Next complete your parents information (#2 and #3), your siblings, etc. Finally, be patient and invest some time in completing this form.)

List Approximate AGE at 1ST DIAGNOSIS

Above Code #	Relation-ship	First Name	Last Name	Age now or at Death	Sex (M F)/Male F/female	(Living or (Dead) (L D)	Year of Birth	Year of Death	Weight (A/O) (Average (Overweight 50 lbs or more	Smoke cigarettes (C F N) (Current Former (Never	Stroke	High Blood Pressure	Heart Attack	Coronary angioplasty (PTCA)	Coronary Bypass Surgery	Asthma	Cancer	What kind of Cancer	If Deceased Cause of Death		
Example	Joseph	Larsan	58	M	L	35		0	F	0	48	0	51	0	0	56	colon	0	0	0	
1. You																					
2. Mother																					
3. Father																					
4. Bro/Sis																					
5. Bro/Sis																					
6. Bro/Sis																					
7. Bro/Sis																					
8. Bro/Sis																					
9. Bro/Sis																					
10. Bro/Sis																					

FIGURE 4.1. Cont.

11. Bro/Sis																													
12. Bro/Sis																													
20. Grand-Father																													
21. Grand-Mother																													
22. Ant/Unc																													
23. Ant/Unc																													
24. Ant/Unc																													
25. Ant/Unc																													
26. Ant/Unc																													
27. Ant/Unc																													
28. Ant/Unc																													
30. Grand-Father																													
31. Grand-Mother																													
32. Ant/Unc																													
33. Ant/Unc																													
34. Ant/Unc																													
35. Ant/Unc																													
36. Ant/Unc																													
37. Ant/Unc																													
38. Ant/Unc																													
40. Spouse																													
41. Son/Dau																													
42. Son/Dau																													
43. Son/Dau																													
44. Son/Dau																													
45. Son/Dau																													
46. Son/Dau																													

FIGURE 4.1. Cont.

together, and arms relaxed at the sides. With the eyes directed straight ahead, the measuring square is adjusted to rest lightly on the scalp, and measurements are recorded to the nearest $1/4$ inch or 0.5 cm.

Body Composition

Although the standard height-weight tables for small, medium, and large frames provide reasonable approximations of the normal weight range for many people, there is considerable interest among health professionals, as well as the general public, in quantifying the relative composition of body weight in terms of percent body fat and lean body mass. The emphasis in today's culture on leanness, fitness, and high-fashion clothing, together with preconceived notions of obesity as defined by standard height-weight tables, often results in obsession in some larger-sized individuals about losing excessive amounts of weight. For many, being "overweight" is not necessarily being "over-fat." Body composition analysis offers a more realistic determination of ideal body weight because the techniques quantify the percent body fat relative to total weight. Problems of both underweight and overweight can be more objectively analyzed by these techniques.

TABLE 4.2. Weight Table for Men (pounds)[a,b]

Height[c] (inches)	Suggested ideal weight[d]	1.1 times ideal weight	1.15 times ideal weight	1.2 times ideal weight
≤60	118	130	136	142
61	121	133	139	145
62	125	137	144	150
63	128	141	147	154
64	132	145	152	158
65	135	149	155	162
66	139	153	160	167
67	143	157	164	172
68	147	162	169	176
69	150	165	173	180
70	154	169	177	185
71	157	173	181	188
72	161	177	185	193
73	164	180	189	197
74	168	185	193	202
75	171	188	197	205
76	175	192	201	210
77	178	196	205	214
78	182	200	209	218
79	185	203	213	222
≥80	189	208	217	227

[a] From Star. Bull. Metro. Life Ins. Co. 40:1–4, Nov–Dec, 1959.
[b] Weight—for partially clothed men (allow 2 pounds for clothes if stripped weight is desired).
[c] Height—without shoes.
[d] "Ideal weight"—0.9 times the average weight of men aged 18 to 34 years as obtained from the National Health Survey: Weight by height and age of adults, United States 1960–1962, Series 11, No. 14. For persons with a height less than or equal to 66 inches the relationship between height and ideal weight is given by the formula Ideal weight = 3.5 Height – 92; for persons taller than 66 inches the relationship is Ideal weight = 3.5 Height – 91.

There are several indirect techniques for assessing body composition that are used in clinical practice. These include (a) hydrostatic (underwater) weighing, (b) skinfold measurements, (c) electrical impedance plethysmography, (d) near-infrared interactance (NIR), (e) body mass index (BMI), and (f) circumference measurements. Each of these methods has advantages and disadvantages in terms of accuracy, cost, convenience, and subject distress. The following section briefly considers these procedures. Readers interested in a comprehensive review of the science of body composition analysis are referred elsewhere (3, 4).

127

TABLE 4.3. Weight Table for Women (pounds)[a,b]

Height[c] (inches)	Average weight[d]	Suggested ideal weight[e]	1.15 times ideal weight
57	114	103	118
58	117	105	121
59	120	108	124
60	123	111	128
61	127	114	131
62	130	117	135
63	133	120	138
64	136	122	140
65	139	125	144
66	142	128	147
67	145	130	149
68	148	133	153
69	151	136	156
70	154	139	160

[a] From Stat. Bull. Metro. Life Ins. Co. 40:1–4, Nov–Dec, 1959.
[b] Weight—for partially clothed women (allow 2 pounds for clothes if stripped weight is desired).
[c] Height—without shoes
[d] "Average weight"—for age group 18 to 34 years.
[e] "Suggested ideal weight"—0.9 times average weight of women aged 18 to 34 years as obtained from the National Health Survey: Weight by height and age of adults, United States 1960–1962, Series 11, No. 14.

Hydrostatic Weighing

Hydrostatic weighing (Fig. 4.2) is a method for determining body density (Db) using Archimedes' principle (5), which states that the loss of weight of an object when submerged in water is equal to the weight of the water displaced by the object. From the weight of the displaced water (Mw) and the known density of water (Dw) at specific temperatures (Table 4.4), the volume of displaced water (Vw) can be computed as follows:

$$Vw = \frac{Mw}{Dw}$$

Since water is not compressible, the volume of displaced water (Vw) is equal to the volume of the submerged object or person (Vb). If the weight of the person in air is Mb, the density of the person (Db) is easily computed:

$$Db = \frac{Mb}{Vb}$$

128

In actual practice the underwater weight consists of two components: the measured weight in water plus the weight of water displaced by air in the lungs, airways, and gastrointestinal system. Many laboratories have the subject expire two-thirds vital capacity, using a spirometer, leaving the remaining one-third vital capacity plus residual volume in the lungs before completely submerging under water. Residual volume can be estimated from prediction equations based on age, sex, and height (6, 7), or it can be directly measured using the helium-dilution or nitrogen-washout techniques (6). The prediction equations for men and women follow:

Men: Residual volume (L) = 0.0216H + 0.207A − 2.840

Women: Residual volume (L) = 0.0197H + 0.201A − 2.421

where H is height (cm) and A is age (years). For most clinical applications estimated residual volumes are adequate. Using this information body density is actually computed from the following equation:

$$Db = \frac{Mb}{\dfrac{Mb - Mw}{Dw}} - (RV + 100 \text{ ml})$$

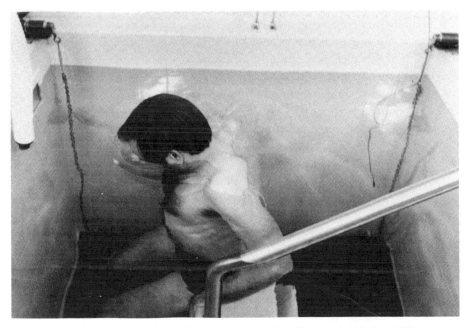

FIGURE 4.2. Hydrostatic weighing technique. The Fitness Institute, LDS Hospital, Salt Lake City, UT.

129

TABLE 4.4. Density of Water at Various Temperatures[a]

Temperature (C)	Density
30	0.99568
31	0.99537
32	0.99506
33	0.99473
34	0.99440
35	0.99406
36	0.99372
37	0.99336
38	0.99299
39	0.99260

[a]Modified from West RC, ed. Handbook of chemistry and physics. 50th ed. Cleveland: The Chemical Rubber Co., 1969.

where RV is the air remaining in the respiratory system (residual volume plus one-third vital capacity), and 100 ml is the estimated volume of air in the gastrointestinal system. Some laboratories have the subject exhale maximally before submerging so that only the residual volume remains in the lungs. This creates somewhat more distress in some individuals.

While the calculation of body density is relatively straightforward, involving few assumptions and fairly simple measurements, the estimation of percent body fat from body density is based on equations derived from the careful dissection of relatively few, fresh, human cadavers. The general assumption in deriving these equations is that the densities of adipose tissue and fat-free lean body mass as measured in these few studies are constant for all individuals and across all population groups. This is probably not a very realistic assumption. Nevertheless, a number of equations for predicting percent body fat from body density have been developed. The equation of Brozek et al. (8)

$$\% \text{ Body fat} = \frac{457}{Db} - 414$$

and that of Siri (9)

$$\% \text{ Body fat} = \frac{495}{Db} - 450$$

are in common clinical usage. Both of these equations provide similar results for adult individuals under 50. For older adults, youth, and children, the equations may overestimate the body fat content because of a lower fat-free body density

130

in these populations (10). In addition, the equations are probably most valid only in subjects ranging from 10 to 30% body fat. Other sources of error have been discussed elsewhere (3, 4, 11, 12).

Skinfold Measurements

Estimating body density from skinfold measurements is based on the assumption that there is a valid mathematic relationship between subcutaneous fat and body density (13). Over the years, many prediction equations have been proposed for body density based on the sum of various skinfolds. Generalized equations have been developed for men and women that take into consideration age, sex, and the curvilinear relationships between body density and skinfold thickness (14, 15). These equations for predicting body density from skinfolds generally correlate well with hydrostatically determined body density, provided that experienced personnel perform the measurements. The advantages of skinfold measurements over hydrostatic weighing are that they require little time, use inexpensive equipment, require minimal space, and need minimal patient cooperation.

Skinfolds are measured with calipers (Harpenden Skinfolds Calipers, British Indicators, Ltd.; Lange Skinfolds Calipers, Cambridge Scientific Instruments, Cambridge, MD) calibrated in divisions of 2 mm, although readings are interpreted to the nearest millimeter. Skinfold measurements should be obtained by the same individual each time, if possible, to reduce interindividual variation. The technique requires that a fold of skin and subcutaneous tissue be picked up between the thumb and forefinger and lifted firmly away from the underlying muscle. The fold should be held between the fingers when the measurement is being made. Measurements should be consistently made on one side of the body. The calipers are applied to the fold 1 cm below the finger, such that pressure on the fold at the point measured is exerted by the calipers' face only and not by the fingers. The calipers are applied to the skinfolds by removing the fingers from the trigger lever. The value registered on the calipers sometimes decreases as one watches the pointer of the dial. This decrease can usually be stopped by taking a firmer pinch. If it continues, the reading must be taken immediately after application of the spring pressure.

A variety of sites for skinfold measurements in men and women have been recommended by various authors using different regression models for predicting body density. The generalized equations developed by Jackson and Pollock (14) seem to minimize the large prediction errors found at the extremes of the body density distribution. Equations based on age, sex, and the sum of three skinfolds are reasonably accurate for most clinical purposes. In women Jackson and Pollock (17) recommend the following three sites for skinfold measurements (Fig. 4.3):

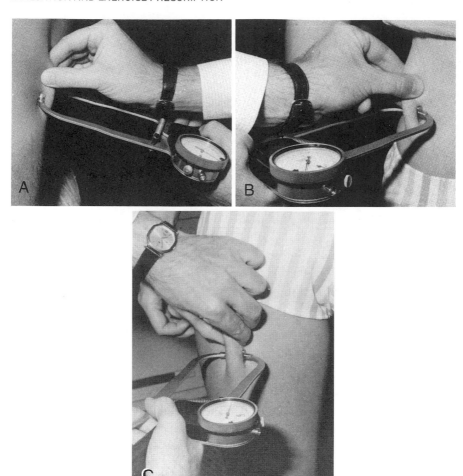

FIGURE 4.3. Skinfold measurement sites for women. **A.** Triceps. **B.** Suprailium. **C.** Thigh.

1. Triceps: A vertical fold on the posterior aspect of the upper arm, half-way between the acromion and olecranon processes. The arm should be extended and relaxed.
2. Suprailium: A diagonal fold above the iliac crest in the anterior axillary line along lines of Linn.
3. Thigh: A vertical fold on the anterior aspect of the thigh halfway between the knee and the hip. A steel tape should be used to measure precisely half the distance between the two points.

Using the sum of these three skinfolds and age, body density can be estimated from the regression equation. The percent body fat is then computed using the formula of Siri (9):

$$\% \text{ Fat} = \frac{495}{\text{Db}} - 450$$

In men Jackson and Pollock (17) recommend the following three sites for skinfold measurements (Fig. 4.4):

1. Chest: A diagonal fold one-half the distance between the anterior axillary line at the axilla and the nipple.
2. Abdominal: A vertical fold 2 cm lateral to the umbilicus.
3. Thigh: Same procedure as that for women (Fig. 4.3C).

Again, body density is determined from the sum of these three skinfolds and age using the generalized prediction equations (14). Tables 4.5 and 4.6 reprinted from Jackson and Pollock (17) provide the percent body fat for women and men, respectively, using age, sum of skinfolds, and the equations previously described.

Other sites for skinfold measurements may also be used. A combination of triceps, suprailiac, and subscapular measurements has been used recently in studies of young and adolescent girls (18), adolescent boys and girls (19), and has previously been recommended for cardiac patients, being used in the National Exercise and Heart Disease Project (20). These three sites are provided in Figures 4.3A, 4.3B, and 4.5 and are positioned as follows:

1. Triceps: Same procedure as that for women (see Fig. 4.3A).
2. Suprailium: Same procedure as that for women (see Fig. 4.3B).
3. Subscapular: Just beneath the inferior angle of the scapular the fold is taken along the lines of Linn at about a 45° angle from the horizontal, going medially upward and laterally downward.

Body fat estimated from these sites is shown in Table 4.7. Other sites should be considered under special circumstances. For some individuals, the thigh or chest skinfolds may be particularly difficult to obtain. Substituting sites in the axilla or subscapular region and using different regression equations would provide an acceptable alternative for estimating body density (11).

Skinfold measurements at select sites have also been used for comparison of fat distributions, although more recent studies have shown that circumference measurements are a stronger indicator of cardiovascular risk (4, 21). Little information is available on the significance of skinfold measurements in boys and girls, although data of adolescents found no significant differences in the correlations between subscapular and triceps skinfolds in relation to cholesterol and blood pressure (22).

133

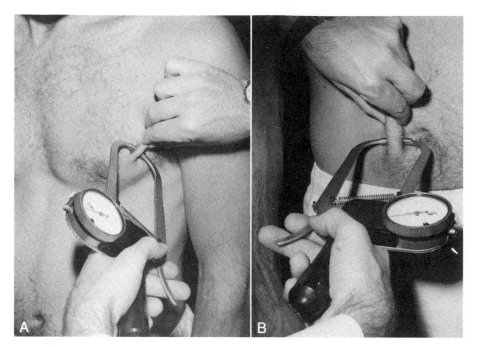

FIGURE 4.4. Skinfold measurement sites for men. **A.** Chest. **B.** Abdomen.

Electrical Impedance Plethysmography

Another procedure for measuring body composition is by impedance ple-thysmography. This relatively simple method is based on the concept that fat-free body mass, because of its high water content, is more highly conductive to electrical current than is adipose tissue. One of two methods is employed: The whole body method, the more common of the two, introduces low amperage alternating current through two electrodes attached to distal skin sites on the wrist and ankle, recording the resistance in ohms from two additional electrodes on the limbs. Because of potential error from several assumptions in the whole body method the segmental method is suggested, which divides the body into respective "cylindrical" segments of arm, leg, and trunk in an attempt to ac-count for differences in body proportions in the different segments. A detailed account of these procedures has been provided by the American College of Sports Medicine (23). In either case the procedure is relatively easy to perform and takes only a few minutes.

Although bioelectric impedance is a relatively new procedure for measuring body composition, a number of studies have summarized its validity and reli-ability (12, 23). Estimates of body composition have generally been reported as accurate, although accuracy may be less for some types of individuals, especially

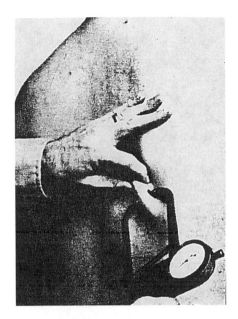

FIGURE 4.5. Subscapular skinfold.

those with abnormal levels or distributions of body fluids (23). Factors affecting body fluids must be taken into careful consideration prior to measurement to maximize accuracy.

Near-Infrared Interactance

The technique of near-infrared interactance (NIR) is a new method of estimating percentage of body fat. NIR is a simple, noninvasive and safe procedure based on the observation that the NIR light beam is absorbed and reflected differently in fat and lean tissues. Optical densities for two wavelengths are measured (Futrex 5000, Futrex, Inc., Gaithersburg, MD) at the biceps to differentiate between subcutaneous fat and muscle. Additional information required to estimate percentage body fat includes height, weight, gender, and physical activity. Currently, few data are available that discuss reliability and validity of the NIR procedure, although information presently available does not support replacing more proven procedures with NIR (24–27). At this time more data are needed before NIR is accepted as a bona fide field measure of body fat.

Body Mass Index

Ideal body weight and obesity are also evaluated by body mass index (BMI):

$$BMI = \frac{weight\ (kg)}{height\ (m^2)}$$

Risk classification based on BMI is presented in Figure 4.6 (4). Body mass index has been adopted as a measure of clinical risk (4), and increased BMI has been shown to be related to risk of cardiovascular disease (28). Mean BMI values are approximately the same in adult men and women (4). Adolescent males and females also have comparable values (18, 22). Because BMI is based on a relationship between height and weight, it has the same limitations as discussed earlier in the Metropolitan tables in classifying individuals with low body fat and high lean body mass.

TABLE 4.5. Percent Body Fat for Women Using the Sum of Triceps, Suprailium, and Thigh Skinfolds[a]

Sum of Skinfolds (mm)	Age (years)								
	<22	23–27	28–32	33–37	38–42	43–47	48–52	53–57	>57
23–25	9.7	9.9	10.2	10.4	10.7	10.9	11.2	11.4	11.7
26–28	11.0	11.2	11.5	11.7	12.0	12.3	12.5	12.7	13.0
29–31	12.3	12.5	12.8	13.0	13.3	13.5	13.8	14.0	14.3
32–34	13.6	13.8	14.0	14.3	14.5	14.8	15.0	15.3	15.5
35–37	14.8	15.0	15.3	15.5	15.8	16.0	16.3	16.5	16.8
38–40	16.0	16.3	16.5	16.7	17.0	17.2	17.5	17.7	18.0
41–43	17.2	17.4	17.7	17.9	18.2	18.4	18.7	18.9	19.2
44–46	18.3	18.6	18.8	19.1	19.3	19.6	19.8	20.1	20.3
47–49	19.5	19.7	20.0	20.2	20.5	20.7	21.0	21.2	21.5
50–52	20.6	20.8	21.1	21.3	21.6	21.8	22.1	22.3	22.6
53–55	21.7	21.9	22.1	22.4	22.6	22.9	23.1	23.4	23.6
56–58	22.7	23.0	23.2	23.4	23.7	23.9	24.2	24.4	24.7
59–61	23.7	24.0	24.2	24.5	24.7	25.0	25.2	25.5	25.7
62–64	24.7	25.0	25.2	25.5	25.7	26.0	26.4	26.7	26.9
65–67	25.7	25.9	26.2	26.4	26.7	26.9	27.2	27.4	27.7
68–70	26.6	26.9	27.1	27.4	27.7	27.9	28.1	28.4	28.6
71–73	27.5	27.8	28.0	28.3	28.5	28.8	29.0	29.3	29.5
74–76	28.4	28.7	28.9	29.2	29.4	29.7	29.9	30.2	30.4
77–79	29.3	29.5	29.8	30.0	30.3	30.5	30.8	31.0	31.2
80–82	30.1	30.4	30.6	30.9	31.1	31.4	31.6	31.9	32.1
83–85	30.9	31.2	31.4	31.7	31.9	32.2	32.4	32.7	32.9
86–88	31.7	32.0	32.2	32.5	32.7	32.9	33.2	33.4	33.7
89–91	32.5	32.7	33.0	33.2	33.5	33.7	33.9	34.2	34.4
92–94	33.2	33.4	33.7	33.9	34.2	34.4	34.7	34.9	35.2
95–97	33.9	34.1	34.4	34.6	34.9	35.1	35.4	35.6	35.9
98–100	34.6	34.8	35.1	35.3	35.5	35.8	36.0	36.3	36.5
101–103	35.3	35.4	35.7	35.9	36.2	36.4	36.7	36.9	37.2
104–106	35.8	36.1	36.3	36.6	36.8	37.1	37.3	37.5	37.8
107–109	36.4	36.7	36.9	37.1	37.4	37.6	37.9	38.1	38.4
110–112	37.0	37.2	37.5	37.7	38.0	38.2	38.5	38.7	38.9
113–115	37.5	37.8	38.0	38.2	38.5	38.7	39.0	39.2	39.5
116–118	38.0	38.3	38.5	38.8	39.0	39.3	39.5	39.7	40.0
119–121	38.5	38.7	39.0	39.2	39.5	39.7	40.0	40.2	40.5
122–124	39.0	39.2	39.4	39.7	39.9	40.2	40.4	40.7	40.9
125–127	39.4	39.6	39.9	40.1	40.4	40.6	40.9	41.1	41.4
128–130	39.8	40.0	40.3	40.5	40.8	41.0	41.3	41.5	41.8

[a]From Jackson AS, Pollock ML. Practical assessment of body composition. Phys Sports Med 1985; 13:76. (Reprinted by permission of the Physician and Sportsmedicine, a McGraw-Hill publication.)

TABLE 4.6. Percent Body Fat for Men Using the Sum of Chest, Abdomen, and Thigh Skinfolds[a]

Sum of Skinfolds (mm)	Age (years)								
	<22	23–27	28–32	33–37	38–42	43–47	48–52	53–57	>57
8–10	1.3	1.8	2.3	2.9	3.4	3.9	4.5	5.0	5.5
11–13	2.2	2.8	3.3	3.9	4.4	4.9	5.5	6.0	6.5
14–16	3.2	3.8	4.3	4.8	5.4	5.9	6.4	7.0	7.5
17–19	4.2	4.7	5.3	5.8	6.3	6.9	7.4	8.0	8.5
20–22	5.1	5.7	6.2	6.8	7.3	7.9	8.4	8.9	9.5
23–25	6.1	6.6	7.2	7.7	8.3	8.8	9.4	9.9	10.5
26–28	7.0	7.6	8.1	8.7	9.2	9.8	10.3	10.9	11.4
29–31	8.0	8.5	9.1	9.6	10.2	10.7	11.3	11.8	12.4
32–34	8.9	9.4	10.0	10.5	11.1	11.6	12.2	12.8	13.3
35–37	9.8	10.4	10.9	11.5	12.0	12.6	13.1	13.7	14.3
38–40	10.7	11.3	11.8	12.4	12.9	13.5	14.1	14.6	15.2
41–43	11.6	12.2	12.7	13.3	13.8	14.4	15.0	15.5	16.1
44–46	12.5	13.1	13.6	14.2	14.7	15.3	15.9	16.4	17.0
47–49	13.4	13.9	14.5	15.1	15.6	16.2	16.8	17.3	17.9
50 52	14.3	14.8	15.4	15.9	16.5	17.1	17.6	18.2	18.8
53–55	15.1	15.7	16.2	16.8	17.4	17.9	18.5	19.1	19.7
56–58	16.0	16.5	17.1	17.7	18.2	18.8	19.4	20.0	20.5
59–61	16.9	17.4	17.9	18.5	19.1	19.7	20.2	20.8	21.4
62–64	17.6	18.2	18.8	19.4	19.9	20.5	21.1	21.7	22.2
65–67	18.5	19.0	19.6	20.2	20.8	21.3	21.9	22.5	23.1
68–70	19.3	19.9	20.4	21.0	21.6	22.2	22.7	23.3	23.9
71–73	20.1	20.7	21.2	21.8	22.4	23.0	23.6	24.1	24.7
74–76	20.9	21.5	22.0	22.6	23.2	23.8	24.4	25.0	25.5
77–79	21.7	22.2	22.8	23.4	24.0	24.6	25.2	25.8	26.3
80–82	22.4	23.0	23.6	24.2	24.8	25.4	25.9	26.5	27.1
83–85	23.2	23.8	24.4	25.0	25.5	26.1	26.7	27.3	27.9
86–88	24.0	24.5	25.1	25.7	26.3	26.9	27.5	28.1	28.7
89–91	24.7	25.3	25.9	26.5	27.1	27.6	28.2	28.8	29.4
92–94	25.4	26.0	26.6	27.2	27.8	28.4	29.0	29.6	30.2
95–97	26.1	26.7	27.3	27.9	28.5	29.1	29.7	30.3	30.9
98–100	26.9	27.4	28.0	28.6	29.2	29.8	30.4	31.0	31.6
101–103	27.5	28.1	28.7	29.3	29.9	30.5	31.1	31.7	32.3
104–106	28.2	28.8	29.4	30.0	30.6	31.2	31.8	32.4	33.0
107–109	28.9	29.5	30.1	30.7	31.3	31.9	32.5	33.1	33.7
110–112	29.6	30.2	30.8	31.4	32.0	32.6	33.2	33.8	34.4
113–115	30.2	30.8	31.4	32.0	32.6	33.2	33.8	34.5	35.1
116–118	30.9	31.5	32.1	32.7	33.3	33.9	34.5	35.1	35.7
119–121	31.5	32.1	32.7	33.3	33.9	34.5	35.1	35.7	36.4
122–124	32.1	32.7	33.3	33.9	34.5	35.1	35.8	36.4	37.0
125–127	32.7	33.3	33.9	34.5	35.1	35.8	36.4	37.0	37.6

[a]From Jackson AS, Pollock ML. Practical assessment of body composition. Phys Sports Med 1985; 13:76. (Reprinted by permission of the Physician and Sportsmedicine, a McGraw-Hill publication.)

TABLE 4.7. Estimation of Percent Body Fat From Three Skinfold Measurements: Triceps, Subscapular, Suprailiac

Total Skinfold (mm)	Fat (% body weight)	
	Males	Females
10.0	2.8	7.8
15.0	7.3	13.3
20.0	10.5	17.2
25.0	13.0	20.3
30.0	15.1	22.8
35.0	16.9	25.0
40.0	18.5	26.9
45.0	19.8	28.6
50.0	21.1	30.2
55.0	22.2	31.6
60.0	23.2	32.8
65.0	24.2	34.0
70.0	25.1	35.1
75.0	25.9	36.2
80.0	26.7	37.1
85.0	27.4	38.0
90.0	28.1	38.9
95.0	28.7	39.7
100.0	29.4	40.5
105.0	30.0	41.2
110.0	30.5	41.9
115.0	31.1	42.6
120.0	31.6	43.3
125.0	32.1	43.9
130.0	32.6	44.5
135.0	33.0	45.1
140.0	33.5	45.7
145.0	33.9	46.2
150.0	34.4	46.7

Circumference Measurements

Measurement of select circumferences provides valuable information about obesity and health risk. In particular the waist/hip ratio (WHR) is widely used. WHR indicates the distribution of upper—and lower body—obesity, android versus gynoid, respectively. Gynoid obesity is characterized as hyperplasia, which is caused by increased cell number, whereas android obesity is a function of fat cell hypertrophy (4), which is more indicative of increased health risk (28).

Girth measurements should be obtained with a steel tape. The waist circumference is taken at the level of the umbilicus whereas hip girth is measured at the broadest part of the gluteal region. A high WHR, >0.8 (females) and >0.9 (males), represents an android fat pattern that is associated with increased health risk in both men and women as shown in Figure 4.7 (4, 29).

Blood Pressure

Hypertension, an often silent disease until major cardiovascular or renal complications appear, is one of the most common and potentially deadly afflictions in adults in our society. Blood pressure screening, therefore, is an important aspect in the evalution of candidates for exercise programs.

Proper technique is essential for obtaining accurate blood pressure measurements. The subject should be sitting upright, legs uncrossed, feet flat on the floor and with arm bared. Rolled-up sleeves should be avoided, since upper arm constriction might affect the validity of the reading. Cuff size is important and has been standardized by the American Heart Association (30). For each cuff size the proper range should be marked on the inside of the cuff so that when the cuff is wrapped around the arm, the index line at the end of the cuff falls within that range. If the index line falls outside the range for that sized cuff, a smaller or larger cuff should be used for that subject. Each testing facility should own standard-sized, large-sized, and pediatric cuffs. Finally, a well-maintained mercury sphygmomanometer should be used for obtaining the blood pressure measurements.

Before taking the subject's pressure, the peak systolic pressure should be estimated by inflating the cuff to a pressure that obliterates the distal radial pulse. The diaphragm of the stethoscope is then positioned over the brachial artery and the cuff inflated approximately 30 mm Hg above the estimated systolic pressure. The cuff is then slowly deflated 2 mm Hg/second until the first Korotkoff's sounds are audible. The systolic blood pressure is defined as the pressure at which the Korotkoff's sounds are heard for two consecutive beats. As the cuff continues to deflate slowly, the diastolic blood pressure is defined as the point when the Korotkoff's sounds completely disappear (phase V). Occasionally, and particularly with exercise, Korotkoff's sounds are present to very low pressures or zero pressure in which case the muffling of sounds should be used (phase IV). The average of two or more blood pressure readings taken from the same arm should be used to determine the subject's initial measurement (30).

The 1993 Report of the Joint National Committee on Detection, Evaluation, and Treatment of High Blood Pressure (31) provides up-to-date guidelines and recommendations for hypertension screening and management (see Chapters 3

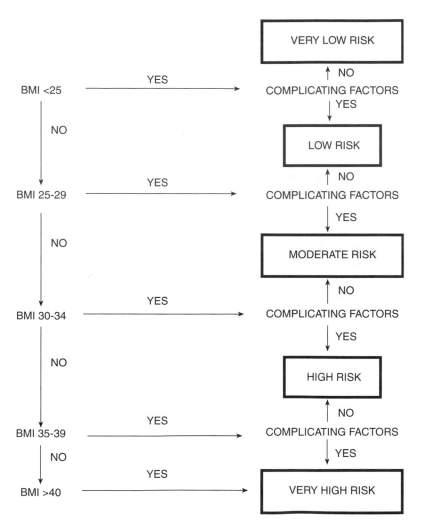

FIGURE 4.6. Risk classification based on body mass index (BMI) and the presence or absence of complicating factors, including elevated waist/hip ratios, diabetes, hypertension, male sex, and age below 40 years. (Adapted from Butler TG, Yanowitz FG. In: Yanowitz FG, ed. Coronary heart disease prevention. New York: Marcel Dekker, 1992; and Bray GA, Gray DS. Obesity. II. Treatment. West J Med 1988; 149:555.)

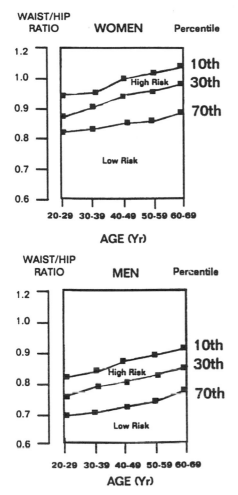

FIGURE 4.7. Percentiles and risk classification for men and women based on waist/hip ratios and age. (Adapted from Butler TG, Yanowitz FG. In: Yanowitz FG, ed. Coronary heart disease prevention. New York: Marcel Dekker, 1992; and Bray GA, Gray DS. Obesity. II. Treatment. West J Med 1988;149:555.)

and 11). It is important to provide individuals with their actual numerical blood pressure values and also to give them the appropriate guidelines for follow-up. Recommendations for managing hypertension in competitive athletes have been published by Walther and Tifft (32).

Muscle Strength, Endurance, and Flexibility

Muscle function tests range from simple field tests to very elaborate laboratory evaluations using expensive muscle testing equipment. These latter tests are generally used by research exercise physiologists, health professionals working with competitive athletes, or medical specialists studying neuromuscular and orthopedic disorders. For the purpose of screening subjects for exercise programs, simple field tests are usually adequate. Other references are recommended for readers interested in more sophisticated testing procedures (33, 34).

Muscle Strength

A battery of tests involving major muscle groups is suggested for evaluating muscle strength. Table 4.8, published by Pollock et al. (11), lists normal reference values for men and women for several muscle-strength tests based on the one-repetition maximal test. Each test consists of a series of trials designed to determine the maximal weight that can be lifted only once before fatigue. If only one test is selected, the one-repetition bench press is recommended (11),

141

since this test most closely correlates with total dynamic strength.

Muscle strength of the hand and forearm can be tested by using a handgrip dynamometer (Harpenden, British Indicators, Ltd., England). After adjusting the grip for the subject's hand size, three attempts at maximal grip strength should be made with each hand, alternately. The highest figure is used for the final score. Table 4.9 illustrates a rating scale for men and women. Muscle strength has been shown to be an important component of adult fitness programs and should be included with all age groups (35, 36).

Muscle Endurance

The testing of muscle endurance is somewhat controversial, since many of the recommended field tests are biased by variations in muscle strength. To standardize for these differences among individuals, a fixed percentage of 70% of the

TABLE 4.8. Normal Reference Values for Strength Testing Based on the One-Repetition Maximal Test[a]

Body Weight (lb)	Bench Press (lb)		Standing Press (lb)		Curl (lb)		Leg Press (lb)	
	Men	Women	Men	Women	Men	Women	Men	Women
80	80	56	53	37	40	28	160	112
100	100	70	67	47	50	35	200	140
120	120	84	80	56	60	42	240	168
140	140	98	93	65	70	49	280	196
160	160	112	107	75	80	56	320	224
180	180	126	120	84	90	63	360	252
200	200	140	133	93	100	70	400	280
220	220	154	147	103	110	77	440	308
240	240	168	160	112	120	84	480	336

[a]From Pollock ML, Wilmore JH, Fox SM. Health and fitness through physical activity. New York: Wiley, 1978.

TABLE 4.9. Handgrip Strength Test

Score	Men	Women
Excellent	65 or above	42 or above
Good	56–63	37–41
Average	44–55	30–36
Fair	36–43	24–29
Poor	30–35	19–23

maximal muscle strength is suggested for testing endurance; that is, determining the maximal number of repetitions that can be carried out by a particular group of muscles at 70% maximal strength. Unfortunately, normal reference values for these tests are not yet available. Norms for more standard endurance tests, such as push-up and sit-up tests, have been published (11).

Joint Flexibility

Accurate tests of muscle flexibility require quantifying the range of motion of the different joints. One useful screening test is the sit-and-reach test, which is used to assess the flexibility of the lower back and posterior thigh muscles. In this test a calibrated flexibility testing bench (e.g., Health Accessories, Seattle, WA) is used as illustrated in Figure 4.8. The subject assumes the sitting position with the knees fully extended, feet together, and soles touching the seat of the bench. On command, the arms are extended and the fingers pointed as the subject reaches forward maximally, pushing a slider along the calibrated back of the bench. Scoring for this test is illustrated in Table 4.10.

Low back flexibility is particularly useful as an indication of potential back injuries and is recommended as a universal screening measure for all ages. Those with poor back flexibility should be assigned to a serious back program.

Submaximal Exercise Testing For Fitness Evaluation

Submaximal exercise testing to estimate maximal aerobic capacity ($\dot{V}O_{2max}$) is a poor substitute for maximal testing (see Chapter 5), although it may be useful in asymptomatic, low-risk subjects for whom a more costly maximal diagnostic test is not needed. These tests can be administered in the field by allied health professionals without ECG monitoring or physician supervision (15) and, as a result, are reasonably inexpensive.

A number of submaximal exercise test protocols have been developed for assessing cardiovascular fitness. The prediction of maximal oxygen uptake from submaximal heart rates and workloads is possible because of the near linear relationship between exercise heart rate and $\dot{V}O_2$, and between $\dot{V}O_2$ and workload (37, 38). It should be noted, however, that there are many limitations to the prediction of $\dot{V}O_{2max}$ from submaximal testing protocols, and at best, these tests provide only approximate measures of cardiovascular fitness.

Leg Ergometry

A stationary bicycle ergometer is often used for submaximal testing, since it is inexpensive, reasonably portable, and the workload can be quantified in watts (W) or kilopond-meters (kpm)/min. Any exercise mode that is quantifiable and calibratable may be used for testing purposes. A widely used single-load submaximal protocol developed by Astrand and Rhyming is as follows (37, 38):

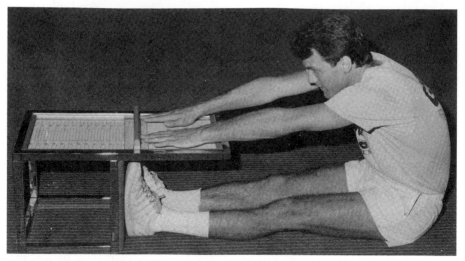

FIGURE 4.8. Sit-and-reach test for muscle flexibility.

TABLE 4.10. Sit-and-Reach Test (inches)

Excellent	+7 or above
Good	+4 to +6
Average	−1 to +3
Fair	−3 to −2
Poor	−4 or less

1. Pedaling speed should be constant at 50 rpm (18 km/hr).
2. A low-level initial workload is selected, usually 50 to 100 W for females and 75 to 150 W for males, depending on the person's size and level of fitness.
3. Heart rates are determined each minute while the workload is progressively increased until a rate of at least 120 to 130 is achieved. Heart rates below 120 to 130 bpm tend to have a curvilinear relationship with workload and may result in overestimating aerobic capacity. The heart rate should not exceed 85% of age-estimated maximum.
4. The workload is then held constant and is continued for 6 minutes. If heart rates during the last 2 minutes are within five beats, the test is terminated. If not, the test is continued until successive heart rates are within five beats.
5. The average heart rate during the last 2 minutes and the respective workload are used to calculate $\dot{V}O_{2max}$ from Table 4.11.
6. The $\dot{V}O_{2max}$ is corrected for age by the respective correction factor, Table 4.12.

7. Table 4.13 is used for an indication and comparison of aerobic fitness.

It should be emphasized that the Astrand-Rhyming test is not valid in individuals taking a variety of medications that affect the heart rate response to exercise (beta-blockers, sympathomimetic agents, some calcium channel blockers). For these people, as well as for older, more high-risk, and/or symptomatic individuals, the maximal exercise test protocols that involve ECG monitoring and physician supervision are recommended. These are fully described in Chapter 5.

Multistage progressive bicycle protocols are also used for submaximal testing to predict functional capacity. Workloads usually start at 25 to 50 W and progress by that amount every 3 to 5 minutes. Pedaling speed is maintained at 50 rpm, heart rates above 120 are plotted against workloads, and a regression line is computed. Maximal oxygen uptake is predicted as illustrated in Figure 4.9. Test results can be compared with normative values (15).

Arm Ergometry

Multistage progressive protocols for arm testing can also be used to predict $\dot{V}O_{2max}$. The arm-crank ergometer is particularly useful for subjects who emphasize upper body activity, as well as for those with vascular or musculoskeletal limitations in the lower extremities. The arm ergometer must be adjusted for the subject prior to testing. An adjustable chest plate is recommended to help standardize arm extension. The arms should be almost extended at the elbow when the pedal is pushed all the way forward. Maintaining continual chest contact with the plate also helps to decrease the usage of ancillary muscle groups of the chest, shoulders, and back.

Arm ergometer tests usually begin at a resistance of 25 W to 50 W and are increased by 12.5 watts per stage every 3 to 4 minutes. A brief pause between stages may be helpful for taking blood pressures and in reducing local muscle fatigue. Heart rates in a steady state at the end of each workload may be plotted against the resistance of that stage, with $\dot{V}O_{2max}$ being estimated in a similar manner to that described in Figure 4.9, except that $\dot{V}O_2$ values will be higher in arm exercise (39, 40). Norms for cardiovascular fitness from arm testing are not available.

Pulmonary Function Screening Tests

Routine spirometry is a useful procedure that is easily performed by allied health personnel. The test may provide the initial evidence for early cardiopulmonary disorders and may identify useful information on physical fitness and training adaptation when considered in units of body size. Individuals complaining of unexplained dyspnea on exertion are especially good candidates for pulmonary function studies, since this common symptom may only reflect deconditioning in some subjects but, in others, may also be a manifestation of

TABLE 4.11. Prediction of Maximal Oxygen Uptake from Heart Rate and Workload on a Bicycle Ergometer (*The value should be corrected for age, using the factor given in Table 4.12.*)[a]

Men

Heart Rate	Maximal Oxygen Uptake, L/min^{-1}				
	300 kpm/min 50W	600 kpm/min 100W	900 kpm/min 150W	1200 kpm/min 200W	1500 kpm/min 250W
120	2.2	3.5	4.8		
121	2.2	3.4	4.7		
122	2.2	3.4	4.6		
123	2.1	3.4	4.6		
124	2.1	3.3	4.5	6.0	
125	2.0	3.2	4.4	5.9	
126	2.0	3.2	4.4	5.8	
127	2.0	3.1	4.3	5.7	
128	2.0	3.1	4.2	5.6	
129	1.9	3.0	4.2	5.6	
130	1.9	3.0	4.1	5.5	
131	1.9	2.9	4.0	5.4	
132	1.8	2.9	4.0	5.3	
133	1.8	2.8	3.9	5.3	
134	1.8	2.8	3.9	5.2	
135	1.7	2.8	3.8	5.1	
136	1.7	2.7	3.8	5.0	
137	1.7	2.7	3.7	5.0	
138	1.6	2.7	3.7	4.9	
139	1.6	2.6	3.6	4.8	
140	1.6	2.6	3.6	4.8	6.0
141		2.6	3.5	4.7	5.9
142		2.5	3.5	4.6	5.8
143		2.5	3.4	4.6	5.7
144		2.5	3.4	4.5	5.7
145		2.4	3.4	4.5	5.6
146		2.4	3.3	4.4	5.6
147		2.4	3.3	4.4	5.5
148		2.4	3.2	4.3	5.4
149		2.3	3.2	4.3	5.4
150		2.3	3.2	4.2	5.3
151		2.3	3.1	4.2	5.2
152		2.3	3.1	4.1	5.2
153		2.2	3.0	4.1	5.1
154		2.2	3.0	4.0	5.1
155		2.2	3.0	4.0	5.0
156		2.1	2.9	4.0	5.0
157		2.1	2.9	3.9	4.9
158		2.1	2.9	3.9	4.9
159		2.1	2.8	3.8	4.8
160		2.0	2.8	3.8	4.8
161		2.0	2.8	3.7	4.7
162		2.0	2.8	3.7	4.6
163		2.0	2.8	3.7	4.6
164		2.0	2.7	3.6	4.5
165		2.0	2.7	3.6	4.5
166		1.9	2.7	3.6	4.5
167		1.9	2.6	3.5	4.4
168		1.9	2.6	3.5	4.4
169		1.9	2.6	3.5	4.3
170		1.8	2.6	3.4	4.3

TABLE 4.11. Cont.

Women

Heart Rate	Maximal Oxygen Uptake, L/min^{-1}				
	300 kpm/min 50W	450 kpm/min 75W	600 kpm/min 100W	750 kpm/min 125W	900 kpm/min 150W
120	2.6	3.4	4.1	4.8	
121	2.5	3.3	4.0	4.8	
122	2.5	3.2	3.9	4.7	
123	2.4	3.1	3.9	4.6	
124	2.4	3.1	3.8	4.5	
125	2.3	3.0	3.7	4.4	
126	2.3	3.0	3.6	4.3	
127	2.2	2.9	3.5	4.2	
128	2.2	2.8	3.5	4.2	4.8
129	2.2	2.8	3.4	4.1	4.8
130	2.1	2.7	3.4	4.0	4.7
131	2.1	2.7	3.4	4.0	4.6
132	2.0	2.7	3.3	3.9	4.5
133	2.0	2.6	3.2	3.8	4.4
134	2.0	2.6	3.2	3.8	4.4
135	2.0	2.6	3.1	3.7	4.3
136	1.9	2.5	3.1	3.6	4.2
137	1.9	2.5	3.0	3.6	4.2
138	1.8	2.4	3.0	3.5	4.1
139	1.8	2.4	2.9	3.5	4.0
140	1.8	2.4	2.8	3.4	4.0
141	1.8	2.3	2.8	3.4	3.9
142	1.7	2.3	2.8	3.3	3.9
143	1.7	2.2	2.7	3.3	3.8
144	1.7	2.2	2.7	3.2	3.8
145	1.6	2.2	2.7	3.2	3.7
146	1.6	2.2	2.6	3.2	3.7
147	1.6	2.1	2.6	3.1	3.6

Heart Rate	Maximal Oxygen Uptake, L/min^{-1}				
	300 kpm/min 50W	450 kpm/min 75W	600 kpm/min 100W	750 kpm/min 125W	900 kpm/min 150W
148	1.6	2.1	2.6	3.1	3.6
149		2.1	2.6	3.0	3.5
150		2.0	2.5	3.0	3.5
151		2.0	2.5	3.0	3.4
152		2.0	2.5	2.9	3.4
153		2.0	2.4	2.9	3.3
154		2.0	2.4	2.8	3.3
155		1.9	2.4	2.8	3.2
156		1.9	2.3	2.8	3.2
157		1.9	2.3	2.7	3.2
158		1.8	2.3	2.7	3.1
159		1.8	2.2	2.7	3.1
160		1.8	2.2	2.6	3.0
161		1.8	2.2	2.6	3.0
162		1.8	2.2	2.6	3.0
163		1.7	2.2	2.6	2.9
164		1.7	2.1	2.5	2.9
165		1.7	2.1	2.5	2.9
166		1.7	2.1	2.5	2.8
167		1.6	2.1	2.4	2.8
168		1.6	2.0	2.4	2.8
169		1.6	2.0	2.4	2.8
170		1.6	2.0	2.4	2.7

From Åstrand I. Aerobic work capacity in men and women with special reference to age. Acta Physiol Scand 1960; 49 (Suppl 169):45–60.

147

TABLE 4.12. Correction Factor for $\dot{V}O_{2max}$ Prediction in Subjects Over Age 35

Age	Factor
25	1.00
35	0.87
40	0.83
45	0.78
50	0.75
55	0.71
60	0.68
65	0.65

TABLE 4.13. Norms for Maximum O_2 Consumption (Aerobic Working Capacity)[a,b]

	Age	Low	Fair	Average	Good	High
Women	20–29	1.69	1.70–1.99	2.00–2.49	2.50–2.79	2.80+
		28	29–34	35–43	44--48	49+
	30–39	1.59	1.60–1.89	1.90–2.39	2.40–2.69	2.70+
		27	28–33	34–41	42–47	48+
	40–49	1.49	1.50–1.79	1.80–2.29	2.30–2.59	2.60+
		25	26–31	32–40	41–45	46+
	50–65	1.29	1.30–1.59	1.60–2.09	2.10–2.39	2.40+
		21	22–28	29–36	37–41	42+
Men	20–29	2.79	2.80–3.09	3.10–3.69	3.70–3.99	4.00+
		38	39–43	44–51	52–56	57+
	30–39	2.49	2.50–2.79	2.80–3.39	3.40–3.69	3.70+
		34	35–39	40–47	48–51	52+
	40–49	2.19	2.20–2.49	2.50–3.09	3.10–3.39	3.40+
		30	31–35	36–43	44–47	48+
	50–59	1.89	1.90–2.19	2.20–2.79	2.80–3.09	3.10+
		25	26–31	32–39	40–43	44+
	60–69	1.59	1.60–1.89	1.90–2.49	2.50–2.79	2.80+
		21	22–26	27–35	36–39	40+

[a]From Åstrand. I. Aerobic work capacity in men and women with special reference to age. Acta Physiol Scand 1960;49 (Suppl 169): 45–60.
[b]Lower figure = ml of O_2/kg body weight.

148

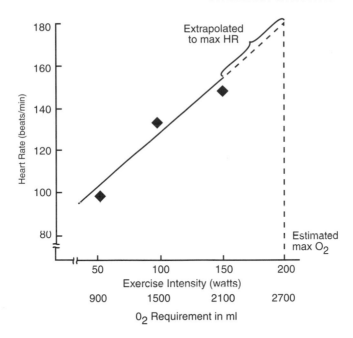

FIGURE 4.9. Heart rates obtained from at least three submaximal exercise intensities may be extrapolated to the age-predicted maximal heart rate. A vertical line to the intensity scale estimates workload. (Adapted from Blair SN. In: Matarazzo JD et al., ed. Behavioral health. a handbook of health enhancement and disease prevention. New York: John Wiley & Sons, 1984.)

serious heart or lung disease. The two spirometric parameters of particular inter-est are the forced vital capacity (FVC) and the forced expiratory volume in one second (FEV_1). Minimal standards for spirometers and the interpretation of spirometric tracings have been published elsewhere (41).

Figure 4.10 illustrates the spirometric lung volumes. The FVC is defined as the maximal volume of air that can be forcefully exhaled following a maximal inhalation. The subject's FVC should be compared to the published normal reference values based on age, sex, and height (41). Those with restrictive lung diseases, characterized by stiff lungs, have reduced lung volumes, including the FVC. Obstructive lung diseases, on the other hand, are characterized by in-creased airways resistance on expiration and reduction in FEV_1. Normally, the FEV_1 is about 80% of the FVC. In obstructive lung diseases, such as asthma, chronic bronchitis, and emphysema, the FEV_1 is less than 75% of the FVC.

Adequate spirometric tracings for analysis require careful attention to details. The following steps published by the Intermountain Thoracic Society are rec-ommended (6):

149

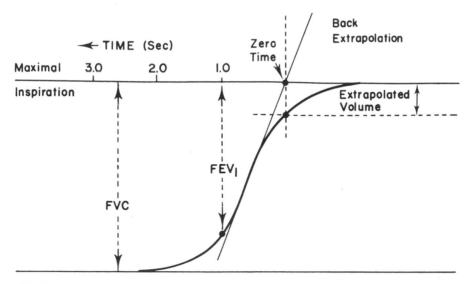

FIGURE 4.10. Measurement of spirometric tracing to determine FEV_1.

1. Have the patient seated comfortably upright.
2. Loosen all tight clothing, including underclothing (belt, girdle, brassiere, etc.).
3. Remove dentures if present.
4. Explain carefully and fully what is to be done prior to starting, demonstrating each phase of the test.
5. Put mouthpiece in patient's mouth, between and beyond the teeth, and be sure no leaks are present.
6. Occlude the patient's nose with a nose clip.
7. Then instruct the patient to slowly but maximally exhale, observing both the patient and the tracing.
8. When the expiration is maximal (residual volume has been reached), then instruct the patient to breathe in as deeply as possible to total lung capacity.
9. When the patient reaches full inspiration, change chart speed to the fast speed (at least 30 mm/sec) and when attained:
   a. Vigorously encourage the patient to blow out the air as rapidly as possible by loudly commanding "blow." (You should be embarrassed by the commotion you must make).
   b. Urge patient to keep exhaling, "blow-blow," until the breath is completed as evidenced by a constant level on the kymograph (straight horizontal line not due to breath-holding).
   c. If the spirogram does not become horizontal, the technician

should not terminate the study but should encourage the patient to continue until he or she is unable to go on. Caution: Hypoxemic patients may become distressed, and in such instances the study should be terminated prematurely.

    d.   At the point where expiration has been assessed to be complete, instruct the patient to maximally and rapidly inhale back to the point of maximal inspiration. Command patient to "suck it in."

10.   Disconnect patient, remove nose clips, let patient relax, and flush out the spirometer.

11.   Repeat study until three acceptable tracings are obtained. Acceptability will be determined by the technician's observation that the subject understood the instructions and performed the test with a smooth continuous exhalation, with apparent maximal effort, with good start, and without the following:

    a.   Coughing.

    b.   A Valsalva maneuver (glottis closure).

    c.   An early termination of expiration. (In a normal patient this would precede completion of the breath; in an obstructed patient this would be assumed to have taken place if the expiration time was less than 5 seconds).

    d.   A leak.

    e.   An obstructed mouthpiece (for example, obstruction caused by the tongue being placed in front of the mouthpiece or false teeth falling in front of the mouthpiece).

    f.   An unsatisfactory start of expiration, characterized by excessive hesitation or false starts. Unsatisfactory starts prevent accurate back extrapolation and determination of time zero. To achieve accurate time zero, the extrapolated volume on the spirogram should be less than 10% of the FVC or 100 ml, whichever is greater.

    g.   An excessive variability among the three acceptable curves. The FVC and FEV_1 of the two best of the three acceptable curves should not vary by more than 5% of reading of 100 ml, whichever is greater.

12.   Record the technician's assessment of patient performance and cooperation (good, fair, poor) with respect to lung function. A maximal effort may be misleading if the patient pits one group of muscles against another. If flow from the mouth is limited by pitting one group of respiratory muscles against another, the value of the spirogram as an indicator of mechanical properties of the lung is reduced.

Once the spirometric tracings have been obtained, the one spirogram representing the subject's best effort should be utilized for performing all calculations. This should be the tracing with the largest absolute sum of the FEV_1 plus the FVC (6). Figure 4.10 illustrates a sample spirogram with the measurements. For the purposes of calculating the FEV_1, zero time is determined by back extrapolation. As seen in Figure 4.10, a line is drawn along the steepest slope and extended back to intersect the maximal inspiratory level. If the "extrapolated volume" (Fig. 4.10) is more than 10% of the FVC or 100 ml, the tracing is considered suboptimal (40).

The FVC and FEV_1 should be expressed in liters to two decimal places, and the ratio FEV_1:FVC to one decimal place. For convenience a transparent spirometric ruler can be used over the tracings to convert the chart displacement in millimeters to volumes. The measured volumes in ambient temperature, pressure, saturated (ATPS) should then be converted to body temperature, pressure, saturated (BTPS) by multiplying the volumes times a conversion factor based on room temperature and barometric pressures (6). The final volumes should be compared to normal reference values based on age, sex, and height (6). Abnormalities should be categorized as mild, moderate, or severe, using published criteria (6).

LABORATORY ASSESSMENT

Selected blood tests might be considered in screening for adult fitness and cardiac rehabilitation. These include blood lipids, electrolytes, fasting blood glucose, and possibly a complete blood count to screen for anemia. The technique of venipuncture is easily learned by allied health personnel, and venous blood samples are readily obtained from most individuals. The use of desktop analyzers that utilize a finger stick to obtain microsamples facilitates the process. These analyzers have been well validated (42) and are being widely used.

Blood Lipids

Blood lipids have become extremely important measurements in recent years because of the following observations:

1. Atherosclerosis continues to be our nation's number-one cause of death and disability (43).
2. The risk of atherosclerosis and coronary heart disease (CHD) appears to be directly proportional to the blood levels of total cholesterol (TC) and low-density lipoprotein cholesterol (LDLC) and inversely proportional to the level of high-density lipoprotein cholesterol (HDLC) (44, 45).

3. Total cholesterol and LDLC levels are influenced in a major way by dietary saturated fat and cholesterol intake (46, 47).
4. Recent scientific evidence strongly suggests that lowering blood cholesterol levels by diet and drug therapy significantly reduces the incidence of CHD in hypercholesterolemic subjects (48).

Since the main objective of adult fitness and cardiac rehabilitation is to improve the cardiovascular health and well-being of participants, it seems reasonable to include lipid screening in the initial evaluation of applicants to these programs (see Chapter 11).

Early cholesterol screening, in childhood or adolescence, is recommended, particularly in those whose parents are known to have elevated values. Recent guidelines have been published for this age group, including the need for follow-up testing (49). Although universal screening is a controversial issue, if undertaken for the purpose of nutritional counseling rather than patient "labeling" there should be few objections. Complete guidelines for managing the hyperlipidemias have been published (49–51).

Blood Glucose

The fasting blood glucose determination is a crude screening test for diabetes mellitus that is not very sensitive unless the fasting glucose is over 150 mg/dl. In asymptomatic subjects over age 40, as well as obese individuals over age 30, it is recommended that a yearly blood glucose be obtained 2 hours after a large breakfast. If the blood glucose value is less than 120 mg/dl, diabetes is ruled out (52).

CONCLUSIONS

Although the physician-administered medical history, physical examination, and maximal exercise stress test are all important in screening individuals at high risk for cardiovascular disease, as well as those with already existing disease, techniques that are usually carried out by allied health professionals are important as well. Not all of these screening tests are necessary for adult fitness or cardiac rehabilitation programs, but they are very likely to improve the overall quality of those programs by providing more comprehensive and individualized data from which to develop the exercise prescriptions.

REFERENCES

1. Metropolitan Life Insurance Company. Four steps to weight control, New York: Metropolitan Life Insurance, 1969.
2. Weigley ES. Average? Ideal? Desirable? A brief overview of height-weight tables in the United States. J Am Diet Assoc 1984;84:417–423.

3. Lohman TG et al. Symposium on body composition. Med Sci Sports Exerc 1984;16:578.
4. Butler TG, Yanowitz FG. In: Yanowitz FG, ed. Coronary heart disease prevention. New York: Marcel Dekker, 1992.
5. McArdle WD, Katch FI, Katch VL. Exercise physiology: energy, nutrition, and human performance. 3rd ed. Philadelphia: Lea & Febiger, 1991.
6. Clinical pulmonary function testing. A manual of uniform laboratory procedures. 2nd ed. Salt Lake City, UT: Intermountain Thoracic Society, 1984.
7. Crapo RO. Lung volumes in healthy nonsmoking adults. Bull Eur Physiopathol Respir 1982;18:419.
8. Brozek J et al. Densitometric analysis of body composition: review of some quantitative assumptions. Ann NY Acad Sci 1963;110:113.
9. Siri WE. Body composition from fluid spaces and density: analysis of methods and techniques for measuring body composition. Washington, DC: National Academy of Sciences National Research Council, 1961.
10. Lohman TG. Body composition methodology in sports medicine. Phys Sports Med 1982;10:47.
11. Pollock ML, Wilmore JH. Exercise in health and disease. Evaluation and prescription for prevention and rehabilitation. 2nd ed. Philadelphia: WB Saunders, 1990.
12. Lukaski HC, Johnson PE, Bolonchuk WW, Lykken GI. Assessment of fat-free mass using bioelectrical impedance measurements of the human body. Am J Clin Nutr 1985;41:810.
13. Martin AD, Ross WD, Drinkwater DT, Clarys JP. Prediction of body fat by skinfold caliper: assumptions and cadaver evidence. Int J Obesity 1985;9:31.
14. Jackson AS, Pollock ML. Steps toward the development of generalized equations for prediciting body composition in adults. Can J Appl Sports Sci 1982;7:187.
15. American College of Sports Medicine. Guidelines for exercise testing and prescription. 4th ed. Philadelphia: Lea & Febiger, 1991.
16. Lukaski HC. Methods for the assessment of human body composition: the traditional and the new. Am J Clin Nutr 1987;46:537.
17. Jackson AS, Pollock ML. Practical assessment of body composition. Phys Sports Med 1985; 13:76.
18. The National Heart, Lung, and Blood Institute Growth and Health Study Research Group. Obesity and cardiovascular disease risk factors in black and white girls: The NHLBI Growth and Health Study. Am J Public Health 1992;82:1613.
19. Fardy PS, White REC, Clark LT, Hurster MM, Magel JR, Amodio G, McDermott KJ. Coronary risk factors and health behaviors in a diverse ethnic and cultural population of adolescents: a gender comparison. J Cardiopulmonary Rehabil 1994;14:52.
20. Project Staff. The National Exercise and Heart Disease Project. Manual of operations. Washington, DC: George Washington University Medical Center, 1974.
21. Bjorntorp P. Classification of obese patients and complications related to the distribution of surplus fat. Am J Clin Nutr 1987;45:1120.
22. Fardy P. Coronary artery disease risk factors (CRF) in multi-ethnic female adolescents. Program book: The National Conference on Cholesterol and High Blood Pressure Control. Washington DC: National Institutes of Health, 1991 (abstract).
23. Baumgartner RN, Chumlea WC, Roche AF. Bioelectric impedance for body composition. In: American College of Sport Medicine, ed. Exercise and Sport Science Reviews. Baltimore: Williams & Wilkins, 1990.
24. Elia M, Parkinson SA, Diaz A. Evaluation of near-infrared interactance as a method for predicting body composition. Eur J Clin Nutr 1990;44:113.
25. Israel RG, Houmard JA, O'Brien KF, McCammon MR, Zamora BS, Eaton AW. Validity of a near-infrared spectrophotometry device for estimating human body composition. Res Q Exerc Sport 1989;60:379.
26. McLean KP, Skinner JS. Validity of Futrex-5000 for body composition determination. Med Sci Sports Exerc 1992;24:253.
27. Kreamer HC, Berkowitz RI, Hammer LD. Methodological difficulties in studies of obesity. I. Measurement issues. Ann Behav Med 1990;12:112.

28. Barakat HA, Burton DS, Carpenter JW, Holbert D, Israel RG. Body fat distribution, plasma lipoproteins and the risk of coronary heart disease in male subjects. Int J Obesity 1988;12:473.

29. Bray GA, Gray DS. Obesity. II. Treatment. West J Med 1988;149:555.

30. Kirkendall WM et al. AHA committee report: recommendations of human blood pressure determination by sphygmomanometers. Circulation 1984;62:1146A.

31. Joint National Committee on Detection, Evaluation and Treatment of High Blood Pressure. The 5th report of the joint national committee on the detection, evaluation and treatment of high blood pressure (JNC-V). Arch Intern Med 1993;153:154.

32. Walther RJ, Tifft CP High blood pressure in the competitive athlete: guidelines and recommendations. Phys Sports Med 1985;13:93.

33. Berger RA. Applied exercise physiology. Philadelphia: Lea & Febiger, 1982.

34. Howley ET, Franks BD. Health fitness-instructor's handbook. 2nd ed. Champaign, IL: Human Kinetics Publishers, 1992.

35. Snow-Harter C, Marcus R. Exercise, bone mineral density, and osteoporosis. In Exercise and sports sciences reviews. Vol 19. American College of Sports Medicine. Baltimore: Williams & Wilkins, 1991.

36. Moffatt RJ, Cucuzzo N. Strength considerations for exercise prescription. In Resource manual for guidelines for exercise testing and prescription. (2nd ed). American College of Sports Medicine. Philadelphia: Lea & Febiger, 1993.

37. Astrand PO, Rhyming I. A nomogram for calculation of aerobic capacity (physical fitness) from pulse rate during submaximal work. J Appl Physiol 1954;7:218.

38. Astrand I. Aerobic work capacity in men and women with special reference to age. Acta Physiol Scand 1960;49 (Suppl 169):1.

39. Fardy PS, Webb D, Hellerstein HK. Benefits of arm exercise in cardiac rehabilitation. Phys Sports Med 1977;5:32.

40. Franklin BA, Scherf J, Pamatmat A, Rubenfire M. Arm-exercise testing and training. Practical Cardiology 1982;8:43.

41. Gardner RM, et al. ATS statement—Snowbird workshop on standardization of spirometry. Am Rev Respir Dis 1979;119:831.

42. Burke JJ, Fischer PM. A clinician's guide to the office measurement of cholesterol. JAMA 1988;259:3444.

43. Heart facts 1992. Dallas: American Heart Association, 1991.

44. Kannel WB, Castelli WP, Gordon T. Cholesterol in the prediction of atherosclerotic diseases New perspective based on the Framingham study. Ann Intern Med 1979;90:85.

45. Kannel WB, Schatzkin A. Risk factor analysis. Prog Cardiovasc Dis 1983;26:309.

46. Levy RI, Rifkind BM, Dennis BH, eds. Nutrition lipids, and coronary heart disease: a global view. New York: Raven Press, 1979.

47. Shekelle, RB, et al. Diet, serum cholesterol and death from coronary heart disease: The Western Electric study. N Engl J Med 1981;304:65.

48. The Lipid Research Clinics Coronary Primary Prevention Trial Results. I. Reduction in incidence of coronary heart disease. Lipid Research Clinic Program. JAMA 1984;251:351.

49. National Cholesterol Education Program. Report of the Expert Panel on Blood Cholesterol Levels in Children and Adolescents. Bethesda, MD: U.S. Department of Health and Human Services, Public Health Service, National Institutes of Health, National Heart, Lung, and Blood Institute. September 1991; NIH pub. no. 91-2732.

50. Brown WV, Goldberg IJ, Ginsberg HN. Treatment of common lipoprotein disorders. Prog Cardiovasc Dis 1984;27:1.

51. Expert Panel on the Detection, Evaluation and Treatment of High Blood Cholesterol in Adults. Summary of 2nd report of the National Cholesterol Education Program (NCEP) expert panel on detection, evaluation and treatment of high blood cholesterol in adults. JAMA 1993;269:3015.

52. Classification and diagnosis of diabetes mellitus and other categories of glucose intolerance. National Diabetes Data Group. Diabetes 1979;28:1039.

5

CLINICAL EXERCISE TESTING: METHODOLOGY, INTERPRETATION, AND APPLICATIONS

EXERCISE TOLERANCE TESTING has become an important assessment tool in the evaluation of individuals participating in adult fitness and cardiac rehabilitation programs (1). In addition, there are many other applications of this technique in the practice of cardiovascular and pulmonary medicine (2–4). This chapter updates and reviews clinical applications of exercise testing that are of interest to physicians and personnel working in cardiac rehabilitation centers, exercise testing laboratories, and wellness and adult fitness programs.

Table 5.1 lists the topics that are discussed in this chapter. Although exercise testing procedures vary somewhat from laboratory to laboratory, depending on needs, personnel, equipment, and particular schools of training, the underlying principles in each of the topics being considered are reasonably standardized within the exercise testing community.

157

TABLE 5.1. Exercise Testing: Indications, Methodology, and Applications

Clinical indications for exercise testing:
    Diagnostic indications
    Evaluation of cardiovascular functional capacity
    Contraindications to exercise testing
    Clinical competence in exercise testing
Exercise testing methodologies:
    Choice of exercise device
    Electrocardiographic lead systems
    Electrodes and skin preparation
    Exercise testing protocols
    Exercise test procedures
Exercise electrocardiography:
    Electrophysiology of myocardial ischemia
    ECG manifestations of myocardial ischemia
    Conduction disturbances during exercise
    Exercise test arrhythmias
Clinical judgment in exercise testing:
    Exercise test accuracy
    Applications of Bayes' theorem to exercise testing
Diagnostic exercise testing:
    Screening of asymptomatic individuals
    Differential diagnosis of chest pain
    Evaluation of syncope and palpitations
Advances in exercise ECG testing:
    The ST/HR slope method
Stress imaging: alternatives to the exercise ECG:
    Thallium perfusion imaging with exercise
    Thallium perfusion imaging with dipyridamole infusion
    Thallium perfusion imaging with adenosine infusion
    Exercise echocardiography
    Dipyridamole stress echocardiography
    Dobutamine stress echocardiography
Risk assessment in coronary heart disease:
    Risk assessment in asymptomatic populations
    Assessment of coronary disease severity
    Risk stratification after acute MI
Functional exercise testing:
    Methods for functional exercise testing
    Clinical applications—patients with disease
    Clinical applications—normal subjects

Like many other areas of scientific investigation, principles of exercise testing are continuously evolving; new ideas, concepts, equipment, protocols, and data frequently appear in the literature that challenge existing methods of practice. Many of these will ultimately be modified or rejected in favor of more traditional methods; some, however, will significantly improve certain aspects of the exercise test. Although change and new ideas are important for the growth of an investigative tool, the cost-benefit issues of each new technology should be carefully resolved before its widespread adoption. In this chapter a number of new and promising approaches to exercise testing are discussed; not all of these recent innovations, however, have proven cost-benefit advantages over more traditional methods.

CLINICAL INDICATIONS FOR EXERCISE TESTING

Many questions regarding the presence or absence of cardiovascular abnormalities can be resolved without exercise testing, using information gleaned from the medical history, physical examination, chest x-ray, and resting electrocardiogram (ECG) (see Chapter 3). The appropriate use of exercise testing therefore requires a careful consideration of the clinical situations where such testing is likely to contribute to patient management in a cost-effective manner. In this section the guidelines for exercise testing are reviewed.

To better define the role of various noninvasive and invasive procedures in the diagnosis and management of patients with known or suspected cardiovascular disease, a joint Task Force of the American College of Cardiology (ACC) and the American Heart Association (AHA) was formed in 1980. The Subcommittee on Exercise Testing published their recommendations in 1986 (5), and these are summarized in Table 5.2. As seen in the table, the "Guidelines" are partitioned into three categories: *Class I*, situations where there is a general consensus that exercise testing is justified; *Class II*, situations where exercise testing is frequently performed but there is some controversy regarding usefulness; and *Class III*, situations where there is general agreement that testing is not justified. In the discussion to follow it is important to keep these three categorical situations in mind.

There are essentially three broad indications for exercise testing: (a) *diagnosis*, (b) *function*, and (c) *prognosis* (Fig. 5.1). Diagnostic testing is performed to resolve questions regarding the presence or absence of myocardial ischemia, which is usually secondary to coronary atherosclerosis. Functional testing, on the other hand, is used to evaluate physical working capacity and often answers questions that are independent of the presence or absence of heart disease. In most clinical situations both diagnostic and functional information contribute to the overall prognostic assessment of the patient and, in addition, permit appropriate therapeutic decisions to be made.

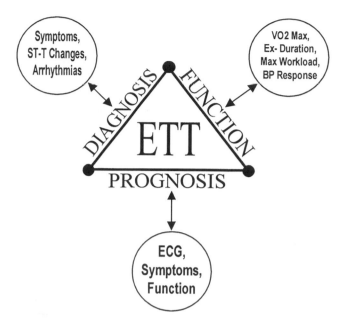

FIGURE 5.1. Three indications for exercise tolerance testing (ETT).

Diagnostic Indications for Exercise Testing

The detection of myocardial ischemia in the adult population is a major challenge to the medical profession, since coronary heart disease (CHD) continues to be the leading cause of death and disability in Western industrialized nations (6). Statistics from the Framingham Heart Study (7) indicate that myocardial infarction (MI) and sudden cardiac death are often the first clinical manifestations of CHD, striking catastrophically in individuals previously asymptomatic of their disease. The task of diagnostic exercise testing therefore is to detect evidence of myocardial ischemia earlier in the natural history of coronary atherosclerosis before these serious complications of advanced disease occur. Unfortunately, as will be discussed, the exercise test is by no means free of diagnostic errors and is only of practical value in certain subsets of the population (Table 5.2).

There is a wide range of opinion regarding diagnostic testing of asymptomatic individuals. With the recent increased public interest in wellness and adult fitness there may be a tendency to overuse the physician-supervised, maximal exercise test in screening asymptomatic men and women for early CHD. In fact, there are no class I indications recommended by the ACC/AHA Task Force "guidelines" in this asymptomatic group (Table 5.2). Nevertheless, it is clear that there is a population of high-risk, asymptomatic men over the age of 40 with two or more coronary risk factors who are at increased risk of

TABLE 5.2. American College of Cardiology/American Heart Association Guidelines for Exercise Testing[a]

Class I:	General agreement that exercise testing is justified.
Class II:	Frequently performed, but varying opinions as to value.
Class III:	General agreement that exercise testing is not justified.

Screening of apparently healthy individuals

Class I: None

Class II: 1. To evaluate asymptomatic males over age 40 in high-risk occupations.
2. To evaluate asymptomatic males over age 40 with ≥2 risk factors (serum cholesterol >240 mg/dl, BP≥160/ ≥90, cigarette smoking, diabetes mellitus, or family history of CHD under age of 55).
3. To evaluate men over age 40 who are sedentary and plan to enter a vigorous exercise program.

Class III: 1. To evaluate asymptomatic, apparently healthy men or women with no CHD risk factors.
2. To evaluate men or women with noncardiac chest discomfort.

Testing in patients with symptoms or signs of CHD or with known CHD

Class I: 1. To diagnose men with atypical symptoms of myocardial ischemia.
2. To assess functional capacity and prognosis in patients with CHD.
3. To evaluate patients with symptoms suggestive of exercise-induced cardiac arrhythmias.

Class II: 1. To diagnose women with typical or atypical anginal symptoms.
2. To diagnose patients taking digitalis or with right bundle branch block.
3. To evaluate function and response to therapy with drugs in patients with CHD or heart failure.
4. To evaluate patients with variant angina.
5. To follow serially (at ≥1-year intervals) patients with CHD.

Class III: 1. To evaluate patients with simple PVCs without CHD evidence.
2. To follow function in cardiac rehabilitation.
3. To diagnose CHD in patients with Wolff-Parkinson-White syndrome or with left bundle branch block.

161

TABLE 5.2. Cont.

Testing soon after myocardial infarction

Class I: 1. To evaluate prognosis and functional capacity in uncomplicated MI.

Class II: 1. To evaluate post-MI patients with baseline ECG changes or co-existing medical problems that might alter the test response.

2. To evaluate complicated post-MI patients.

Class III: 1. To evaluate patients with acute ischemic syndromes.

2. To evaluate post-MI patients with unstable rhythm, conduction, or heart failure conditions.

Use after specific procedures

Class I: 1. To evaluate patients after coronary bypass or angioplasty procedures.

Class II: 1. To evaluate asymptomatic patients yearly after revascularization.

Testing in patients with valvular heart disease

Class I: None

Class II: 1. To evaluate functional capacity in patients with valvular heart disease.

Class III: 1. To evaluate patients with symptomatic aortic stenosis or obstructive cardiomyopathy.

Testing in patients with hypertension or cardiac pacemakers

Class I: None

Class II: 1. To evaluate BP response in patients being treated for hypertension who wish to engage in static or dynamic exercise training.

Class III: 1. To evaluate patients with severe, uncontrolled hypertension.

2. To evaluate BP response to exercise in patients with hypertension who are not engaging in vigorous exercise activities.

3. To evaluate pacemaker function in patients with cardiac pacemakers.

Testing in children

Class I: 1. To evaluate functional capacity in selected patients with congenital heart disease.

Class II: 1. To evaluate functional capacity in patients with valvular heart disease.

[a] From Subcommittee on Exercise Testing. J Am Coll Cardiol 1986; 8:725–738.

developing symptomatic CHD and meet class II guidelines for exercise testing. Exercise testing is also frequently performed in asymptomatic men over age 40 who are sedentary and plan to initiate a *vigorous* exercise program (1). As seen in Table 5.2, however, diagnostic exercise testing is generally *not* recommended in asymptomatic, apparently healthy women of any age because of the high false-positive rate in this population.

Symptoms of chest discomfort are among the most frequent reasons adults seek medical attention. As discussed in Chapter 3, the physician can often determine whether the symptoms represent angina pectoris from the patient's description of chest discomfort. Chest pain descriptors such as quality of discomfort, location, duration, predictability, and precipitating and relieving factors will usually enable the symptoms to be classified as *typical angina pectoris* or *nonanginal chest pain*. At times, however, the symptoms will be only suggestive . of ischemic heart disease, and exercise testing can help in the differential diagnosis. The ACC/AHA guidelines (Table 5.2) recommend exercise testing to evaluate men with atypical symptoms (class I), but there is a difference of opinion as to the efficacy of the exercise test in diagnosing women with chest pain (class II).

Exercise testing is frequently used to make prognostic and therapeutic decisions in post-MI patients either just prior to hospital discharge or shortly thereafter. The identification of ischemic ECG abnormalities is usually indicative of multivessel coronary artery disease and suggests an increased risk for reinfarction and mortality in the first year following acute MI (8). The absence of such abnormalities, however, coupled with a reasonable exercise tolerance and blood pressure response, identifies a very low risk subgroup of patients who are able to return to productive lifestyles soon after discharge (9, 10). Similar indications for exercise testing apply to evaluating patients following coronary artery bypass graft (CABG) and percutaneous transluminal coronary angioplasty (PTCA).

In addition to detecting myocardial ischemia, exercise testing is also used to evaluate the cause or mechanisms of sudden loss of consciousness (syncope) and palpitations, especially when these symptoms occur during exertional activities. Exercise testing is often used in conjunction with ambulatory ECG monitoring in the workup of these patients for arrhythmias and conduction abnormalities (11).

Evaluation of Cardiovascular Functional Capacity

The second major indication for exercise testing is assessing cardiorespiratory function capacity in various clinical situations (Table 5.3). Questions regarding the need for further diagnostic studies, therapeutic decisions, and prognosis can often be resolved by knowing the functional capacity of the patient. For many patients with heart disease, knowledge of an adequate functional cardiac status is an important factor in their psychologic well-being and productivity.

TABLE 5.3. Indications for Functional Exercise Testing

I. Assessment of patients with cardiovascular diseases
   A. Evaluation of physical working capacity for occupational or leisure activities
      1. Stable angina pectoris
      2. After myocardial infarction
      3. After cardiac surgery
      4. After coronary angioplasty
   B. Prognostic stratification of CHD patients into high- and low-risk subgroups
   C. Therapeutic considerations:
      1. Evaluating the need for surgery
      2. Selection of optimal therapy
      3. Assessing therapeutic response
   D. Exercise prescription for cardiac rehabilitation program

II. Differential diagnosis of dyspnea: respiratory vs. cardiac vs. deconditioning

III. Assessment of patients with known or suspected disabilities

IV. Assessment of athletic performance

In coronary disease functional exercise testing often provides information needed for optimal management (Table 5.3). Data derived from functional testing are used to determine the type of physical activities that can be safely performed during work and recreation. In general, patients feel reassured knowing their particular exercise limitations (12).

Identification of high-risk subsets of coronary patients is frequently emphasized in the literature, since many new interventional therapies are now available that promise to improve long-term outlook. In fact, the management of high-risk patients has so preoccupied the medical community that insufficient attention has been given to the recognition of low-risk patients, who probably represent the majority of the CHD population. Changing economic forces in medicine will likely result in more emphasis on low-risk patients, since these patients can be encouraged to lead productive lifestyles without the need for costly diagnostic and treatment procedures. Of all the uses of exercise testing discussed in this chapter, the identification of low-risk coronary patients is likely to be the most cost-effective.

The decision to treat or not to treat and the choice of therapy are frequently determined by the patient's functional capacity and exertional symptoms.

Coronary patients with good functional capacity and minimal symptoms during exercise are usually not candidates for interventional therapy. The multiplicity of drugs available today for the treatment of angina, arrhythmias, and heart failure requires careful assessment of the functional consequences of various therapies to optimize dosages and types of drugs needed to manage particular problems.

Exercise testing prior to phase II cardiac rehabilitation is, of course, an important prerequisite for the successful implementation of an exercise prescription. The design of an exercise program and the rate of progression during the program will depend, in part, on the exercise test results (1). Exercise testing, however, is not recommended to follow patients serially in rehabilitation because of the high costs associated with these tests (Table 5.2) (5).

There are many other indications for functional exercise testing in evaluating patients with other cardiovascular and pulmonary diseases. Decisions regarding the need for cardiac catheterization, the choice and assessment of various drug therapies, and the optimal timing for operative interventions can all be enhanced by evaluation of a patient's exercise tolerance. Exercise testing is also used in the assessment of disability claims involving a variety of conditions associated with work intolerance. The test provides an objective evaluation of cardiorespiratory functional capacity, which helps in determining the extent to which an individual is able to perform physically demanding tasks. Furthermore, the extent of impairment of the cardiovascular, respiratory, and musculoskeletal systems can often be determined and recommendations given for appropriate rehabilitation.

Contraindications to Exercise Testing

Although there are many indications for exercise testing in clinical practice, the test is not without potential risk or discomfort to the patient. Each patient therefore should be assessed prior to testing to determine if the benefits of testing clearly outweigh the possible risks and if the test results will contribute to patient management. Most of the contraindications listed in Table 5.4 are relative, since there may be occasions when low-level exercise testing is conducted under careful supervision to answer specific questions needed for optimal management. Many of the noncardiac contraindications listed in Table 5.4 can be resolved prior to testing; testing may not even be appropriate under some of these circumstances. Common sense is usually sufficient to resolve most of these issues.

Clinical Competence in Exercise Testing

An important aspect of assessing the quality of a physician's practice in a hospital is the granting of clinical staff privileges based on presumed competencies. The evaluation of clinical competencies is usually accomplished by peer review

TABLE 5.4. Contraindications to Exercise Testing

Unstable or severe cardiovascular disorders

1. Recent acute myocardial infarction
2. Unstable angina pectoris
3. Uncontrolled cardiac arrhythmias
4. Severe congestive heart failure
5. Severe aortic stenosis
6. Active myocarditis, pericarditis, or endocarditis
7. Dissecting aortic aneurysm
8. Recent pulmonary or systemic emboli
9. Resting blood pressure $\geq 200/\geq 120$ mm Hg
10. Acute thrombophlebitis

Noncardiovascular conditions

1. Active infections
2. Severe emotional distress
3. Uncontrolled metabolic disease such as thyrotoxicosis, myxedema, or diabetes mellitus
4. Neuromuscular, musculoskeletal, and arthritic conditions that preclude exercise
5. Other systemic illnesses that would make exercise difficult

of the physician's knowledge and skills in performing particular procedures. In exercise testing, a joint task force of the American Heart Association, the American College of Physicians, and the American College of Cardiology has developed guidelines to assist in evaluating competencies (14). The task force felt that a minimum of 50 exercise procedures supervised by a physician qualified in exercise testing be required. This experience could be obtained during residency or fellowship training. Alternatively, physicians already out of their training programs could qualify for competencies in exercise testing by being supervised while performing tests or by having more than three years of experience doing exercise tests. The cognitive skills needed to perform exercise testing that were developed by the task force are listed in Table 5.5. The task force report emphasized that just attending a short course or workshop in exercise testing with limited hands-on experience is clearly insufficient to result in competence.

EXERCISE TEST METHODOLOGIES

In this section the methodologic aspects of exercise testing are discussed. It is important to emphasize that procedures vary from laboratory to laboratory

TABLE 5.5. Competencies for Performing Exercise Testing Procedures[a]

Knowledge of indications, contraindications, and risks for exercise testing

Knowledge to recognize and treat complications of exercise testing

Competence in basic and advanced cardiac life support (AHA guidelines)

Knowledge of specificity, sensitivity, and predictive accuracy of exercise
testing in different patient populations (i.e., applications of Bayes' theorem)

Knowledge of various exercise testing protocols and their indications

Knowledge of basic cardiovascular and exercise physiology

Knowledge of resting and exercise electrocardiography

Knowledge of cardiac arrhythmias and treatment of serious arrhythmias

Knowledge of cardiovascular drugs and their effects on exercise testing

Knowledge of false-positive and false-negative errors in exercise testing

Knowledge of age and disease effects on the hemodynamic and ECG response
to exercise testing

Knowledge of exercise testing methodology, including lead placement and skin
preparation

Knowledge of the prognostic value of exercise testing

Knowledge of alternative procedures to exercise testing

Knowledge of exercise test end points and indications for terminating exercise

Knowledge of metabolic equivalents (METs) and estimations of exercise
intensity in different modes of exercise

Ability to communicate exercise test results and other relevant information to
the patient, the medical record, and other physicians

Understanding of the principles of informed consent

[a] From Schlant R et al. J Am Coll Cardiol 1990;16:1061–1065.

without necessarily affecting the quality of the testing. Every attempt is made in this review to conform to standards developed by the AHA (13) and the American College of Sports Medicine (ACSM) (1).

Choice of Exercise Device

The stationary bicycle ergometer and the motor-driven treadmill are the two most common modalities for clinical exercise testing. Each has advantages and disadvantages, and many laboratories have the flexibility of using either device, depending on the particular needs of the patient. In North America the treadmill is more popular because this exercise device has more appeal to physicians and the public. Treadmill protocols are more flexible than bicycle protocols, since speed and grade can be varied independently to increase the workload. Unlike the bicycle, the treadmill is not patient dependent, and therefore it is more reproducible. In addition, workloads are more accurately measured on the treadmill than on the bicycle, where pedaling frequency is an important determinant of the total work.

The bicycle, on the other hand, is less expensive, requires less space, and is more portable, less likely to break down, and less noisy. At high workloads it is easier to obtain good ECG data free of motion artifact. Blood pressures are also more easily measured on the bicycle because upper body motion is reduced. Some patients such as the very obese may be less anxious on the bicycle because they are more in control of their exercise efforts and can stop at any time. For individuals who have difficulty walking because of age, debilitating illnesses, or orthopedic problems, the bicycle may be the only method of assessing exercise tolerance. Arm crank ergometry may also be carried out with these devices to assess the cardiovascular effects of upper extremity exercise (15). This may be particularly useful in coronary disease patients who do physically demanding upper extremity work or have lower extremity limitations.

The bicycle ergometer may be positioned for supine leg exercise during cardiac catheterization or noninvasive imaging studies using ultrasound or nuclear techniques. Important differences exist, however, between the body's response to exercise in the supine and upright positions (13). In patients with heart disease left ventricular filling pressures and volumes often increase abnormally during supine exercise because of the increased venous return from the lower extremities. Heart rates are higher and maximal workloads lower in the supine position; angina and ST-segment depression also occur at lower double products.

Regardless of which exercise device is used for testing, it is important to understand the methods for calibrating the workloads. The treadmill varies its workload by changing speed (mph) and elevation (percent grade). The accuracy of the speedometer is checked by placing a visible marker on the treadmill belt and counting the number of belt revolutions in one minute. The belt speed is calculated using the following formula:

$$S = C \times R/1056$$

where S is speed in mph, C is the belt circumference measured in inches, and R is the number of belt revolutions in one minute. If the calculated speed is not the same as that indicated by the speed meter, the meter should be adjusted as described in the "owner's manual" for that particular treadmill.

The percent grade of the treadmill is calculated by measuring the vertical heights from the floor to the treadmill belt at two different points. If the horizontal difference between the two points on the floor is x, and the difference in vertical heights at the two points is y, then the percent grade is $y/x(100)$. If the elevation meter is different from the calculated grade, the meter should be adjusted appropriately.

Calibrating the bicycle ergometer is more complicated and depends on whether the ergometer is mechanically braked or electrically braked. Methods for calibration have been described in the literature (16), as well as in the manuals for each type of ergometer.

Electrocardiographic Lead Systems

The ideal ECG lead system for exercise electrocardiography has yet to be defined. Most agree, however, that multiple leads are preferable to single leads in the detection of myocardial ischemia. By far the most popular of the lead systems is the modified 12-lead system first described by Mason and Likar in 1966 (17) and illustrated in Figure 5.2. Although originally the arm electrodes were placed below the clavicles just medial to the deltoid muscles, it has been shown that this lead placement results in a significant rightward shift in QRS axis; this can mask ECG evidence for old inferior wall myocardial infarction and mimic

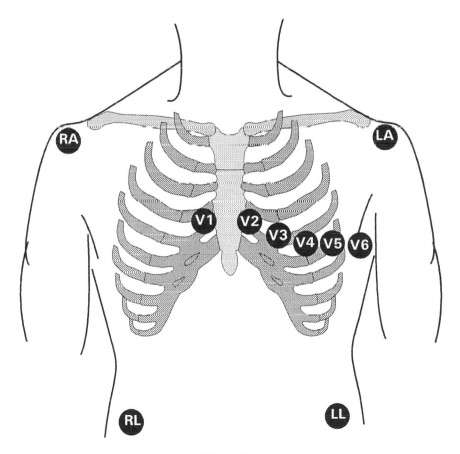

FIGURE 5.2. The Mason-Likar modified 12–lead system for exercise testing. (From Mason RE, Likar I. Am Heart J 1966;71:196–204.)

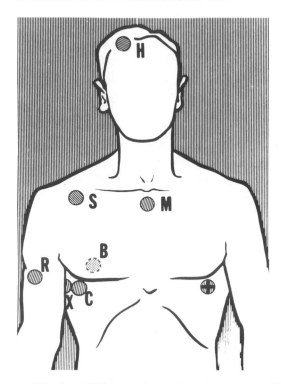

FIGURE 5.3. Bipolar lead sites for exercise testing. The positive pole for each of the bipolar leads is located in the standard V_5 chest position. (From Froelicher VF et al. Chest 1976;70:611.)

lateral infarction by causing false Q waves to appear in lead aVL (18). These changes can be minimized by moving the arm electrodes to the base of the shoulders against the deltoid border 2 cm below the clavicles. The leg electrodes should be placed below the umbilicus near the iliac crests; the six chest electrodes are in their usual positions as for the standard 12-lead ECG (see Chapter 3).

Bipolar ECG leads have the advantages of being simpler, requiring less time to set up, and they are less costly and less noisy in terms of motion artifact. Several commonly used bipolar lead sites are illustrated in Figure 5.3. Most of the leads use the V_5 chest position for the positive pole and somewhat resemble standard lead V_5, but with larger QRS voltages. It has been suggested that these leads are more sensitive to ischemic ST-segment changes than standard leads. The bipolar lead CM5, with the negative electrode placed on the manubrium (M), is frequently added to the standard 12-lead system in calculating the ST-segment/heart rate (ST/HR) slope, a more quantitative descriptor of ischemia than ST-segment depression (19).

Electrodes and Skin Preparation

The ECG detection of myocardial ischemia during progressive exercise becomes more difficult with increasing heart rates. Unless special attention is given to electrodes and skin preparation, the deteriorating signal:noise ratio with increasing exercise will preclude obtaining adequate ECG data for interpretation. Motion artifact accounts for most of the electrical noise that is superimposed on the ECG signal during exercise. Although considerable bioengineering efforts have been implemented to reduce unwanted artifact using expensive computer-processing techniques, the simplest and most effective method is still careful skin preparation prior to testing.

The patient should be supine while electrodes are being placed to ensure accurate location of the electrode sites. Male patients will often need to be shaved around the chest electrode sites before skin preparation. The patient should be informed of this prior to shaving to avoid unnecessary distress. It should also be explained that there will likely be some minimal chest wall irritation for several weeks following the test as the hair regrows. The actual electrode sites will depend on the particular lead system. Sites over large muscles should be avoided to minimize artifact caused by myoelectric potentials. In some older patients with loose or sagging skin electrode sites will have to be adjusted when assuming the upright position. In heavy breasted women the chest electrodes should be positioned as accurately as possible under the breast in the correct interspace.

Tam and Webster (20) have studied the possible causes of motion artifact by measuring potential drops at the electrode-paste interface and the skin-paste interface, concluding that the latter was the major source of artifact. They also showed how skin abrasion to remove the superficial horny layer of epidermis (stratum corneum) could significantly lower the electrical impedance across the skin/paste interface and improve the signal:noise ratio. Skin abrasion can best be accomplished using an abrading paste rubbed over the electrode sites; alternatively, one can also use fine-grain sandpaper. Special care is needed to avoid abrading into the superficial capillaries immediately below the stratum corneum. It is usually a good idea to clean the sites with alcohol or acetone prior to electrode application.

Many excellent exercise test electrodes are now available that are specially designed to minimize motion artifact. Most of these electrodes incorporate a recessed silver-silver chloride disk adjacent to a sponge soaked with electrolyte solution, which forms a low-resistance interface between electrode disk and skin. An adhesive pad surrounds the disk and holds it to the skin. In some individuals who sweat excessively during exercise, the adhesive does not hold, and it may be necessary to wrap the electrodes to the chest and abdomen with an Ace bandage or to use an elastic vest. It is generally not necessary to check the impedance across each electrode-skin interface with an ohmmeter to verify that the impedance is less than 5000 ohms. Tapping each electrode while observing the oscilloscopic ECG signal for noise will usually identify bad electrodes needing replacement. This is most often caused by drying out of the electrolyte sponge in the electrode. Finally, it is important to make sure that the electrode wires are not pulling on the electrodes when the patient is sitting or standing, since deformation of the skin can cause spurious shifts in ECG baseline.

Exercise Testing Protocols

Most clinical indications for exercise testing require an incremental protocol beginning at a low workload and progressing to higher workloads until either a

171

predetermined end point is reached (target heart rate or workload) or until signs or symptoms develop that preclude further exercise. If the limiting symptoms are reflective of the person's functional capacity, the test is called *maximal*. Steady state or constant workload protocols are sometimes used in the evaluation of suspected pulmonary disorders, but they are not commonly used in clinical cardiology testing.

In clinical practice the progressive workload protocols are usually continuous with the workload increasing in a series of stages without intermittent rest periods. Although intermittent protocols are sometimes used in research studies because they enable subjects to achieve higher maximal workloads, they are not practical for routine testing because of the long time required to complete the protocol.

It is important for exercise test personnel to have a working knowledge of different protocols to have the flexibility to accommodate different patient populations. In any particular patient, a protocol should be chosen that best answers the clinical questions being asked with minimal risk to the patient. Serial testing in a given patient should usually follow the same protocol to enable comparisons to be made over time. This is especially important when assessing the threshold for myocardial ischemia, since ischemic thresholds have been shown to be protocol dependent, as well as dependent on the extent and severity of the coronary artery disease (21). For maximal testing, standardized protocols are preferred, since comparisons can be made between patients, and normal reference values for different age groups have been published in the literature (2).

Protocols for Upright Bicycle Testing

Before beginning exercise the seat height and handle bar should be adjusted for patient comfort and efficiency of pedaling. The seat height should be set so that there is only minimal (5 degree) flexion at the knee when the foot is at its lowest position on the pedal. Pedaling frequency should be 50 to 60 rpm to achieve valid workloads; this can be monitored with a metronome or an rpm meter.

The optimal bicycle protocol is one that matches the duration of exercise to the subject's functional capacity. Buchfuhrer et al. (22) have shown that treadmill or bicycle exercise tests of short duration (<8 min) with large incremental steps or of long duration (>18 min) with small incremental steps are associated with lower measures of functional capacity ($\dot{V}O_{2max}$) than tests of 8 to 17 minutes' duration. They recommend that the work rate increment be selected to bring the subject to maximal effort in 10 ± 2 minutes. This implies that subjects be assessed prior to testing to estimate their functional ability to exercise to determine their optimal, incremental work rate. Each person should be questioned about habitual physical activity and classified as active or inactive based on the amount of recreational or occupational physical activities performed on a weekly basis. Body weight should also be taken into consideration, since larger individuals may have a performance advantage on the bicycle because of large leg muscles.

Exercise should begin with the person pedaling against minimal resistance for several minutes as a warm-up. Thereafter the work rate can be increased in increments of 15 watts (90 kpm/min) to 25 watts (150 kpm/min) every 1 to 2 minutes, depending on the subject's heart rate response, aiming for a test duration of 10 ± 2 min. Extremely sedentary subjects or individuals with cardio-pulmonary disorders may require even smaller increments.

Protocols for Treadmill Testing

A number of continuous incremental treadmill protocols have achieved popularity in the United States and elsewhere. Many of these have been evaluated and compared in the literature, with data published relating work rate and time to the subject's maximal oxygen uptake (23–28). Protocols vary in terms of percent grade, speed, duration of stages, and size of increments between stages. Several commonly used protocols are outlined in Table 5.6.

The standard Bruce protocol is probably the best known of treadmill protocols, resulting in large part from the many important contributions to exercise testing made by Dr. Robert Bruce at the University of Washington (23). In this protocol both speed and grade are increased every 3 minutes in rather large increments. Because the initial work rate may be too strenuous for many individuals, many exercise laboratories use a modified Bruce protocol that adds several easier levels of exercise to the protocol (i.e., stage 0 and stage 1/2). The primary advantage of the standard Bruce protocol is the relatively short duration needed for most subjects to reach maximal effort, although for some this may be a disadvantage, because the large increments may be too great to accurately assess functional capacity. In addition, subjects who exercise beyond stage III may have to run to keep up, making "clean" ECG recordings and blood pressure measurements more difficult to achieve.

Another modification of the Bruce protocol, the Cornell protocol, was developed by Okin et al. (28) for use in the computerized ST/HR slope determination, an improved method for quantitative exercise electrocardiography. In this protocol each of the standard Bruce stages is divided into two stages of smaller increments and two-minute durations to enable the computer to sample more data points and make a more accurate assessment of the ST/HR slope. Several of the commercially available treadmill exercise testing vendors provide this protocol with their computerized analyses programs. The diagnostic advantage of this computerized approach to exercise ECG data will be discussed in a later section.

The modified Naughton protocol was developed to assess the cardiovascular status of post-MI patients before hospital discharge or shortly after discharge

173

Table 5.6. Treadmill Exercise Protocols in Clinical Practice

Protocol	Stage	Grade (%)	Speed (mph)	Total Time (min)	O₂ Uptake (ml/kg/min)	METs[a]
Bruce (23)	(1/2)	5	1.5	3	11	3
	I	10	1.7	6	17	4
	II	12	2.5	9	25	7
	III	14	3.4	12	35	10
	IV	16	4.2	15	47	13
	V	18	5.0	18	56	16
Cornell (28)	1	0	1.7	2	7	2
	2	5	1.7	4	11	3
	3	10	1.7	6	17	4
	4	11	2.1	8	19	5.5
	5	12	2.5	10	25	7
	6	13	3.0	12	30	8.5
	7	14	3.4	14	35	10
	8	15	3.8	16	40	11.5
	9	16	4.2	18	47	13
Naughton (27)	1	0	2.0	2	7	2
	2	3.5	2.0	4	10.5	3
	3	7.0	2.0	6	14	4
	4	10.5	2.0	8	17.5	5
	5	14.0	2.0	10	21.0	6
	6	17.5	2.0	12	24.5	7
	7	12.5	3.0	14	28	8
	8	15.0	3.0	16	31.5	9
Balke[b] (24)	1	0	3.3	1	14	4
	3	3	3.3	3	17	5
	6	6	3.3	6	21	6
	9	9	3.3	9	26	7
	12	12	3.3	12	31	9
	15	15	3.3	15	36	10
	18	18	3.3	18	41	12
USAFSAM (25)	I	0	3.3	3	14	4
	II	5	3.3	6	21	6
	III	10	3.3	9	28	8
	IV	15	3.3	12	36	10
	V	20	3.3	15	46	13
	VI	25	3.3	18	52	15

[a] Metabolic equivalents.
[b] Not all stages listed.

(27). This protocol has been used extensively in recent years to classify patients into high-risk and low-risk categories (risk stratification) that have important prognostic and therapeutic implications. The protocol is also used in the functional assessment of patients with chronic congestive heart failure who are being managed medically or are under consideration for cardiac transplantation (3). The work rate increments are small, increasing each stage by 1 metabolic equivalent (1 MET = resting oxygen requirements ~3.5 ml O_2/kg/min).

The Balke protocol was originally developed to assess physical fitness in reasonably healthy military personnel and not for cardiovascular screening (24). In this protocol the speed remains constant at 3.3 mph with 1% increases in grade every minute. The major disadvantage in healthy subjects is the long duration of exercise required to achieve maximal effort. In older or more diseased individuals the 3.3-mph speed may be too fast. There have been a number of modifications of this protocol to improve its applicability to clinical testing. Speeds of 2.0 mph and 3.0 mph are often substituted for the original speed. Another practical modification of the Balke Protocol was designed by the U.S. Air Force School of Aerospace Medicine (USAFSAM) for screening the apparently healthy Air Force population. Like the Balke protocol, subjects walk at a constant speed of 3.3 mph, but with 5%-grade increments every 3 minutes. Oxygen uptakes, blood pressures, and heart rates are comparable for the two protocols (25).

Exercise Test Procedures

The preparation of a patient for exercise testing begins with an explanation of the purpose for the test and the various procedures that will be carried out during the test. Every effort should be made to familiarize the patient with the test procedures and relieve any anxieties or concerns. The specific instructions prior to testing will vary from one laboratory to another. When scheduling tests, patients should be advised not to eat, smoke, or consume alcoholic drinks for several hours prior to testing. They should be told to bring or wear comfortable clothes and walking shoes to the testing facility. Women should wear a loose-fitting blouse that buttons in front, along with shorts or slacks. A snug-fitting bra is recommended to secure the breasts and minimize electrical interference while exercising. The laboratory should also have hospital gowns available for patients who dress inappropriately for exercise.

Informed consent implies that the patient is aware of the potential benefits and occasional risks of the test and agrees to be tested. Most often this is accomplished by having the patient read and sign a consent form after all questions have been answered to the patient's satisfaction. Sample consent forms have been published by the AHA (29) and the ACSM (1). Each exercise testing laboratory should design a consent form that is compatible with state and local laws governing consent, as well as the hospital or other institutional review board

---

THE FITNESS INSTITUTE'S EXERCISE TEST CONSENT FORM

NAME: _____DATE: _____

AGE: _____SEX: _____PHYSICIAN: _____

INFORMED CONSENT: In order to evaluate the functional performance and capacity of the heart, lungs, and blood vessels, each individual consents, voluntarily, to perform an exercise test. Before being tested, she/he is questioned and examined by a physician, and has an electrocardiogram recorded (to show whether or not testing should proceed), after which he/she walks on a treadmill, with speed and incline increased every three minutes, until the limits of fatigue, breathlessness, chest pain, and/or other symptoms are of such severity that he/she should stop the effort. Blood pressure and electrocardiogram are monitored while he/she is exercising. In some instances expired air will be collected and oxygen uptake determined.

RISKS of testing including occasional changes in the rhythm of the heart beats and the possibility of excessive changes in blood pressure. There is a remote chance of fainting and even a more remote chance of a heart attack. Professional supervision protects against injury, by providing appropriate precautionary measures, and in the unlikely event that these precautions are insufficient, emergency hospital treatment is available.

BENEFITS of testing include quantitative assessment of working capacity and critical appraisal of the disorders or diseases that impair capacity, the knowledge of which facilitates better treatment and more accurate prognosis for future cardiac events.

Both the right to withdraw from the test at any time with impunity and the right to withhold confidential information from nonmedical persons (such as employers and insurance agents) without consent are assured. The welfare of each person will be protected.

In addition to participating in this exercise test, each person permits his/her name to be registered for future follow-up studies.

CONSENT:

Having read the information statement above and had the opportunity to ask questions, I hereby willingly consent to be tested.

DATE: _____SIGNED: _____

TIME: _____WITNESS: _____

FIGURE 5.4. Consent form for exercise testing.

(Fig. 5.4). It is unlikely, however, that signed consent will offer any legal protection to a laboratory if an exercise complication is the result of negligence or improper procedures.

Patient Interview and Examination

If the patient is being tested for a known or suspected cardiovascular problem, a brief examination by a physician or physician assistant is necessary to rule out any contraindications to testing (Table 5.4) and to gather information that will facilitate interpreting the test results. In some laboratories a preliminary history and review of cardiovascular risk factors is obtained by the exercise test technologist as the patient is being prepared for the test. Alternatively, a self-administered questionnaire may be completed by the patient prior to testing. If the patient has a history of chest discomfort, the symptoms should be reviewed and classified as typical angina pectoris, atypical angina, or nonanginal chest pain (see Chapter 3).

A brief cardiovascular examination should be performed with special attention given to detecting heart murmurs and gallops. Severe aortic stenosis, for example, is a contraindication to maximal exercise testing. This is recognized as a harsh, systolic ejection murmur at the base with delayed upstroke of the carotid artery pulse and diminished pulse volume. Findings of mitral valve prolapse, including a midsystolic click and late systolic murmur, are also important to recognize, since this common condition may be associated with resting ST-T-wave abnormalities and false-positive exercise ECG results.

ECG Data Collection

The resting 12-lead ECG should be reviewed by the supervising physician or physician assistant prior to testing. Although uncommon, ECG findings of acute MI have been observed in patients referred for chest pain evaluation (see Chapter 3). These patients need intensive coronary care, not exercise testing. In addition, diagnostic ECG stress testing cannot be performed if left bundle branch block or other ECG abnormalities with marked ST-T-wave changes are present. These patients might be better evaluated using stress radionuclide or echocardiographic imaging techniques.

The resting ECG should be obtained in the supine and standing positions. Some laboratories routinely hyperventilate all patients for 30 seconds to look for ST-T-wave changes that mimic ischemia. However, if there are no labile, positional ST-T-wave changes that occur with standing, it is unlikely that hyperventilation will cause significant changes.

Blood Pressure Measurements

Blood pressures should be obtained at rest in the supine (or sitting) and standing positions and during the last minute of each exercise stage. Some practice is necessary to accurately measure exercise blood pressures, especially during treadmill testing where ambient noise and patient movement often interfere with the measurements. For ease of measurement the arm should be straightened and the hand placed on the shoulder or in the axilla of the person taking the blood pressure. Automated blood pressure recording devices have been designed for exercise testing and may offer significant advantages over manually obtained measurements. One such device, using a microphone pickup of Korotkoff's sounds and ECG-assisted microprocessing of unwanted noise, has been favorably evaluated in the literature (30). Disadvantages of these devices are that they are expensive, take longer to measure the blood pressure (30–45 sec), and may be uncomfortable for the patient because of the slow deflation time.

Observations During Exercise

During exercise the patient should be carefully observed and periodic assessments made of symptoms, ECG data, blood pressure, and any untoward physical signs. Continuous observation of ECG rhythm and waveform on the oscilloscope is essential. Most commercial exercise ECG monitors have delay memory capabilities that permit playback of arrhythmic events noted on the oscilloscope. The 12-lead ECG should be obtained for waveform analysis at the end of each stage and at peak exercise.

Chest pain during exercise is an important observation, especially if the patient is being evaluated for suspected or known coronary artery disease. Careful observation of the patient's facial expression and color, the ECG, and the blood pressure will usually enable the symptoms to be classified as anginal or nonanginal chest pain. It may not be necessary to stop the test at the onset of chest pain if the intensity of pain is mild, if the patient's blood pressure is stable or rising, and if the ECG does not yet show significant ST-T-wave abnormalities. Indications for terminating the test include (a) increased pain intensity, (b) fall in systolic blood pressure, (c) marked ST-segment depression or elevation, and (d) increasing ventricular ectopic activity.

Exercise Test End Points

The decision to stop an exercise test is sometimes determined by the patient (limiting symptoms), sometimes by the physician (abnormal findings), and sometimes by the protocol (submaximal end points). A list of these various end points is given in Table 5.7.

The patient's request to stop should always be a serious consideration for terminating the test. At times, however, when the patient seems poorly motivated and is clearly in no distress, the supervising physician may encourage the patient to continue exercising until more limiting signs or symptoms are noted. In general, a diagnostic test that fails to achieve 85 to 90% of the patient's predicted maximal heart rate (i.e., 220 − age) without chest pain or ischemic ECG findings is considered inadequate to rule out ischemic heart disease. For this reason it is sometimes important to urge the patient to continue exercising until a more appropriate heart rate response is achieved (assuming the patient is not taking heart-rate slowing drugs). Patients who are not accustomed to exercise may misinterpret their symptoms as limiting when, in fact, they are clearly submaximal. Careful preparation of the patient before testing and kind encouragement during testing will often improve the exercise response.

Physician-determined end points may be absolute or relative, depending on the particular circumstances. Clinical judgment, experience, and knowing the patient being tested are all important factors in safely completing the exercise test. Rate-dependent bundle branch block, for example, may not always be an

TABLE 5.7. Exercise Test End Points

Patient-determined end points
  Patient wants to stop
  Significant chest discomfort
  Marked fatigue
  Severe dyspnea
  Other limiting symptoms (dizziness, leg cramps, joint discomfort, etc.)
Physician-determined end points
  Patient does not look good (e.g., ataxia, confusion, pallor, cyanosis, etc.)
  ECG end points
    Marked ST-segment depression or elevation
    New bundle branch block or AV junctional heart block
    Ventricular tachycardia or fibrillation
    Increasing frequency of PVCs or couplets
    Onset of supraventricular tachyarrhythmias
  Exertional hypotension (systolic BP falls below standing BP)
  Systolic BP >250 mm Hg
  Diastolic BP >120 mm Hg
  Equipment failure
Protocol-determined end points (submaximal tests)
  Heart rate determined (e.g., 120 bpm)
  Workload determined (e.g., 5 METs)

AV, atrioventricular; *PVCs*, premature ventricular complexes, *METs*, metabolic equivalents.

indication to terminate a test if this was a previously recognized abnormality and not related to myocardial ischemia.

The protocol-determined end points are related to the submaximal protocols designed for low-level exercise testing. The predischarge exercise test after acute MI may be terminated when the patient's heart rate achieves 70% of predicted maximal heart rate or when the workload reaches 5 METs.

Procedures After Exercise

After a brief cool-down period, while the patient is still standing on the treadmill or sitting on the bicycle, the ECG should be recorded. Patients on the treadmill should hold onto the rails, because venous pooling may cause light-headedness. If the test is a diagnostic test and if significant ECG abnormalities did *not* develop during exercise, the patient should return to the supine position for the recovery period. The increased venous return that occurs when supine may aggravate borderline ischemic myocardium because of increased

179

end-diastolic pressure and result in diagnostic ECG changes. Lachterman et al. (31) have shown that ST-segment changes limited to the recovery period were as predictive of underlying coronary disease as changes that occur during exercise. For patients who develop ECG abnormalities during exercise, however, it may be safer to have the patient sit during recovery to minimize the risk of ischemic ventricular arrhythmias. Regardless of patient position, the ECG should be continuously monitored and records obtained every two minutes.

During recovery the patient should be examined for new gallops and murmurs that indicate myocardial dysfunction. An S-4 gallop may be indicative of decreased ventricular compliance associated with myocardial ischemia. A new systolic murmur is usually caused by papillary muscle dysfunction and mitral regurgitation. These are usually transient findings associated with reversible myocardial ischemia.

Exercise Test Data Forms

Figure 5.5 represents a two-page exercise test report form that is modified from Koppes et al. (32). The form attempts to capture all the clinically important information needed for interpreting the exercise test results. The first page asks for clinical data, cardiovascular risk factors, reasons for testing, description of the resting ECG, and exercise test data from each stage of exercise and recovery. The second page documents physical findings before and after exercise, reasons for stopping, specific ECG abnormalities, prognostic indicators, and interpretive statements. This form is most applicable to diagnostic exercise testing of patients with known or suspected coronary heart disease. Other forms may be substituted for functional testing where more physiologic parameters need to be assessed. Many of the commercially available exercise testing configurations generate summary reports of the exercise ECG information and physiologic parameters.

Life-Threatening Complications of Exercise Testing

Although rare, exercise testing may be associated with untoward events. In a 1980 survey of the exercise testing community, Stuart and Ellestad (33) analyzed data from over 500,000 exercise tests and found that, for every 10,000 tests, there were approximately 3.5 MIs, 4.8 serious arrhythmias, and 0.5 deaths. Table 5.8 lists the requirements for minimizing exercise test complications. Periodic inservice training should be given to the exercise testing staff to review emergency treatment procedures, so that any potentially serious or life-threatening complications can be recognized early and managed appropriately.

INTERMOUNTAIN HEALTH CARE, INC.
A community hospital system serving the intermountain west

CARDIOLOGY DIVISION
LDS HOSPITAL
325 8th Ave., S.L.C., Utah (801) 350-1185

REPORT OF TREADMILL EXERCISE TEST
(PAGE ONE)

PATIENT IDENTIFICATION
Hospital No. ....
Name: ....
Address ....
PVT MD: .... Phone: ....

SEND REPORT TO

TREADMILL NO.	AGE	SEX	WT. (KG.)	HT. (CM)

☐ INPATIENT
☐ OUTPATIENT
DATE (MO., DAY, YR.) 24 HR. TIME

PREVIOUS TEST NO.
☐ NO ☐ YES, LAST:
HOURS SINCE LAST MEAL
LAST CIGARETTE

MEDICATIONS
☐ DIGITALIS ☐ NITRATES
☐ BETA-BLOCKER ☐ QUINIDINE/PRONESTYL
☐ DIURETIC ☐ OTHER

CARDIAC RISK FACTORS

HISTORY OF HYPERTENSION ☐ YES ☐ NO ☐ SUSP
NOW ELEVATED ☐ YES ☐ NO
ON TREATMENT ☐ YES ☐ NO

CIGARETTE SMOKING ☐ NO ☐ PAST ONLY ☐ YES
NO. YEARS AGO QUIT
PACK-YEARS, PACKS/DAY

CHOLESTEROL LEVEL ☐ Not Known
☐ NORMAL ☐ HIGH:
FAMILY HISTORY PREMATURE ASHD ☐

ACTIVITY STATUS
☐ Sedentary ☐ Active Recreation
☐ Recent Bed Rest ☐ Active Occupation ☐ Athlete

OTHER RISK FACTORS

CLINICAL REASONS FOR TEST

EVALUATION OF ATYPICAL SENSATION OR PAIN POSSIBLY DUE TO ASCVD (Explain)
☐

EVALUATION OF ANGINA: ONSET:
☐ TYPICAL ☐ ATYPICAL ☐ UNSTABLE

ARRHYTHMIA EVALUATION ☐ SUSPECT ONLY
☐ PVDs ☐ SVT ☐ OTHER:

OTHER HEART DISEASE ☐ VALVULAR ☐ OTHER:
☐ MITRAL PROLAPSE ☐ CONGENITAL

EVALUATION POST AMI ☐
TIME SINCE LAST INFARCT: WEEKS MONTHS YEARS

CORONARY ANGIOGRAM: DATE

SCREENING ASYMPTOMATIC INDIVIDUAL ☐
☐ FUNCTIONAL CAPACITY EVALUATION
☐ EXERCISE PRESCRIPTION

CORONARY BYPASS SURGERY (DATE AND TYPE)

☐ OTHER

RESTING ECG ☐ NORMAL ☐ ABNORMAL
DESCRIBE

STAGE	MPH/ GRADE	METS	MIN/SEC IN STAGE	HR (AT END OF STAGE)	BP	DESCRIBE: CHEST PAIN/ARRHYTHMIAL/ST CHANGES/LEADS
Supine	3.5 cc O_2/Kg/Min = 1 MET					
HV For 30 Sec	(BASAL)					
Stand						
1/4	1.7 /0%	2				
1/2	1.7 /5%	3				
I	1.7/10%	4				
II	2.5/12%	7				
III	3.4/14%	10				
IV	4.2/16%	14				
V	5.0/18%	16				
						PREDICTED MAX HEART RATE 220- = /Min.
Immed	MAX SBP (______) X					
1 min.	MAX HR (______) =					
3 min.	.... x 10^3					
5 min.	$\dot{V}O_2$ MAX {est. = / mxed. =					
7 min.						
.... min.						

CARDIOLOGY 18-78

FIGURE 5.5. Data form for diagnostic exercise testing used at The Fitness Institute, LDS Hospital, Salt Lake City, Utah. (Modified from Koppes G, McKiernan D, Froelicher VF. Curr Prob Cardiol 1977;7:34.)

INTERMOUNTAIN HEALTH CARE, INC.
A community hospital system serving the Intermountain West
CARDIOLOGY DIVISION

LDS HOSPITAL
325 8th Ave., S.L.C., Utah (801) 350-1185

REPORT OF
TREADMILL EXERCISE TEST
(PAGE TWO)

PATIENT IDENTIFICATION

| PROBABILITY OF CAD | ☐ Unlikely | ☐ Probable | EXPLAIN |
| PRIOR TO TEST = % | ☐ Possible | ☐ Very Probable | |

| PHYSICAL | PRE | S3 | ☐ YES ☐ NO | S4 | ☐ YES ☐ NO | MURMUR ☐ YES ☐ NO | TYPE |
| EXAM | POST | S3 | ☐ YES ☐ NO | S4 | ☐ YES ☐ NO | SIGNS/SYMPTOMS CHF ☐ | MURMUR ☐ YES ☐ NO | TYPE |

REASONS FOR STOPPING 1. Primary 2. Secondary 3. Tertiary	CHEST PAIN	DYSPNEA	FATIGUE/ WEAKNESS	CLAUDI-CATION	GENERAL APPEARANCE	CNS SYMPTOMS
	HYPER-TENSION	HYPO-TENTION	ST CHANGES	ARRHYTHMIA	TECHNICAL PROBLEM	PHYSICAL DISABILITY
	POOR PATIENT COOPERATION	LEG FATIGUE	OTHER:			

ECG RESPONSE	ARRHYTHMIA	NO	FEW PVD's	FREQ PVD's	VT	FREQ PAD's	SVT
		OTHER	EXPLAIN:				
	CONDUCTION	NORMAL	LBBB	RBBB	BLOCK	AXIS SHIFT
		EXPLAIN:				
	ST SEGMENT	NORMAL	BORDERLINE	DEPRESSION	ELEVATE	NORMALIZE
		EXPLAIN:				
	T & U WAVES	NORMAL	T-INVERSION	TALL T	U-INVERSION	PROMINENT U
		EXPLAIN:				

| PATIENT RESPONSE | MAX HR ☐NL ☐HI ☐LO | SYSTOLIC BP ☐NL ☐HI ☐FALL | FUNCTIONAL CAPACITY ☐EXCELLENT ☐NORMAL ☐LOW | FAI = % ☐ VERY LOW |
| | ANGINA ☐ YES ☐ NO | ATYPICAL PAIN ☐ YES ☐ NO | CHF SIGNS ☐ YES ☐ NO | OTHER COMPLICATIONS ☐ YES ☐ NO | MAXIMAL EFFORT ☐ YES ☐ NO |

| PROG-NOSTIC INDI-CATORS | ONSET ST-DEPRESSION STAGE: HR= | MAX ST-DEPRESSION MM LEADS: | MAX EXERCISE STAGE: HR= | POST-EXERCISE DURATION OF ST DEPRESSION min. | ANGINA ONSET HR= |
| | OTHER | | | | |

INTERPRETATION

NORMAL MAXIMAL TEST	COMMENTS	
NORMAL SUBMAXIMAL TEST	% MAX HR = %	COMMENTS
BORDERLINE ABNORMAL	EXPLAIN	
ABNORMAL ST DEPRESSION	LOW RISK / HIGH RISK	EXPLAIN
ABNORMAL ST ELEVATION	COMMENTS	
OTHER ABNORMALITIES	EXPLAIN	
NEW PROBABILITY OF CAD AFTER TEST = %	COMMENTS:	

Interpreted By: _____ Date _____

Approved By: _____ Date _____

CARDIOLOGY 1A-78

FIGURE 5.5. Cont.

TABLE 5.8. Minimizing the Risks of Exercise Testing

Trained personnel (testing, treatment, CPR expertise, etc.)
Physician attendance during testing
Continuous ECG monitoring during and after exercise
Pretest history and physical examination
Resting ECG interpretation before exercise begins
Patient awareness of signs and symptoms
Emergency resuscitation equipment and drugs
Attention to exercise test end points (Table 5.7)
No shower until cool-down finished

CPR, cardiopulmonary resuscitation.

EXERCISE ELECTROCARDIOGRAPHY

Electrophysiology of Myocardial Ischemia

Although the ECG has great utility in the recognition of myocardial ischemia, the underlying cellular electrophysiologic events that are responsible for the ECG abnormalities are only partially understood. Nevertheless, before discussing exercise ECG changes, it is appropriate to review the pathophysiology of myocardial ischemia and the various mechanisms responsible for ischemic ECG changes.

Myocardial ischemia (silent or symptomatic) results whenever there is an imbalance between myocardial oxygen supply and demand that leaves myocardial cells deprived of oxygen (Fig. 5.6). In the setting of significant fixed coronary artery obstructions myocardial ischemia occurs during exercise or other stressful events that increase heart rate, heart size (ventricular volume), blood pressure (ventricular pressure, wall tension), or myocardial contractility—all major determinants of myocardial oxygen demand. Ischemia of this type is usually called *secondary* because it is caused by factors that increase oxygen requirements. Alternatively, myocardial ischemia may result when the myocardial oxygen supply is briefly interrupted as occurs during coronary artery spasm. This type of ischemia is called *primary* because it is independent of any changes in myocardial oxygen demands. Most patients with CHD have *mixed* ischemia with episodes resulting from either increased demand, decreased supply, or both.

Regardless of the type of myocardial ischemia, however, what follows is a well-recognized sequence of events, initially reversible, that have mechanical, metabolic, electrophysiologic, and, at times, symptomatic consequences (Fig. 5.7). An *ischemic cascade* has been described in which mechanical abnormalities appear first, followed next by metabolic and electrophysiologic changes, and

183

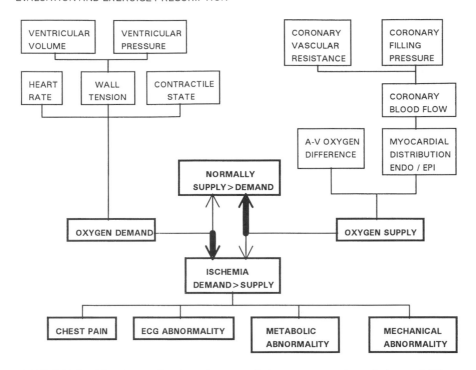

FIGURE 5.6. The determinants of myocardial oxygen supply and demand. The major determinants of oxygen demand are illustrated on the left, and the factors influencing oxygen supply and coronary blood flow are shown on the right. Normally, the oxygen supply matches the demand. Myocardial ischemia occurs whenever the demand for oxygen exceeds the supply. Ischemia manifestations are expressed as mechanical, metabolic, electrocardiographic, and symptomatic abnormalities.

ending with anginal symptoms, although symptoms need not always be present (*silent ischemia*) (34). The mechanical consequences are the result of the inability of hypoxic myocardial cells to contract or relax normally. They are recognized using various imaging techniques that detect segmental wall motion abnormalities and decreased ventricular ejection fractions. Metabolic abnormalities include abnormal lactate production by hypoxic cells that can be detected during cardiac catheterization by sampling blood from the coronary sinus. The electrophysiologic consequences are responsible for the ischemic ECG changes and, at times, the precipitation of cardiac arrhythmias and conduction abnormalities. The following discussion focuses on the mechanisms for ischemic ECG changes.

Figure 5.8 illustrates the relationship between the intracellular action potential of ventricular muscle cells and the surface ECG. The QRS complex represents the time sequence of ventricular muscle depolarization (phase 0 of the

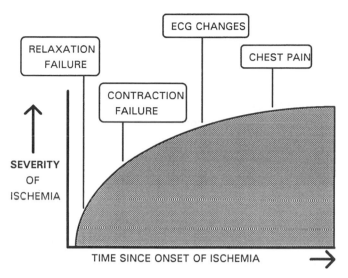

FIGURE 5.7. The ischemic cascade. The manifestations of myocardial ischemia are determined by the severity of the ischemic process (*ordinate*) and the time since the onset *(abscissa)*.

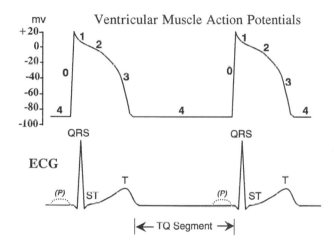

FIGURE 5.8. Relationship between intracellular action potentials of ventricular muscle *(top)* and the body surface ECG *(bottom)*. See text.

action potential waveform). The ST segment represents the plateau or phase 2 of ventricular muscle repolarization, and the T wave reflects the time sequence of repolarization potentials during phase 3. In this diagram the P waves are superimposed waveforms, since they are independent of ventricular muscle depolarization and repolarization. It is important to observe that the resting membrane potential, phase 4, is represented by the TQ segment of the surface

ECG. As will be seen, the TQ segment has a prominent role in the ECG manifestations of ischemia (35–37).

During myocardial ischemia the intracellular action potentials become markedly altered in the ischemic zone. Several changes occur within seconds of oxygen and blood flow deprivation that alter action potential shape and duration. The earliest and most specific change is a decrease in resting membrane potential (phase 4) caused by failure of the membrane sodium-potassium pump and accumulation of extracellular potassium (38). The second and less specific change is a shortening of action potential duration and amplitude as repolarization accelerates during phases 2 and 3.

The corresponding ECG changes in myocardial ischemia are determined by the relationship between the ECG lead orientations and the location of the ischemic zone in the ventricular myocardium. The simplest relationship to understand, in the setting of exercise-induced ischemia, is illustrated in Figure 5.9. In this example a *subendocardial* zone of left ventricular myocardium becomes ischemic during exercise because a high-grade coronary lesion limits oxygen delivery to this vulnerable zone. The overlying *subepicardial* zone of myocardium remains normal.

Figure 5.9*A* depicts a normal section of the ventricular wall that is divided into an outer (subepicardial) and inner (subendocardial) region. An intracellular action potential from each region is diagrammed along with a hypothetical ECG waveform recorded from a typical unipolar precordial chest lead. Since electrical activation (depolarization) spreads from endocardium to epicardium and recovery (repolarization) moves in the opposite direction, action potentials begin in the subendocardial region earlier than those in the subepicardial region but terminate later. The normal upright QRS complex reflects the depolarization wavefront moving toward the positive ECG electrode. During early repolarization (phase 2) the action potentials from both regions are approximately at the same level of potential, and the corresponding ST segment is therefore close to the baseline. The upright T wave, however, reflects the earlier recovery in the subepicardial zone and the resulting potential difference between the inner and outer zones during late repolarization (phase 3). During phase 4 the resting membrane potentials are similar in the two zones and the corresponding TQ segment is therefore on the baseline.

In Figure 5.9*B*, the inner subendocardial zone has now become ischemic and the affected myocardial cells have a decrease in resting membrane potential (phase 4). As illustrated, depolarization still spreads from endocardium to epicardium, repolarization from epicardium to endocardium, and during phase 2 the action potentials are still at the same level of potential. Although the ST segment remains close to baseline, the TQ segment shifts upward because a new *diastolic current of injury* has developed between the ischemic inner zone and the normal outer zone during phase 4, or ventricular diastole. What the

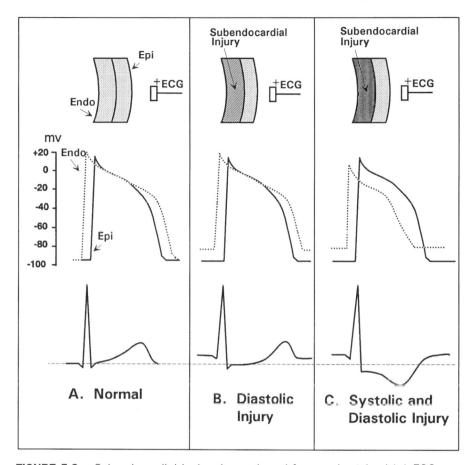

FIGURE 5.9. Subendocardial ischemia as viewed from a chest lead (+) ECG electrode. **A.** Normal ECG waveform and action potentials from endocardial and epicardial regions. **B.** Diastolic (phase 4) current of injury from subendocardial ischemia resulting in TQ-segment elevation on ECG waveform. **C.** Systolic and diastolic currents of injury from subendocardial ischemia resulting in TQ-segment elevation and ST-segment depression.

clinician sees, however, is ST-segment depression, because modern ECG recorders are designed (i.e., condenser coupled) to detect and correct baseline shifts in the ECG signal, which are often caused by artifact (i.e., low frequency noise). When the upward displaced TQ segment is electronically moved back to the original baseline, however, the ST segment becomes artificially depressed below baseline. This is not considered "true" ST-segment depression, because it is not the result of an abnormality in phase-2 repolarization.

In Figure 5.9*C*, additional alterations in action potential morphology associated with continued subendocardial ischemia have developed. Both the

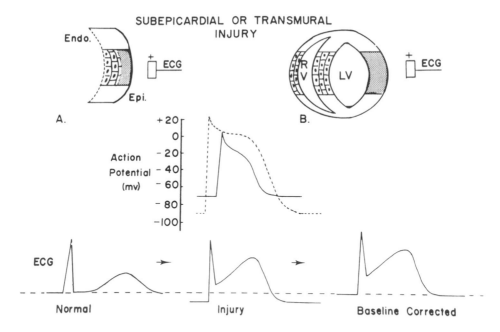

FIGURE 5.10. Subepicardial (**A**) and transmural (**B**) injury as viewed from a chest lead (+) ECG electrode. Systolic and diastolic currents of injury are generated between the injured (ischemic) and normal myocardial cells. The resulting ECG changes in both cases include TQ-segment depression and ST-segment elevation.

amplitude and the duration of the ischemic action potentials are now reduced, resulting in a *systolic current of injury* between the inner and outer layers of myocardium. The ECG manifestations of these alterations include "true" ST-segment depression and inversion of the T wave caused by earlier recovery of the ischemic subendocardium and reversal of the direction of repolarization. The ECG changes seen in Figure 5.9, *B*, and *C*, are typical of the changes recorded during and after exercise in patients with exercise-induced ischemia.

Figure 5.10 illustrates the effects of an ischemic process involving either an outer epicardial region or a full-thickness transmural region of myocardium. Isolated epicardial injury rarely occurs in coronary disease, but it is found in pericarditis. In either case, systolic and diastolic currents of injury exist between the ischemic and nonischemic regions of myocardium that result in ST-segment elevation and increased T-wave amplitude in ECG leads facing the ischemic zone. For reasons discussed previously but now in a different direction, ST-T-wave deflections are caused by both TQ-segment depression, which artificially elevates the ST segment, and "true" ST-T-wave elevation.

In summary, the displacement of ST segments above or below the isoelectric baseline during myocardial ischemia is the result of two very distinct electrophysiologic events. The most specific change is a diastolic current of injury caused by a decrease in resting membrane (phase 4) potential in ischemic myocardium that affects primarily the TQ segment. The second mechanism is related to a systolic current of injury that develops between ischemic and normal myocardium that results in true ST-T-wave changes. The magnitude and direction of the ST-T-wave changes are determined by the location of the ischemic region relative to the position of the (+) ECG electrodes on the body surface. ST-segment elevation occurs when the ischemic myocardium and ECG electrodes are in close proximity without intervening nonischemic myocardium. ST-segment depression is more likely to reflect subendocardial ischemia with normal heart muscle situated between the ischemic tissue and the ECG electrodes. It should be understood that this explanation is an oversimplification of a very complex geometric relationship between ventricular anatomy and ECG leads (39). Nevertheless, it should suffice to facilitate a better appreciation of the actual ECG changes in myocardial ischemia that are seen during exercise testing.

ECG Manifestations of Myocardial Ischemia

From the preceding discussion it is clear that the most important ischemic ECG changes are related to shifts in the TQ and ST segments. Unfortunately, the more specific changes in TQ segment cannot be differentiated from those that primarily affect the ST-T wave. Primary ST-T-wave abnormalities that mimic ischemia may be caused by many other conditions, including an assortment of drugs, electrolyte abnormalities, mitral valve prolapse, and other heart disease states, all of which contribute to false-positive errors in exercise electrocardiography (35).

Figure 5.11 diagrams the various ST-T- and U-wave abnormalities that are recognized to be associated with exercise-induced myocardial ischemia. The normal resting ECG waveform as recorded in lead V_5 is illustrated in Figure 5.11A. Note the smooth transition from the ST segment to an asymmetric T wave followed by a small positive U wave. During exercise the initial portion of the ST segment often becomes depressed below the baseline, as illustrated in Figure 5.11B, but the smooth ST-T transition persists with return of the ST segment to baseline rather quickly. This normal response is called *J junctional* or *J point* depression, since the J point defines the onset of the ST segment.

In Figure 5.11, the diagrams *C, D,* and *E* show the various types of ST-segment depression seen in subendocardial ischemia that characterize the "positive" exercise test response. During exercise "upsloping," ST depression appears first, followed by "horizontal" and sometimes "downsloping" ST-segment changes, usually the latter only seen after exercise as the heart rate slows. Generally the left precordial leads V_{4-6} or unipolar leads using the V_5

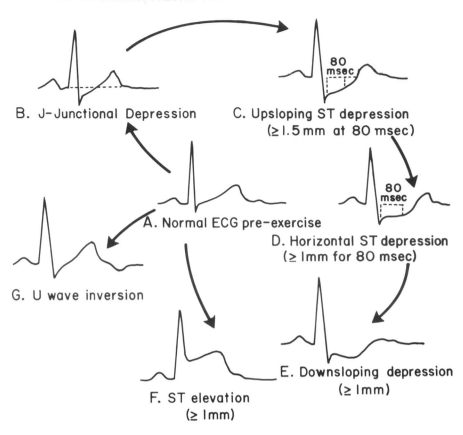

FIGURE 5.11. ECG changes during exercise testing.

location are the most sensitive recording sites for detecting ischemic ST-segment depression. Rarely, however, the inferior limb leads II and aVF are the only leads to exhibit ischemic-looking ECG changes. These patients may have single-vessel right coronary artery disease (40), although most often isolated ST depression in the inferior leads is a false-positive response (41).

The ECG waveform diagrammed in Figure 5.11*F* shows ST-segment elevation, which is an unusual manifestation of exercise-induced myocardial ischemia and reflects transmural or full-thickness myocardial ischemia. This is a more serious abnormality because a larger mass of heart muscle is involved. Three clinically different subsets of patients may present with this abnormality (42). One group has the unusual syndrome of *variant* or *Prinzmetal's angina* characterized by chest pain episodes mostly at rest, ST-segment elevation during pain, and coronary artery spasm (43). In this syndrome exercise-induced ST elevation occurs in 10 to 30% of patients presumably because of α-adrenergic-induced coronary vasoconstriction (44). A second group has severe, often multivessel, coronary artery disease such that transmural ischemia is more likely than localized subendocardial ischemia because of the marked reduction of coronary blood flow to that segment of myocardium (45). These patients are clearly candidates for coronary angiography and consideration for revascularization therapy. The third group of patients has had previous myocardial infarctions, and ST-segment elevation is seen in leads showing infarct Q-wave abnormalities. This is often not an ischemic finding but a reflection of an underlying, myocardial-wall motion abnormality in the infarcted left ventricle (46). This is a common finding in post-MI patients and, unless associated with other abnormal findings, should not be considered a sign of severe ischemia.

The most unusual and least understood ECG manifestation of ischemia is U-wave inversion, illustrated in Figure 5.11G. Although originally described in the early exercise testing literature of the 1940s, this interesting finding did not reappear in the literature until 1979 when Gerson et al. (47) published their data. They described 36 patients with U-wave inversion after exercise testing in a population of 248 patients undergoing coronary angiography. Thirty-five patients (97%) had significant CHD by angiography, and in 33 patients (92%) the disease involved either the left main or left anterior descending coronary artery. Although the probability of U-wave inversion in patients with coronary disease was quite low (15%) in this study, it was a very specific diagnostic marker for disease. In support of these findings Yano et al. (48) have observed transient negative U waves during percutaneous transluminal coronary angioplasty procedures before detectable ST-segment elevation. Inverted U waves are best recognized during the post-exercise recovery period as the heart rates are slowing down. The recognition of U-wave inversion requires finding a discrete negative deflection between the T and P waves relative to the "isoelectric" PR segment. The inverted U waves usually become upright after several minutes, which is helpful in verifying that U-wave inversion truly occurred. U-wave inversion in resting ECG tracings is sometimes seen, but it is not a specific marker for coronary disease.

Examples of actual exercise ECG data illustrating the previously described ischemic abnormalities are shown in Figures 5.12 to 5.14.

Conduction Disturbances During Exercise Testing

Although unusual, atrioventricular (AV) and intraventricular heart block may occur during exercise testing. These abnormalities are not necessarily manifestations of myocardial ischemia unless accompanied by anginal symptoms or preceded by ST-T-wave changes.

AV heart block is rare during exercise testing. In the resting state type I second-degree AV block, or Wenckebach, is often a benign condition that is associated with increased vagal tone. It has been reported in very athletic individuals but has no clinical significance. It usually disappears during activity as

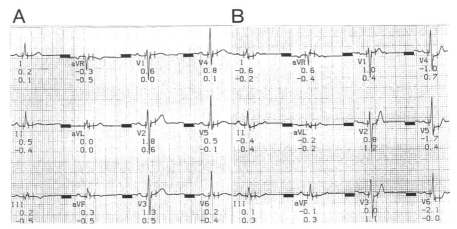

FIGURE 5.12. Exercise-induced ST-segment depression. **A.** Computer averaged resting 12-lead ECG showing normal ST-T waves. **B.** Computer-averaged 12-lead ECG at peak exercise showing ≥ 1 mm ST-segment depression in leads V$_{4-6}$. In each lead the top number indicates the ST-segment level (mm) at 80 msec after the J point; the bottom number reflects the ST-segment slope. Coronary angiographic findings revealed an 80% obstruction of the left anterior descending coronary artery.

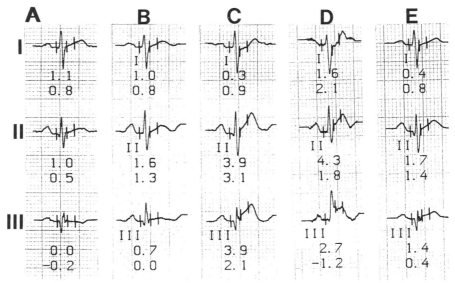

FIGURE 5.13. Exercise-induced ST-segment elevation. **A.** Computer-averaged leads I, II, and III at rest. **B.** Exercise Stage I. **C.** Maximal exercise. **D.** One minute of recovery after exercise. **E.** Nine minutes of recovery after exercise. In each lead the top number indicates the ST-segment level (mm) at 80 msec after the J point; the bottom number reflects the ST-segment slope. Increasing ST-segment elevation is seen in leads II and III. Coronary angiography revealed a 95% obstruction of the right coronary artery.

192

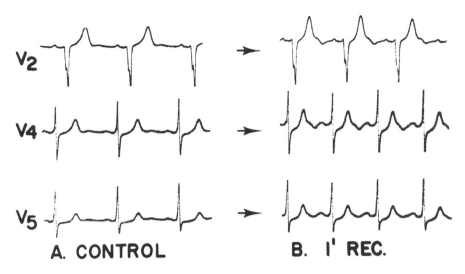

FIGURE 5.14. Exercise-induced U-wave inversion in leads V_2, V_4, and V_5.
A. Resting ECG showing small upright U waves following the T waves. **B**. One minute after exercise illustrating U-wave inversion most obvious in leads V_2 and V_4. This patient had multivessel coronary artery disease, including a high-grade left anterior descending coronary lesion.

vagal tone diminishes and sympathetic tone increases. It may be seen during the recovery period when vagal tone returns. Type II second-degree AV block, or Mobitz II, is a more serious manifestation of conduction system disease and usually is seen in the presence of preexisting bundle branch block. It may be associated with presyncopal or syncopal episodes and is frequently a precursor to complete AV block. When detected during exercise testing or ambulatory monitoring, a permanent artificial pacemaker is indicated.

Exercise-induced bundle branch block is most often rate related, becoming apparent when the heart rate exceeds a critical threshold. When first seen it often causes anxiety for the laboratory staff, because the sudden transition from narrow to wide QRS complexes at fast heart rates mimics ventricular tachycardia. Unless the patient is known to the staff for this problem, the exercise test should be terminated to determine the cause for the sudden QRS change. Unlike ventricular tachycardia, however, the P to QRS relationship in bundle branch block is maintained, and as the heart rate slows down, the recognition of sinus rhythm becomes obvious. The heart rate at which the bundle branch block disappears during recovery is always significantly lower than the heart rate at which it appeared during exercise.

The diagnostic implications of exercise-induced left bundle branch block (LBBB) have been the subject of several recent publications (49, 50). Although CHD is always suspect in this situation, patients without chest pain during

193

FIGURE 5.15. Schematic drawing of rest and exercise lead V$_5$ in left bundle branch block (LBBB) and right bundle branch block (RBBB).

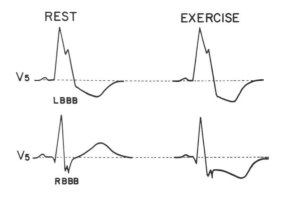

exercise and whose LBBB appear only at heart rates greater than 125 beats/min are unlikely to have significant coronary disease (49). In addition, the absence of clinical findings of heart disease is usually associated with an excellent prognosis.

The recognition of myocardial ischemia in the presence of intraventricular conduction abnormalities may be difficult, especially in left bundle branch block. Ventricular conduction defects cause the sequence of muscle activation to be altered, thus changing the shape and duration of the QRS complex. This change in activation sequence necessitates an obligatory change in the sequence of recovery, resulting in "secondary" ST-T-wave changes. As a general rule, the direction of the ST-T deflection in bundle branch block is opposite to the terminal or main direction of the QRS complex. Figure 5.15 illustrates right and left bundle branch block at rest and during exercise as seen in lead V$_5$. In left bundle branch block (LBBB), the ST-T deflection is normally depressed below the baseline in this lead, which prevents recognition of myocardial ischemia with any degree of certainty. In right bundle branch block (RBBB), however, the ST-T deflection in V$_5$ is similar to the normal ECG, and significant ST depression during exercise may be indicative of myocardial ischemia. Such is not the case in the right precordial leads (V$_{1-2}$) in RBBB, since the ST-T deflection at rest is normally depressed in these leads (opposite to the prominent rSR' QRS complex); further depression during exercise is not specific for ischemia. Because of these difficulties in recognizing ischemic ECG changes in bundle branch block, it may be more cost-effective to utilize stress radionuclide or echocardiographic techniques.

Exercise Test Arrhythmias

One of the most challenging aspects of exercise testing is the recognition and management of exercise-induced cardiac arrhythmias. Various supraventricular and ventricular arrhythmias have been observed in clinically healthy subjects, as well as in patients with heart disease. Their occurrence should not be considered a specific manifestation of any particular disease process such as myocardial ischemia, although it is well recognized that patients with ischemic heart disease are at greater risk for exercise-induced arrhythmias.

There are three generally recognized electrophysiologic mechanisms of cardiac arrhythmias: (a) abnormal automaticity, (b) triggered activity, and (c) reentry (51). Exercise may contribute to the genesis of arrhythmias by facilitating one or more of these mechanisms. Increased sympathetic activity and circulating catecholamines during exercise may promote spontaneous automaticity (increased slope of phase-4 depolarization) of ectopic pacemakers in the atria, AV junction, or ventricular tissues. This may lead to premature beats and ectopic tachycardias. Sympathetic activity and catecholamines also contribute to delayed after-depolarizations (triggered automaticity), which are thought to be responsible for some cases of exercise-induced ventricular tachycardia (52). These delayed afterpotentials and related tachyarrhythmias may be prevented by treatment with beta-blocker drugs or verapamil (53). Exercise-induced myocardial ischemia may lead to reentrant arrhythmias by increasing the temporal dispersion of recovery potentials or by causing delayed conduction in the Purkinje system. Ischemia also potentiates enhanced automaticity of ectopic pacemaker cells.

Exercise may also suppress atrial and ventricular arrhythmias present at rest because of the increase in sinus rate, although suppression of a particular arrhythmia should not be used as evidence that the arrhythmia is benign. Conversely, an increase in frequency of ectopic beats with exercise is not necessarily an indication that the arrhythmia is caused by serious underlying heart disease. Each arrhythmia should be analyzed according to the clinical context within which it occurs.

Table 5.9 lists the common arrhythmias that may occur during exercise testing. It is essential that exercise testing personnel become familiar with the ECG characteristics of these arrhythmias both as they appear on the oscilloscope, as well as on hard-copy rhythm strips. A brief atlas of common cardiac arrhythmias is presented in Chapter 3.

Supraventricular Arrhythmias

Exercise-induced premature atrial complexes (PACs) are quite common and generally pose no serious threat to the patient. Occasionally, however, they may precipitate paroxysmal supraventricular tachycardia (PSVT), atrial fibrillation, or atrial flutter. When this occurs the test should be terminated. Most often these tachyarrhythmias are transient and resolve within minutes. The restoration of sinus rhythm in patients with sustained PSVT may be facilitated by having the patient perform a Valsalva maneuver or by carefully massaging the right or left carotid sinus (assuming clinical competency in performing this technique). Rarely will it be necessary to use pharmacologic intervention with intravenous verapamil or adenosine (54).

Atrial fibrillation and atrial flutter are unusual exercise-induced arrhythmias and rarely occur in healthy individuals. These arrhythmias are usually caused by

TABLE 5.9. Exercise-Induced Cardiac Arrhythmias

Supraventricular arrhythmias

    Premature atrial complexes (PACs)

        Isolated

        Couplets

        With or without aberration

        P-on-U phenomenon

    Paroxysmal supraventricular tachycardia (PSVT)

    Atrial fibrillation

    Atrial flutter

Ventricular arrhythmias

    Premature ventricular complexes (PVCs)

        Isolated

        Couplets

        Unifocal or multifocal

        R-on-T phenomenon

    Ventricular tachycardia

        Nonsustained (i.e., <30 sec duration)

        Sustained (i.e., ≥30 sec duration)

    Ventricular fibrillation

---

cardiac dysfunction that is associated with dilatation of the atria. If they do not resolve spontaneously with cessation of exercise, it may be necessary to treat pharmacologically with digoxin, beta-blocker, or verapamil (55). Rarely will it be necessary to electrically cardiovert these arrhythmias.

Ventricular Arrhythmias

Exercise-induced premature ventricular complexes (PVCs) are extremely common and have received a great deal of attention in the literature (56–58). Although more frequent in CHD, these arrhythmias are found in all populations undergoing exercise testing. They are more common with increasing age and at increasing heart rates during exercise. In CHD, however, they may occur at lower heart rates and workloads. Patients with recent MIs, multivessel disease, and left ventricular dysfunction are at greatest risk for PVCs and more serious ventricular arrhythmias (58). In general, the more severe the disease, the greater the frequency of ventricular arrhythmias. Multifocal PVCs and R-on-T phenomena are considered to be more serious, although they are frequently found in both healthy and diseased populations. It is usually not necessary to terminate exercise in patients with frequent PVCs unless associated with limiting symptoms, ischemic manifestations, or exertional hypotension. In some patients PVCs occur during a particular heart rate range, above and below which they disappear.

Ventricular tachycardia, defined as three or more consecutive PVCs at a rate greater than 100 beats/min, is extremely uncommon in normal subjects during maximal exercise testing (59). When seen therefore this arrhythmia is always of great concern and usually necessitates immediate termination of the test. Ventricular tachycardia may only last several seconds or may become sustained for many minutes and require therapeutic intervention. In patients with heart disease ventricular tachycardia is often associated with left ventricular dysfunction or multivessel coronary artery disease with ischemia. When related to ischemia, ventricular arrhythmias are especially prone to develop during the postexercise period. It is recommended therefore that patients with ischemic ECG abnormalities be monitored for longer periods of time after exercise (8 to 10 minutes). In addition, the sitting position after exercise may be less arrhythmogenic than the supine position in these patients.

Sustained ventricular tachycardia (>30 seconds in duration) usually reverts spontaneously to normal sinus rhythm soon after exercise is stopped. Occasionally, however, emergency cardiac support may become necessary. For patients who are hemodynamically stable, intravenous lidocaine is the treatment of choice. If unstable with hypotension, obtundation, or severe chest pain, direct-current (DC) cardioversion should be carried out under physician supervision. It is important that the exercise-testing staff have written policies regarding the management of life-threatening arrhythmic emergencies and periodic in-service programs to review these treatment plans.

The prognostic significance of ventricular tachycardia (VT) during exercise testing does not appear to be ominous. Yang (60) retrospectively reviewed 3351 patients undergoing routine testing and identified 55 (1.6%) patients with exercise-induced ventricular tachycardia. Fifty of these patients had nonsustained VT and only 5 had sustained VT (one of which died suddenly 7 months after testing). When followed for an average of 2 years, the total mortality in the VT group was not significantly different from the mortality of the entire group (3.6% versus 5.1%), suggesting that VT, especially the nonsustained variety, is not a marker of poor prognosis.

Exercise-induced ventricular fibrillation, although the most serious of cardiac arrhythmias, is extremely uncommon in the exercise-testing laboratory. When it occurs, it is always a humbling experience for the laboratory staff since it is so unexpected. The clinical setting is usually that of far-advanced coronary heart disease with ischemia and left ventricular dysfunction.

Figure 5.16 shows an occurrence of postexercise ventricular fibrillation in a 57-year-old male physician with stable angina pectoris 5 years after an anterior wall myocardial infarction. One year prior to this episode he exercised into stage

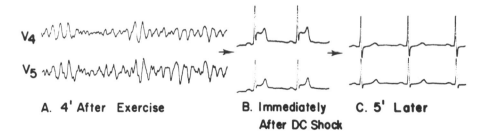

FIGURE 5.16. **A**. Ventricular fibrillation 4 minutes after exercise in patient with known CHD. **B**. Immediately after defibrillation there is ST-segment elevation in leads V$_4$ and V$_5$. **C**. Resolution of ST-segment abnormalities 5 minutes later. Following this procedure the patient underwent a 6-vessel coronary artery bypass operation.

IV of the Bruce protocol with ischemic ST-segment depression, U-wave inversion, and mild angina pectoris. Because of his normal functional capacity and mild symptoms, he elected to remain on medical therapy. One year later, with stable symptoms, he again exercised into stage IV with similar ST-segment and U-wave abnormalities. In the fourth minute of recovery after his symptoms had subsided, ventricular fibrillation occurred very unexpectedly. Within seconds he was successfully defibrillated, and several minutes later his ECG was back to the resting control configuration. This patient subsequently underwent multi-vessel coronary artery bypass surgery but has refused to undergo further exercise testing.

CLINICAL JUDGMENT IN EXERCISE TESTING

There is considerable controversy in the medical community regarding the diagnostic accuracy of exercise ECG testing in screening for CHD. Of particular concern is the extent to which the exercise test improves our ability to recognize coronary disease over that of the routine clinical assessment. In Chapter 3 the logical sequence for establishing a cardiovascular diagnosis was emphasized—medical history, physical examination, and additional tests as necessary to answer *clinically important* questions. The detection of CHD in high-risk asymptomatic individuals is of major concern to our society, since the complications of this disease are the leading causes of death and disability in this country. Clearly, there is a hierarchy of diagnostic tests for detecting significant coronary atherosclerosis, ranging from the low-cost, low-risk clinical assessment to the high-cost, technically complex coronary angiogram. Exactly where the exercise ECG test fits into this hierarchy is the subject of this section.

Exercise Test Accuracy

The diagnostic accuracy of the exercise ECG test can only be discussed within a predefined, clinically relevant framework. If an abnormal or positive ECG response to exercise is to be considered evidence for significant coronary atherosclerosis, the definitions of "abnormal" and "significant" must first be agreed on.

The ECG manifestations of myocardial ischemia have been described in the preceding section. The usual criteria for an "abnormal" ECG response to exercise are summarized in Table 5.10 and generally assume that the resting ECG is within normal limits. In the evaluation of a *diagnostic* test's accuracy it is necessary to have a "gold standard" measure of the disease under consideration. For most published studies coronary angiographic anatomy has been the gold standard for defining coronary heart disease rather than a more direct measure of myocardial ischemia. Unfortunately more direct measures of ischemia are not readily available. Most studies correlating exercise ECG findings with coronary angiography have focused primarily on ≥1 mm horizontal or downsloping ST-segment depression as evidence for an abnormal test response. This is clearly an oversimplification of the diagnostic utility of the exercise ECG test, although a useful starting point for discussion.

The definition of a "significant" coronary obstruction on angiography is also somewhat arbitrary and, unfortunately, is based on an inaccurate standard—visually determined percent diameter stenosis. There is a general consensus, however, that coronary blood flow is not impaired at rest until 90% or greater reduction in cross-sectional area of a major coronary artery occurs. This corresponds to a 75% reduction in luminal diameter. During exercise, when myocardial oxygen demands are increased, a 75% reduction in cross sectional area (50% diameter reduction) may be sufficient to impair oxygen delivery to the myocardium. A number of other factors such as anemia, coronary collaterals, lesion location, and superimposed coronary spasm may complicate the relationship between lesion size and adequacy of myocardial blood flow.

Table 5.10. Usual ECG Criteria for an "Abnormal" Exercise Test[a]

ST-segment depression
    Upsloping: ≥1.5 mm (0.15 mV) depression at 80 msec from J point
    Horizontal: ≥1.0 mm (0.1 mV) depression lasting ≥80 msec
    Downsloping: ≥1.0 mm (0.1 mV) depression at J point
ST-segment elevation
    ≥1.0 mm (0.1 mV) elevation above control resting ST segment
New U-wave inversion during or after exercise

---

[a] Assumes resting ECG is within normal limits.

TABLE 5.11. Treadmill-Angiographic Correlation in 102 patients[a]

Treadmill Test	CAD+ (%)	CAD- (%)	Totals
Abnormal (T+)	36 (80%)	8 (14%)	44
Normal (T-)	9 (20%)	49 (86%)	58
Totals	45 (100%)	57 (100%)	102

[a] Unpublished data from LDS Hospital in Salt Lake City, UT.
CAD+, significant coronary lesions on angiogram; CAD-, no significant coronary lesion on angiogram; T+, positive treadmill test; T-, negative treadmill test.

These confounding factors plus the well-recognized limitations of angiographic assessment of lesion size make any absolute definition of what is a "significant" lesion almost impossible. Nevertheless, it is clinically important to evaluate the exercise ECG test in terms of its ability to differentiate patients with significant coronary disease from those with insignificant lesions or normal arteries. Recent studies using a Doppler catheter to measure coronary flow reserve in partially occluded coronary arteries have demonstrated that exercise ECG testing is an accurate method for detecting physiologically significant coronary lesions (61). Reduced coronary flow reserve may become a better marker for identifying physiologically significant coronary lesions than quantitating lesion size on angiography.

Table 5.11 illustrates a standard 2 × 2 contingency table for determining the diagnostic accuracy of the exercise ECG test using traditional coronary angiographic techniques for identifying disease. Data from 102 patients undergoing diagnostic studies for CHD at the LDS Hospital in Salt Lake City are shown. For this study the angiographic definition of coronary disease (CHD+) was ≥75% reduction in luminal diameter of a major coronary artery. An abnormal exercise ECG response (T+) was defined as ≥0.1 mV horizontal or downsloping ST-segment depression lasting 80 msec or longer. There were 45 patients with angiographically defined CHD of which 36 (80%) had an abnormal exercise ECG response. Nine CHD+ patients (20%) had a normal exercise test (T-). Similarly, there were 57 subjects who did not have significant CHD on coronary angiography (CHD-) of which 49 (86%) had a negative exercise test and 8 (14%) had a positive ECG response to exercise.

The accuracy of the exercise ECG test in this small study is reflected by four parameters: sensitivity (true positives), specificity (true negatives), false positives, and false negatives. The *sensitivity* of a diagnostic test represents the fraction of patients with documented disease who have abnormal test findings (Table 5.12). In the preceding example 80% (36/45) of CHD+ patients had abnormal ST-segment depression during exercise; the sensitivity or true-positive rate was 0.80. The remaining 20% (9/45) of CHD+ patients had a

TABLE 5.12. Sensitivity, Specificity, and Predictive Value of Positive Test

Treadmill Test	CAD+	CAD-	Totals
Abnormal (T+)	TP	FP	TP + FP
Normal (T-)	FN	TN	FN + TN
Totals	TP + FN	FP + TN	TP + FN + FP + TN

Sensitivity = True positives/CAD+ = TP/(TP + FN)
Specificity = True negatives/CAD- = TN/(FP + TN)
Predictive value+ = True positives/all positives = TP/(TP + FP)

TP, true positives; *FP*, false positives; *FN*, false negatives; *TN*, true negatives.

negative exercise test; the *false-negative* rate was 0.20. Note that the true positives and false negatives add up to 1.0 or 100% of the CHD+ population.

In contrast, the *specificity* of a diagnostic test is a measure of the test's ability to rule out disease in nondiseased individuals (Table 5.12). This represents the fraction of nondiseased subjects that have negative test results. In the preceding example 86% (49 of 57) of CHD- patients had a normal ECG response to exercise; the specificity or true-negative rate was 0.86. Eight of 57 CHD- subjects (14%) had abnormal ST-segment depression during exercise; the false-positive rate was 0.14. Note again that the true-negative and false-positive rates add up to 1.0 or 100% of the CHD- population.

Although the preceding data are comparable to some studies published in the literature, there is wide variability in the reported accuracy of the exercise ECG. Gianrossi et al. (62) carried out a meta-analysis of 147 consecutively published studies comparing exercise-induced ST-segment depression with coronary angiographic findings in 24,074 subjects. This analysis revealed a mean sensitivity of 0.68 (range 0.23 to 1.0) and a mean specificity of 0.77 (range 0.17 to 1.0). The authors concluded that the wide variability in test accuracy, unfortunately, could not be explained by the data presented in these studies, but was most likely the result of incomplete reporting of important methodologic factors and clinical descriptors of the test populations. It is also likely that the inherent limitations of coronary angiographic analyses contribute to variability in test accuracy (61).

There are other serious limitations to exercise test-angiographic correlation studies. Most, if not all, patients participating in these studies were symptomatic (or else they would have not undergone angiographic procedures). The applicability of these data to the general population and especially to asymptomatic patients with coronary disease is open to question (63, 64). In addition, the exercise ECG is designed to detect myocardial ischemia, whereas the coronary angiogram identifies anatomic lesions; that is, we're comparing apples and oranges. A more ideal comparison would be to correlate exercise ECG findings with another independent measure of myocardial ischemia, for example, reversible thallium perfusion defects. Unfortunately, other tests of myocardial ischemia are not accurate enough to serve as a "gold standard," and they still rely on the coronary angiogram to define disease. Lastly, the exercise ECG test is limited to those patients whose resting ECGs are normal; patients with resting ECG abnormalities such as left bundle branch block or diffuse ST-T changes need non-ECG-based provocative tests to detect myocardial ischemia.

Having defined the accuracy of the exercise test in terms of sensitivity and specificity, however, permits the identification of two types of errors. The false-negative error refers to the percentage or fraction of "nonischemic" tests obtained in patients with significant coronary disease; in contrast, the false-positive error reflects the percentage of abnormal ischemic tests seen in the nondiseased population. Like sensitivity and specificity, both of these errors depend on the criteria chosen for ischemic ECG abnormalities, as well as the definition of "significant" coronary disease on angiography. Table 5.13 lists the causes of false-negative and false-positive errors.

False-negative errors occur in 20 to 40% of the coronary disease population and depend somewhat on the clinical and angiographic characteristics of the patients being studied. Because the coronary angiogram is used as the gold standard for defining disease, many so-called errors may come from patients with coronary disease who do not, in fact, have myocardial ischemia. This is especially likely to happen in single-vessel coronary disease where adequate collaterals may protect the myocardium from ischemia during exercise. The inclusion of post-MI, post-bypass surgery, or post-PTCA patients in studies of exercise test accuracy also confounds the false-negative error, since these patients may no longer have exercise-induced ischemia even though significant lesions are still seen on coronary angiography. Finally, overestimation of angiographic lesion size may lead to a diagnosis of "significant" disease in patients who do not have ischemic symptoms or manifestations. Fortunately, the prognosis for these "diseased" patients with false-negative exercise test errors is quite good, especially if they are asymptomatic and have adequate exercise tolerance.

There are, however, patients who have significant coronary disease, myocardial ischemia, *and* normal exercise ECG findings. This represents a potentially more serious false-negative error, since these patients are truly misdiagnosed by the exercise test. One reason for this error is failure of the ECG lead system to detect the ischemia that is present. The standard placement of the ECG leads, especially the chest leads, may be inadequate to detect a small ischemic region caused by a single-vessel coronary lesion. Attempts to improve the ECG detection of ischemia by adding additional chest leads (65) or by body surface ECG mapping (66) have received mixed reviews in the exercise testing literature. At the present time there is not much enthusiasm to further explore these cumbersome multilead ECG systems because there are better imaging-based provocative tests for ischemia detection such as radionuclide perfusion and exercise echocardiographic studies. In some cases there may not be sufficient ischemia to affect the ECG waveform, although ischemic abnormalities may still be recognized with other more sensitive imaging techniques. This often occurs in patients with preexisting ECG abnormalities at rest or in those taking beta-blocking drugs.

The false-positive error occurs in 10 to 20% of nondiseased patients undergoing exercise testing. Again, the percentage of errors is related to the characteristics of the population being studied. One group of false-positives are patients with other forms of heart disease who get ischemic ECG changes when

TABLE 5.13. Errors in Exercise Electrocardiography

False-negative errors
    CHD without exercise-induced myocardial ischemia
        Single-vessel disease with adequate collaterals
        Post-MI patients without ischemia
        Post-coronary bypass surgery patients
        Post-coronary angioplasty patients
        Overestimation of angiographic lesions
    Myocardial ischemia without ECG abnormalities
        Inadequate number of ECG leads to detect ischemia
        Preexisting ST-T-wave abnormalities on resting ECG
        Insufficient intensity of ischemia to affect the ECG waveform
False-positive errors
    Myocardial ischemia without significant angiographic coronary lesion
        Underestimation of lesion size on angiogram
        Other conditions that can cause exercise-induced ischemia
            Valvular heart disease with left ventricular hypertrophy
            Hypertensive heart disease
            Cardiomyopathies
            Severe anemia
    ECG changes that mimic ischemia
        Digoxin therapy
        Hypokalemia
        Hyperventilation-induced ST-T-wave changes
        Mitral valve prolapse syndrome
        Pectus excavatum chest wall deformity
        Neurocirculatory (vasoregulatory) asthenia

---

increased myocardial oxygen demands exceed the available supply. Valvular heart disease, severe hypertension with left ventricular hypertrophy, and cardio-myopathies all have been associated with exercise-induced ischemia. Severe anemia may also be associated with ischemic ECG abnormalities caused by in-adequate oxygen-carrying capacity in the coronary blood. In general, patients with these disorders are easily recognized and do not undergo diagnostic exer-cise testing.

Other patients with false-positive abnormalities are those whose ECG find-ings mimic ischemia but who truly do not have myocardial ischemia. Drugs and electrolyte abnormalities are frequent causes of false-positive errors. Digoxin is the major offending drug in this category. The characteristic resting ECG changes in digitalized patients consist of sagging or scooped ST-segment depression with flat to slightly inverted T waves and shortened QT intervals. During exercise the ST segments become more depressed, often meeting crite-ria for ischemia. Unlike true ischemic changes, however, patients on digoxin usually have more ST depression early in exercise and less as the heart rate and workload increase (67). If possible, patients should be taken off digoxin at least 3 weeks prior to diagnostic testing. Alternatively, exercise radionuclide or echo studies are more appropriate methods of detecting ischemic abnormalities.

The major electrolyte abnormality associated with false-positive errors is hypokalemia, frequently the result of excessive diuretic therapy. The resting ECG findings in hypokalemia include the triad of ST depression, flat or slightly inverted T waves, and prominent upright U waves, These same ECG abnor-malities, however, may also be seen in other disorders. Patients with hypo-kalemia are easily recognized by the history of taking diuretics and by the characteristic resting ECG abnormalities. Diagnostic exercise ECG testing should be postponed until the potassium and often accompanying magnesium deficiencies are corrected.

Mitral valve prolapse is a common and often benign abnormality of the mitral valve apparatus with characteristic auscultatory and echocardiographic findings (68). Listening at the cardiac apex in these patients reveals a midsystolic click with or without a late systolic murmur. The murmur is caused by mitral regurgi-tation associated with the prolapsed mitral valve leaflet. For reasons that are unclear, these individuals may have resting and exercise ST-T-wave abnormali-ties that mimic ischemia and vague chest discomfort symptoms. There is also an increased occurrence of cardiac arrhythmias. Mitral prolapse is more common in women and may account for a portion of the false-positive exercise ECG tests observed in women.

Another group of patients with false-positive exercise tests are those with labile, positional, and/or hyperventilation-induced ST-T-wave changes. This also occurs more commonly in women and in people who have a vertically ori-ented frontal plane QRS axis (+90 degrees). Ellestad (69) believes that some of these patients may have ECG changes because of alterations in sympathetic tone and has labeled this phenomenon "Reynolds syndrome." A somewhat related condition associated with sympathetic nervous system imbalance is called neurocirculatory (or vasoregulatory) asthenia. Also known as the hyperkinetic heart syndrome, these patients often complain of dyspnea, palpitations, nervousness, and vague nonanginal chest pains. Friesinger et al. (70) have described exercise ECG abnormalities in these patients that mimic ischemia. Beta-blocking drugs may be effective in eliminating these findings, further supporting a sympathetic nervous system etiology. These patients generally do not experience anginal symptoms during exercise testing, and their ECG abnormalities are minimal.

Application of Bayes' Theorem to Exercise Testing

The sensitivity and specificity of the exercise ECG test define how well the test differentiates patients with angiographically significant coronary disease from individuals without significant disease. As discussed in the preceding section, the presence of false-positive and false-negative errors makes it necessary to interpret exercise test findings in probabilistic terms rather than definitive statements regarding the presence or absence of disease.

The sensitivity (the percent of true positives) is an expression of the probability that a patient with known coronary disease will have an abnormal exercise test. This is expressed as a *conditional probability*, P(T+ | CHD+); i.e., the probability of a positive test *given* the diagnosis of CHD. Similarly the specificity (the precent of true negatives) represents the probability that an individual without significant CHD will have a normal test, P(T- | CHD-). The false-negative probability is expressed as P(T- | CHD+), and the false-positive probability is expressed as P(T+ | CHD-). In all of these probabilities the condition that is known is the angiographic status of the population being tested (i.e., either CHD+ or CHD-), and the unknown is whether the test will be positive or negative. Although these probabilities are useful in characterizing the diagnostic accuracy of the exercise test in known populations, they do not answer the diagnostic questions being asked when an individual whose diagnosis is uncertain undergoes an exercise test.

When a patient undergoes diagnostic exercise testing, the known condition is the outcome of the test, which is either "positive" or "negative" for ischemia based on ECG criteria discussed previously. The unknown is the presence or absence of significant coronary artery disease on angiography. The "posterior" probability, P(CHD+|T+), is called the *predictive value of a positive test* and is the probability that coronary disease is present if the exercise test is abnormal. Similarly, the *predictive value of a negative test* can be expressed as P(CHD- |T-), which is the probability that coronary disease is not present when the test is negative for ischemia.

Bayes' theorem of conditional probabilities states that the predictive value of a test depends on the descriptors of test accuracy (sensitivity and specificity) *and* the prevalence of disease in the population being tested (71). Using the previously described terminology, this important formula can be expressed as follows:

$$P(CHD+|T+) = \frac{P(CHD+) \; P(T+|CHD+)}{P(CHD+) \; P(T+|CHD+) + P(CHD-) \; P(T+|CHD-)}$$

The terms P(CHD+) and P(CHD-) are called *pretest* or *prior* probabilities and reflect the probability of coronary disease (CHD+) or no coronary disease (CHD-) before testing. From a population perspective, these terms define the prevalence of disease in that particular population. Together, they add up to 100% of the population being considered for testing. For example, if 10% of the population has underlying coronary disease, P(CHD+) is 0.1 and P(CHD-) is 0.90.

A similar Bayes' theorem formula can be expressed for the predictive value of a negative test:

$$P(CHD-|T-) = \frac{P(CHD-) \; P(T-|CHD-)}{P(CHD-) \; P(T-|CHD-) + P(CHD+) \; P(T-|CHD+)}$$

These two equations for predictive value can best be understood from a population example illustrated in Table 5.14. In population A only 10% have coronary disease; the predictive value of a positive test is 0.39 or 39% (61% of the positive tests are false positives). The predictive value of a negative test is 0.97 or 97% (only 3% of the negative tests are false negatives). The same test applied to population B, where coronary disease prevalence is 90%, yields strikingly different predictive values. The predictive value of a positive test is now 0.98 (98%) with 2% false positives; the predictive value of a negative test is 0.32 (32%) with 68% false negatives.

From this example it can be seen that the number of false positives and false negatives in a particular population depends greatly on the characteristics of the population. If there is very little disease in a population, there will be few positive tests and most of them will be false positive. In a population of high disease prevalence, however, most of the negative tests will be false negative. In both of these extremes the test adds little to the pretest probability of disease.

How does all this apply clinically to an individual undergoing a diagnostic exercise test? The prevalence of coronary disease in the population is not of immediate concern. What is of interest, however, is the person's pretest probability of coronary disease, P(CHD+). This should be assessed prior to exercise testing from the patient's medical history, which includes coronary risk factors and any symptoms of chest discomfort. In a classic publication Diamond and

TABLE 5.14. The Predictive Value of a Positive and Negative Exercise Test in Two Hypothetical Populations

Test accuracy:

Sensitivity = $P(T+|CHD+)$ = 80%
False negatives = $P(T-|CHD+)$ = 20%
Specificity = $P(T-|CHD-)$ = 86%
False positives = $P(T+|CHD-)$ = 14%

Population A: Coronary disease prevalence of 10%

$P(CHD+)$ = 10%
$P(CHD-)$ = 90%

$$P(CHD+|T+) = \frac{10 \times 80}{(10 \times 80) + (90 \times 14)} = \frac{800}{2060} = 39\%$$

$$P(CHD- \, T-) = \frac{90 \times 86}{(90 \times 86) + (10 \times 20)} = \frac{7740}{7940} = 97\%$$

Population B: Coronary disease prevalence of 90%

$P(CHD+)$ = 90%
$P(CHD-)$ = 10%

$$P(CHD+|T+) = \frac{90 \times 80}{(90 \times 80) + (10 \times 14)} = \frac{7200}{7340} = 98\%$$

$$P(CHD- \, T-) = \frac{10 \times 86}{(10 \times 86) + (90 \times 20)} = \frac{860}{2660} = 32\%$$

Forrester (71) show how age, sex, risk factors, and symptoms can be used to determine an individual's pretest probability of coronary disease. If the patient is asymptomatic, $P(CHD+)$ can also be estimated from updated tables derived from the Framingham heart disease study (72). Although the Framingham equations used to construct these tables predict future occurrence of CHD based on age, sex, and risk factors, Diamond and Forrester (71) suggest that these probabilities can be equated to the actual prevalence of disease in the population. For example, an asymptomatic patient with a 10% probability of developing clinical manifestations of coronary disease in 6 years also has approximately the same likelihood of having angiographically significant disease at the time of study. The use of these tables will be discussed in the next section.

207

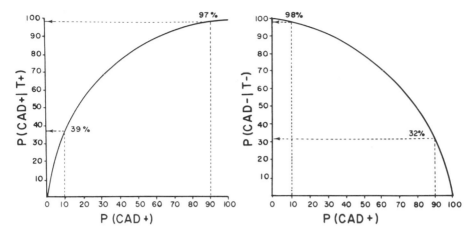

FIGURE 5.17. Bayesian analysis of diagnostic exercise ECG testing. The pretest probabilities are on the abscissa; the predictive values for a positive test *(left)* and negative test *(right)* are on the ordinate. See text.

Figure 5.17 illustrates a graphic representation of Bayes' theorem relating pretest probabilities of coronary disease to the predictive value of a positive or negative test. The actual shape of the two curves depends on the sensitivity and specificity of the test. For this example, sensitivity (80%) and specificity (86%) were chosen to correspond to data presented in Table 5.12. The two examples shown in Table 5.14 are also indicated on the predictive value curves.

It should be apparent that Bayes' theorem is applicable to just about every diagnostic test in medicine. The message of Bayes' theorem is that the diagnostic significance of any positive or negative test result depends on *both* the accuracy of the test (sensitivity and specificity) *and* the patient's pretest probability of disease assessed before the test is performed. For patients with very low pretest risk (<10%), an abnormal test is likely to be false positive; for patients with a very high pretest risk (>75%), a normal test is likely to be false negative. The diagnostic test offers the most information in patients with an intermediate risk for disease. In screening for silent CHD, for example, the exercise test is most useful in patients with significant risk factors (pretest risk >10%). The test is also useful in the differential diagnosis of atypical chest pain symptoms.

The preceding examples using Bayes' theorem represent rather simplistic illustrations of the application of information theory to diagnostic testing. In these examples the exercise test response was dichotomized into "positive" or "negative" categories based on a single criterion of 0.1 mV ST-segment depression. A mathematically more sophisticated version of Bayes' theorem has been described by Diamond et al. (73), which permits calculating the predictive values for different degrees of ST-segment depression. This approach significantly improves the diagnostic content of the exercise ECG when the specific magnitude of the ST-segment depression is used instead of categorical criteria such as 0.1 mV depression. The predictive value of a positive test becomes progressively greater with increasing degrees of ST-segment depression.

Rifkin and Hood (74) have also analyzed exercise test data published in the literature and constructed Bayesian graphs relating pretest probabilities to predictive values for half-millimeter partitions of ST-segment depression. They concluded that the predictive value depends on the degree of ST-segment depression. They also thought that the terms *positive* and *negative* are inappropriate descriptors of exercise test results; instead they suggested that the test be interpreted as a continuum of risk based on the degree of ST-segment abnormality.

These concepts have important implications for relatively low-risk, asymptomatic subjects who are being screened for CHD as part of a wellness program. A positive test in this population should be interpreted only as *another risk factor* for coronary disease that increases that person's probability of disease. If a person with a 10% pretest risk has a degree of ST-segment depression such that the predictive value for CHD becomes 40%, this represents a fourfold increase in risk. Because there is still considerable uncertainty as to diagnosis, another test such as a radionuclide study can be performed with a new pretest risk of 40%.

Patterson et al. (75) have published nomograms for diagnosing CHD based on sequential Bayesian analyses applied to a series of tests. Using this approach, a cost-effective strategy can be designed for each patient undergoing diagnostic testing, beginning with the low-cost risk factor assessment and symptom classification, moving next to the exercise ECG test and then, if necessary, to the more expensive exercise thallium test. Each test result becomes the new pretest probability for the subsequent test until a degree of certainty has been achieved that allows for the appropriate treatment decision to be made.

DIAGNOSTIC EXERCISE ECG TESTING

The decision to perform a diagnostic test in medicine is one that should be made only after careful consideration of the cost:benefit ratio to the patient. This is especially important in cardiovascular medicine, where recent technologic advances have given us a plethora of new and expensive procedures. As these procedures become increasingly more available, there is a natural tendency to want the most up-to-date quantitative assessment for every patient.

Exercise ECG testing, although less expensive than many cardiovascular procedures, has become rather routine in screening for coronary disease. There is some concern that the test may be overutilized, especially in low-risk populations (76). The following sections will focus on the diagnostic applications of exercise testing and indicate those clinical situations where exercise testing is likely to contribute to patient management.

Screening of Asymptomatic Individuals

This is the most controversial area of diagnostic testing because of the false-positive problem. Bayes' theorem implies that the lower the pretest risk, the more likely an abnormal test result is a false positive. Yet, clinical CHD often strikes catastrophically with acute MI or sudden cardiac death as the first manifestations. The challenge in screening the asymptomatic population for coronary disease therefore is to first identify a high-risk subset most likely to benefit from exercise testing.

As discussed earlier in this chapter and summarized in Table 5.2, there are no class I (i.e., universally accepted) indications in the recently published ACC/AHA Task Force Guidelines (5) for exercise testing in healthy, low-risk asymptomatic individuals. The arguments against routine screening in this population were stated by Sox et al. (76) in their cost-effectiveness analysis of exercise testing: (a) most asymptomatic individuals do not have coronary disease; (b) most positive tests in this population are false positive; and (c) most coronary disease in asymptomatic subjects is mild and not likely to be benefited by coronary angiography and revascularization.

Class II indications represent conditions for which exercise ECG testing might be of value in patient management, although there is divergence of opinion among physicians regarding the necessity for such testing. In asymptomatic men over age 40, class II indications include the presence of two or more coronary risk factors (serum cholesterol ≥240 mg/dl, blood pressure ≥160/≥90, cigarette smoking, diabetes mellitus, or family history of CHD with onset under age 55), special occupations (firemen, pilots, police officers, bus or truck drivers, railroad engineers), and sedentary individuals who plan to begin *vigorous* exercise training (5). The new ACC/AHA Guidelines caution that a positive test in an asymptomatic man should be interpreted only as an increase in probability (i.e., predictive value) of coronary disease and not a definitive diagnosis. The potential for costly follow-up testing and other iatrogenic problems resulting from screening should always be considered. A positive test, however, should provide a strong incentive to motivate high-risk individuals to adopt preventive health behaviors to reduce their coronary risk.

In the advent of a positive ECG response to exercise in an asymptomatic man, a reasonable follow-up strategy should be implemented. Although the majority of positive tests in these individuals are false positives, a small subset of patients may require further diagnostic testing. There are basically three categories of abnormal test responses that need to be differentiated: (a) the "high-risk" positive test; (b) the "intermediate-risk" response; and (c) the "low-risk" response. One basis for this classification was published by McNeer et al. (77) in a study of over 1400 patients undergoing exercise testing, coronary angiography, and long-term follow-up. The ability to exercise into stage IV of the Bruce protocol (>10 METs) *or* achieve a maximal heart rate greater than 160 bpm was associated with an excellent prognosis and a low probability for three-vessel or left main coronary disease. In contrast, patients who develop ischemic ECG changes in stage I or II *or* at heart rates less than 120 bpm had a poor prognosis with a high probability of advanced three-vessel or left main coronary disease. The intermediate-risk group fell between these two extremes.

Based on these data, it seems reasonable to recommend coronary angiography for those patients with high-risk abnormalities, since they are more likely to be candidates for revascularization procedures. In contrast, patients with low-risk test findings can be managed conservatively with serial exercise testing and treatment of identifiable coronary risk factors. The intermediate-risk patients should probably undergo further noninvasive testing such as thallium-201 scintigraphy and, if positive, coronary angiography. Patients with three-vessel or left main coronary disease are good candidates for coronary by-pass surgery even when asymptomatic because survival is better with surgery than with medical management (78).

For asymptomatic men and women who have no significant coronary risk factors there is a consensus of opinion that diagnostic exercise testing is of no clinical benefit (5). Not only is the predictive value of a positive test very low in this population, but also positive findings often lead to expensive and unnecessary follow-up testing, including nuclear imaging procedures and coronary angiography. Frequently, exercise tests in these individuals are carried out as part of the battery of screening tests offered in a wellness program designed to assess and modify cardiovascular risk. There is a temptation in these programs to promote the exercise ECG test as an integral and necessary component in the screening of all men and women who reach some arbitrary age cutoff such as 40 years. Furthermore, many participants in wellness programs are requesting these tests for themselves because of the erroneous belief that they are legitimate screening methods for the early detection of coronary disease regardless of pretest risk. It is for these reasons that organizations such as the American Heart Association, the American College of Cardiology, and the American College of Sports Medicine have established guidelines for clinical exercise testing (1, 5). Major efforts are under way to educate health professionals and the general public regarding the proper use of exercise tests and other diagnostic procedures.

Differential Diagnosis of Chest Pain

In the symptomatic population the exercise test is of proven value. Diamond and Forrester (71) have provided data on pretest probabilities for men and women whose symptoms can be categorized as nonanginal chest pain, atypical angina, and typical angina (Table 5.15). In men over age 40 and women over age 60, symptoms of *typical angina* are associated with pretest probabilities of 90% or greater. Exercise testing would not be expected to add significant diagnostic

TABLE 5.15. Pretest Probability (%) of Coronary Disease According to Age, Sex, and Symptoms[a]

Age	Nonanginal Chest Pain		Apical Angina		Typical Angina	
	Men	Women	Men	Women	Men	Women
30–39	5	1	22	4	70	26
40–49	14	3	46	13	87	55
50–59	22	8	59	32	92	79
60–69	28	19	67	54	94	91

[a]Modified from Diamond GA, Forrester JS. N Engl J Med 1979;300:1350–1358.

information in these patients, although testing might be useful in assessing cardiovascular function and disease severity or prognosis.

When symptoms are less than typical for angina, or when typical angina occurs in younger patients, the exercise test can contribute important diagnostic information. Patients able to achieve high workloads and heart rates greater than 85% of their age-predicted maximum without significant chest discomfort or ECG abnormalities are very unlikely to have fixed obstructive coronary lesions as the basis for their symptoms (77). On the other hand, patients who develop anginal symptoms during exercise along with diagnostic ECG changes have a very high probability of underlying CHD. Further treatment decisions can be made after classifying the abnormal responses into low-risk, intermediate-risk, and high-risk abnormalities as defined by McNeer et al. (77). Symptomatic patients with low-risk abnormalities have a good short-term prognosis and can usually be managed conservatively with antianginal medications and risk factor modification. The intermediate-risk and high-risk responders who have exercise-induced angina and ECG abnormalities should proceed directly to coronary angiography and be considered for revascularization therapy.

The subset of symptomatic patients who have exercise-induced chest pain *without* ECG abnormalities is uncommon. Weiner et al. (79) determined that the predictive value of exercise-induced angina for coronary disease was 90% in their series of 302 patients. This is comparable to the predictive value of typical angina by history as reported by Diamond and Forrester (71) for men over age 40 and women over age 60. In Weiner's study (79) exercise-induced angina was also as predictive as ST-segment depression and therefore can be used as another criterion for a positive test. Using a similar management strategy as described for asymptomatic subjects and symptomatic patients with ECG abnormalities, high-risk patients whose symptoms are limiting at low workloads (≤4 METs) and/or low heart rates (<120 bpm) should undergo coronary angiographic studies. Low-risk patients with good exercise tolerance and normal exercise heart rates can be followed with periodic exercise testing and antianginal medication. The intermediate-risk subgroup should undergo further noninvasive testing and, if abnormal, followed by coronary angiography.

Evaluation of Syncope and Palpitations

Although ambulatory ECG monitoring is usually the preferred diagnositc test for evaluating patients with symptoms of syncope, presyncope, or palpitations, exercise testing is useful if the symptoms are clearly exercise related. Many patients complaining of intermittent palpitations do not have significant cardiac findings on history or physical examination; the symptoms can often be related to episodes of sinus tachycardia or simple premature beats. These patients usually do not need sophisticated diagnostic studies.

In patients with known heart disease, especially those with ischemic manifestations, provocative testing to induce arrhythmic events is often necessary for optimal management. Many of these patients are at risk for sudden death and require complex, arrhythmia evaluations that may include exercise testing, ambulatory ECG monitoring, and invasive electrophysiologic testing. Arrhythmias associated with ST-segment abnormalities or left ventricular dysfunction are signs of poor prognosis and indicate the need for aggressive management strategies, including cardiac catheterization and surgical procedures.

There are no particular exercise testing methods that are specifically designed for evaluating arrhythmias or transient conduction defects. The exercise protocol should be chosen according to the patient's ability to exercise and clinical status. The decision to terminate an exercise test because of an arrhythmic event is determined by the characteristics of the arrhythmia and the clinical state of the patient. Serious arrhythmias such as ventricular tachycardia, frequent multifocal PVCs, couplets or R-on-T phenomenon, and rapid atrial tachyarrhythmias require terminating the test prematurely. Isolated PVCs that develop during exercise in the absence of other ECG or clinical abnormalities do not necessitate ending the test.

The interpretation of an exercise test prematurely stopped by an arrhythmia is often difficult. If the patient achieved at least 85% of the predicted maximal heart rate without ST-T changes or chest pain, it is unlikely that the arrhythmia was caused by myocardial ischemia. Terminating the test at lower workloads makes the test inadequate to evaluate ischemia, unless there are already ischemic ECG abnormalities. If the patient has no other manifestations of heart disease and the arrhythmia is not reproducible on repeat testing, it is unlikely that the arrhythmia is clinically important.

Occasionally, serious exercise-induced ventricular arrhythmias have been observed in clinically healthy individuals who have either smoked cigarettes or consumed caffeine-containing drinks prior to testing. Repeat testing after avoiding these noxious stimulants for several hours often fails to reproduce the

TABLE 5.16. Advances in Diagnostic Exercise ECG Testing

---

1. Computer analysis of the exercise ECG (used routinely)
2. Quantitative ST-segment analysis (used routinely)
3. ST/HR slope and index (some clinical use)
4. Multivariate analysis of exercise ECG data (some clinical use)
5. Body surface ECG mapping (research only)

---

arrhythmias, and further cardiac workup usually fails to uncover underlying heart disease.

ADVANCES IN EXERCISE ECG TESTING

In the preceding sections the diagnostic utility of the exercise test was discussed primarily from the viewpoint of ST-T-wave changes visually analyzed in selected ECG leads. This was the state-of-the-art in exercise testing up to the 1970s and is still the primary method of exercise ECG interpretation. Unfortunately, the false-positive and false-negative errors are substantial and limit the use of diagnostic exercise testing in many subsets of patients. In recent years, however, there have been a number of interesting advances in exercise ECG testing that suggest an improved predictive accuracy for detecting CHD. In studies of selected patient populations these advanced methods have resulted in more accurate detection of myocardial ischemia, as well as more quantitative assessment of ischemic size and location. Although most exercise ECG testing laboratories continue to rely primarily on visual ST-T-wave analysis, it is likely that some of these new concepts will eventually become incorporated into clinical exercise testing.

Table 5.16 lists several important advances that have improved the diagnostic accuracy of the exercise test. The applications of computers to ECG signal processing and interpretation are well known. Most manufacturers of exercise test equipment now include basic computerized ECG processing and quantitative ST-segment analysis. Other more sophisticated algorithms have been developed with varying degrees of success. One of these advances, the ST/HR slope method, has generated considerable interest in the literature and is discussed in the following section.

The ST/HR Slope Method

Perhaps the most provocative and controversial of the advanced exercise ECG techniques is the "*ST/HR slope*" method first proposed by Elamin et al. from Leeds, England in 1980 (80). The scientific rationale for this method appeared logical: the degree of ST-segment depression relative to heart rate change should be proportional to the extent of exercise-induced myocardial ischemia. The Leeds group therefore carefully measured the amount of ST-segment depression, 80 msec after the J-point, to the nearest 0.1 mm using a calibrated magnifying glass in each of 13 ECG leads and for each stage of exercise. Plots of ST depression versus heart rate were then derived for each lead. If a statistically significant linear regression line could connect three or more data points beginning at maximal exercise and working backwards, the slope of that line was computed and called the "ST/HR slope" for that lead. The maximal slope from all the leads was defined as the "*maximal ST/HR slope*," and that became the "score" of the exercise test. What was extraordinary about this early work was the perfect correlation found between maximal ST/HR slopes and coronary angiographic results in over 300 patients. Not only did the ST/HR slope values completely differentiate patients without coronary artery disease from those with disease, it also enabled a perfect separation of patients with one-, two-, and three-vessel coronary artery disease (80).

After publication of the Leeds studies there was general disbelief in the exercise testing community, and subsequent attempts to replicate this very provocative study were unsuccessful (81). One of the problems in the follow-up studies, however, was the unwillingness of other investigators to faithfully reproduce the methods of the Leeds group, because it took an average of 2.5 to 3 hours per test to visually analyze the data and manually compute the maximal ST/HR slopes (personal communication). One modification of the very time-consuming methodology was to substitute the "*ST/HR Index*" or $\Delta ST/\Delta HR$, where ΔST is the difference in ST-segment amplitude between rest and maximal exercise, and ΔHR is the change in heart rate (82). This simple substitution, unfortunately, did not improve the diagnostic accuracy of the exercise test for either the presence or the severity of coronary disease compared to the more traditional ST-segment analysis.

The application of computer techniques to exercise ECG interpretation paved the way for more serious attempts to study the ST/HR slope method. This effort was initially carried out by Kligfield and his associates at Cornell University (83). The computerized version of the ST/HR slope method differed from the original Leeds method in several ways. Treadmill exercise testing was substituted for bicycle ergometry. A new treadmill exercise protocol, the "Cornell protocol," described earlier (Table 5.6), was designed to produce smaller heart rate increments between stages, which enabled more accurate calculation of the ST/HR slopes (28). The bipolar lead, CM_5, was used in addition to the standard 12 leads. A commercial treadmill ECG system, the Marquette Case II, was used for data acquisition, and ST-segment amplitudes were measured to the nearest 10 μV, 60 msec after the J-point, from each signal-averaged ECG lead. Figure 5.18 illustrates a commercial version of this computerized program in a patient with definite coronary artery disease.

215

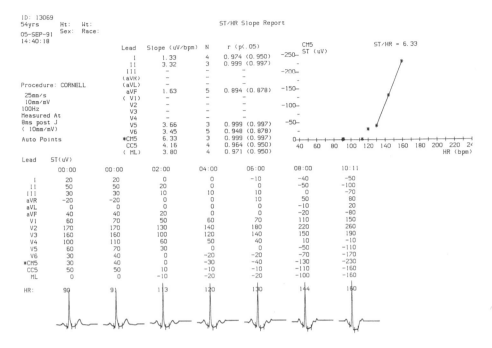

FIGURE 5.18. ST/HR slope report. The maximal ST/HR slope *(graph)* is 6.33 mV/bpm in lead CM$_5$. Representative lead CM$_5$ ECG waveforms from stages of exercise are shown at the bottom.

The normal range for the maximal ST/HR slope was established from a study of 150 subjects who were clinically classified as "low likelihood of coronary artery disease," although they did not undergo coronary angiography (84). The upper limit of normal, 2.4 µV/beats/min, was chosen to include 95% of these normal subjects (i.e., specificity = 95%). Using this partition, 95% of 150 patients with a "high likelihood of coronary artery disease" (based on either coronary angiographic findings of symptoms of angina pectoris) had maximal ST/HR slopes >2.4 µV/beats/min (i.e., sensitivity = 95%). In this population the sensitivity of standard ST-segment criteria was only 68%, comparable to previously published data (84). Equally impressive, moreover, was the test sensitivity relative to the extent of coronary artery disease. Although perfect separation of one-, two-, and three-vessel disease was not seen, 89% of those with one-vessel disease, 94% of those with two-vessel disease, and 100% of three-vessel disease patients had maximal ST/HR slopes >2.4 µV/beats/min. In addition, maximal ST/HR slopes ≥6 µV/beats/min identified three-vessel disease with a sensitivity of 89% and specificity of 88% (83). Thus the accuracy of the ST/HR slope method in this study was far superior to the standard methods for interpreting exercise ECG data.

216

Unfortunately, the above studies from one group of investigators are limited by the rather small database used to establish the accuracy of the method and by the lack of an independent "gold standard" for myocardial ischemia other than symptoms and coronary angiographic findings in a small subset of patients. A number of conflicting studies have appeared in the literature that disputes the Cornell data (85, 86). It is expected that future studies will clarify the utility of this interesting new method of ECG analysis for routine diagnostic exercise testing. Until such studies are reported, it is reasonable to conclude that the ST/HR slope method is a promising but unproved advance over more traditional methods of exercise ECG interpretation. Although several commercial exercise equipment manufacturers now include this computerized method as an optional module, it is important to continue analyzing exercise ECG data using standard criteria for ischemia until such time as the computerized methods have been adequately validated.

STRESS IMAGING: ALTERNATIVES TO THE EXERCISE ECG

There are a number of limitations to exercise ECG testing that have led to the development of newer and more expensive diagnostic techniques for detecting myocardial ischemia (Table 5.17). As already discussed, the ECG response to exercise suffers from a relative lack of sensitivity and specificity in many clinical situations where ischemia is suspected. In particular, patients with resting ECG abnormalities such as left bundle branch block, left ventricular hypertrophy, or diffuse ST-T-wave changes are poor candidates for exercise ECG studies because the baseline ECG changes enhance the likelihood of false-positive ST-segment responses to exercise. In these patients stress imaging using nuclear or ultrasound techniques are clearly preferable because the marker for ischemia (i.e., segmental wall motion abnormality) is more sensitive and independent of the ECG. In addition, there are patients who are unable to exercise because of

TABLE 5.17. Limitations of the Exercise ECG Test

1. ECG evidence of right or left ventricular hypertrophy
2. Bundle branch blocks or other intraventricular conduction defects
3. Previous myocardial infarction patterns on resting ECG
4. Hyperventilation-induced ST-T-wave changes
5. Drug effects on the ECG (e.g., quinidine, digoxin, beta-blockers)
6. Electrolyte abnormalities (e.g., hypokalemia)
7. Wolff-Parkinson-White preexcitation syndrome
8. Artificial pacemaker rhythms
9. Nonspecific ST-T-wave changes on resting ECG

advanced age, neurologic abnormalities, or orthopedic abnormalities. In these patients pharmacologic, stress-imaging techniques have been developed to detect suspected myocardial ischemia. It is beyond the scope of this chapter to comprehensively review these different imaging techniques. A comparison of several nuclear and ultrasound techniques are briefly discussed in the following section.

Thallium Perfusion Imaging With Exercise

Thallium 201 (^{201}TI), a potassium analog, is a perfusion-limited radioactive tracer that is distributed within the myocardium in proportion to myocardial blood flow and cellular viability (87). In normally perfused heart muscle there is rapid accumulation of thallium in an evenly distributed pattern throughout the myocardium when imaged with a scintillation camera. Because ischemic myocardium is underperfused, it appears as a defect or "cold spot" surrounded by normally perfused muscle. In exercise-induced myocardial ischemia the defect is usually transient; after several hours there is delayed uptake of thallium into the previously ischemic zones and efflux of thallium from the nonischemic zones. Repeat imaging during this "redistribution" phase will show a uniform distribution of the radiotracer within the myocardium. Ischemic myocardium is thus differentiated from scar tissue (old MI) which is identified by a persistent defect on the redistribution scans.

In this procedure symptom-limited exercise testing is carried out on a bicycle ergometer or treadmill. At approximately one minute before maximal exercise is reached, 2 mCi ^{201}TI is administered intravenously. Immediately after exercise the patient is placed supine and imaging is begun. Images are obtained in several views, including the anterior, left anterior oblique, and left lateral positions. Repeat nuclear scanning is done 3 to 4 hours later to obtain the redistribution patterns. Interpretation involves both visual analyses of the immediate and delayed images as well as computer-processed quantification of regional ^{201}Tl activity and kinetics. Recently, more advanced imaging technology, single photon emission computerized tomography (SPECT), has yielded images with higher contrast resolution for more accurate localization and sizing of perfusion defects. Figure 5.19 illustrates immediate and redistribution thallium scans in a patient with coronary artery disease. In 1993 the average costs of thallium exercise tests were $1200 to $1800.

Abnormal findings on imaging include (a) reversible perfusion defect (cold spot)—ischemia; (b) fixed defect (present on delayed images)—scar; (c) defect present but smaller on redistribution images—indicates viable myocardium intermixed with scar tissue. For visual analysis of ^{201}TI images, the sensitivity for CHD detection in patients with chest pain symptoms is 80 to 85%, and the specificity is 75 to 80% (87). Using quantitative, computer-assisted methods, the sensitivity and specificity are improved to approximately 90%. SPECT

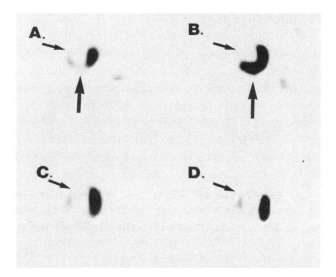

FIGURE 5.19. Immediate postexercise and redistribution thallium scans in a patient with coronary artery disease. **A.** Midventricular short-axis tomographic view immediately after exercise. Note marked reduction in count activity in the anterior wall and septum *(small arrow)* and inferior wall *(large arrow)*. **B.** Corresponding view after 3-hour delay. Note the persistent defect in the anterior wall and septum *(small arrow)* representing infarction *(scar)* and the redistribution of thallium in the inferior wall *(large arrow)* demonstrating reversible ischemia. **C.** Midventricular horizontal long-axis tomographic view immediately after exercise. Note the marked reduction in count activity in the anterior wall and septum *(small arrow)* **D.** Corresponding view after 3-hour delay showing the same defect in the anterior wall *(small arrow)* representing infarction.

imaging has a sensitivity of 90 to 95% and a specificity of 70 to 80% (87). High-risk ^{201}Tl abnormalities for left main or multivessel disease include (a) multiple reversible defects; (b) defects in two or three major arterial distributions; (c) transient left ventricular cavity dilatation; and (d) increased lung ^{201}Tl uptake, which is indicative of left ventricular failure.

Thallium Perfusion Imaging With Dipyridamole Infusion

In those people who are unable to exercise, dipyridamole infusion can be used to create an imbalance of myocardial oxygen supply and demand; the resulting ischemic zone can be detected with ^{201}Tl perfusion imaging (88). Dipyridamole potentiates the action of adenosine, a potent coronary vasodilator produced in the body, and leads to a "coronary steal" effect when significant coronary obstructive lesions are present. The adenosine-induced vasodilation of normal coronary arteries shunts blood away from regions of myocardium that are supplied by diseased arteries, thus creating ischemic zones. In other words the drug

219

robs oxygenated blood from poorly perfused areas and gives it to well-perfused myocardium (i.e., a "reverse Robin Hood" effect). Candidates for this procedure include the elderly, as well as patients with severe arthritis, claudication, cerebrovascular disease; and other orthopedic abnormalities that limit exercise. Pulmonary patients taking xanthine bronchodilators (e.g., aminophylline) are not suitable for dipyridamole testing because these drugs block adenosine receptors in the body.

The testing procedure involves the intravenous administration of 0.56 mg/kg dipyridamole over four minutes followed by 2.0 mCi ^{201}TI given three minutes later (88). The immediate images are obtained shortly thereafter, and the delayed images, 3 to 4 hours later. Aminophylline (80 to 240 mg) may be given IV if necessary to counteract the ischemic and other side effects of dipyridamole. The diagnostic accuracy, safety, and costs are similar to those for exercise thallium testing.

Thallium Perfusion Imaging With Adenosine Infusion

Although still an experimental technique, this procedure has some advantages over dipyridamole-thallium stress testing (89). Adenosine administered intravenously has a rapid onset of action with near maximal coronary vasodilation and a short half-life, thereby allowing a more consistent pharmacologic effect in most patients. The initial drug dose of 50 µg/kg/min is increased in stepwise increments to a maximal rate of 140 µg/kg/min. Early and delayed images are obtained as is done with dipyridamole testing. The disadvantage of this technique is that patients experience frequent minor side effects such as chest and jaw pain, flushing, and headache, which last only for a few minutes. The costs are likely to be similar to those for other thallium stress-testing procedures.

Exercise Echocardiography

Another imaging modality that has utility in the detection of exercise-induced myocardial ischemia is echocardiography (90). The most sensitive and specific ultrasound markers for ischemia (or infarction) using this technology are regional wall motion abnormalities (dyssynergy). Three forms of dyssynergy have been described: (a) hypokinesis, reduction of systolic motion; (b) akinesis, absence of systolic motion; and (c) dyskinesis, paradoxical (i.e., outward) systolic motion. Reduced regional systolic wall thickening, left ventricular cavity dilation, and Doppler signs of global systolic or diastolic dysfunction may also reflect evidence for myocardial ischemia or infarction.

Echocardiographic images are obtained at rest and immediately after symptom-limited exercise. The exercise activity is usually performed in the supine position using a specially designed bicycle ergometer imaging table. Segmental wall motion abnormalities induced by exercise are considered to be ischemia and are the primary findings of interest to the physician. The sensitivity and specificity of this technique for coronary artery diseases detection are both approximately 85%. Satisfactory studies require an adequate exercise performance by the patient. Mild ischemic abnormalities that recover soon after exercise is terminated may be missed with this technique.

Dipyridamole Stress Echocardiography

Dipyridamole can be used as an alternative to exercise in stress echocardiography studies (88, 91). The intravenous dose is 0.56 mg/kg over four minutes, followed by four minutes of no drug, and then 0.28 mg/kg for two additional minutes. Echocardiographic images are recorded continuously during infusion and for ten minutes afterwards; multiple views are obtained to look for regional wall motion abnormalities. A positive test is defined as the detection of transient dyssynergy that was absent or of a lesser degree during baseline exam. The sensitivity of this test is approximately 53% for single-vessel disease and 88% for multivessel disease. The specificity is approximately 95%. This procedure has a significant cost advantage over dipyridamole [201]TI imaging. In addition, images are obtained in real time by the physician doing and interpreting the test. Delayed images are not required as they are for [201]TI imaging.

Dobutamine Stress Echocardiography

Dobutamine is predominately a beta$_1$ sympathetic nervous system agonist but with some β_2 and α adrenergic effects on the cardiovascular system. Myocardial oxygen requirements are raised as a result of drug-induced increases in contractility, systolic blood pressure, and heart rate. The procedure involves the intravenous administration of dobutamine, beginning at 2.5 to 5.0 µg/kg/min with increases of 5 µg/kg/min every 3 to 5 minutes until 20 to 40 µg/kg/min are given or until systolic blood pressure increases over 220 mm Hg, diastolic blood pressure increases over 120 mm Hg, or until serious ventricular arrhythmias occur (88, 91, 92). Adverse effects can be reversed with intravenous propranolol (0.1 mg/kg).

Echocardiographic images are performed continuously during and for 20 minutes after the dobutamine infusion, looking in various anatomic views for new wall motion abnormalities. The accuracy of the test based on a summary of 524 patients from 7 published studies in 1991 and 1992 suggests a sensitivity of 88% and a specificity of 81% (92). Although dobutamine has a greater arrhythmogenic potential compared to dipyridamole, the costs are comparable, and, unlike dipyridamole, the drug can be used in patients taking xanthine type bronchodilators.

RISK ASSESSMENT IN CORONARY HEART DISEASE

In patients with known CHD the question is no longer the presence or absence of disease but the prognosis for future morbidity and mortality from the disease. This is the task of *risk stratification*, and it is an important prerequisite for effective preventive and therapeutic interventions. There are many different testing strategies for identifying high-risk and low-risk patients. The following discussion addresses three clinical areas of interest where exercise testing provides valuable prognostic information: (a) risk assessment in asymptomatic individuals; (b) assessment of CHD severity; and (c) risk stratification after acute MI. In each of these three areas various management decisions are likely to be influenced by the results of the exercise test.

Risk Assessment in Asymptomatic Populations

From Bayes' theorem it was shown that the predictive value of exercise-induced ST-segment abnormalities was dependent on the pretest or prior probability of CHD (75). In apparently healthy, low-risk individuals the predictive value of isolated ST-segment depression for diagnosis of CHD is quite low, since the majority of positive tests are false positives. From the prognostic perspective, however, the question concerns whether a person with a positive test is at greater risk for future coronary disease events (MI, angina pectoris, or sudden death) than someone with negative results.

There have been many reports investigating the prognostic value of exercise test findings in clinically healthy individuals (76, 93–95). Although these studies suggest that isolated ST-segment depression without angina may be an independent risk factor for future coronary disease events, the clinical relevance of these findings to patient care is uncertain (76). This uncertainty has great financial implications for the growing "wellness" industry, since exercise ECG testing is often carried out in the workup of asymptomatic participants. The controversy concerns the concept of *silent ischemia*, the objective evidence of myocardial ischemia in the absence of symptoms (34, 96).

There are several aspects to this controversy. First, not all patients with asymptomatic coronary artery disease have silent ischemic episodes. They may have adequate coronary collateralization that prevents ischemia from occurring, or they may be post-MI patients without ischemic manifestations (e.g., single-vessel disease). Second, most ischemic-looking ST-segment responses to exercise testing in otherwise healthy, asymptomatic adults are not ischemia but are false positives. When healthy, symptomatic middle-aged men with positive exercise tests have undergone coronary angiography, only 2.5 to 10% (average, 4%) had significant coronary artery disease (96). In asymptomatic women, moreover, it is likely that the percentage of abnormal exercise tests that are true positive is much lower. The challenge therefore is to identify a high-risk subset of asymptomatic people for whom exercise testing to identify silent ischemia is cost-effective. One possible strategy is to restrict asymptomatic exercise testing to men over age 40 with two or more major coronary risk factors (96). This was a "class II" indication for stress testing in the ACC/AHA guidelines discussed earlier (i.e., considerable difference of opinion as to its value) (see Table 5.2) (5).

From an epidemiologic perspective, however, studies show that asymptomatic men with positive exercise tests do have increased CHD morbidity and mortality during long-term follow-up (93–95). Giagnoni et al. (94) observed that the "positive" test responders had a risk ratio for future cardiac events of 5.5:1 when compared to "negative" responders. In the Lipid Research Clinics follow-up study (97), the 8-year mortality was 11.2% in asymptomatic "positive" responders compared to 1.2% with negative exercise test results. Comparable data for women are not yet available.

The management of asymptomatic men with ST-segment depression on routine exercise testing is also very controversial. Certainly the majority of these individuals do not need to be followed up with expensive coronary angiographic studies. What about slightly less expensive thallium perfusion studies? It may be reasonable to follow up asymptomatic positive exercise ECG tests with exercise thallium studies to identify the subset of patients with silent ischemia. These persons would then be candidates for preventive interventions that might include diet and drug therapy for hyperlipidemia, smoking cessation, and possibly antiischemic therapy with beta-blocking agents. An alternative, less expensive strategy that avoids the problem, however, is to restrict screening exercise ECG testing to individuals who have a higher pretest likelihood for coronary disease (e.g., men with two or more coronary risk factors) to minimize the false-positive error. This would reduce the number of unnecessary follow-up thallium studies, coronary angiograms, and revascularization procedures.

Assessment of Severity of Coronary Disease

The diagnosis of CHD is only the first step in the process of developing an effective management plan. Many of the techniques used for diagnostic studies including the history, physical examination, noninvasive procedures, and invasive investigations, also provide information regarding disease severity. The ECG and hemodynamic and clinical responses to exercise testing can be used to distinguish high-risk from low-risk patients (98–101). Table 5.18 lists exercise test abnormalities that have been associated with severe CHD, usually defined angiographically as left main or triple-vessel disease. A test is considered to be strongly indicative of severe disease when one or more of these findings are detected. Such abnormalities are usually the basis for recommending coronary angiographic studies to further define the extent of disease and the potential for revascularization.

Table 5.18. Exercise Test Parameters Predictive of Severe Coronary Heart Disease

---

ECG parameters
  ST-segment depression
    Marked (≥ 3 mm) ST-segment depression
    Early onset (i.e., at workloads ≤ 4 METs)
    Downsloping ST-segment configuration
    ST-segment depression lasting ≥ 7 minutes during recovery
    Multiple-lead ST-segment depression (global ischemia)
  ST-segment elevation (indicator of transmural ischemia)
  U-wave inversion
Low maximal workload (≤ 4 METs)
Abnormal blood pressure response
  Inadequate blood pressure rise with exercise
  Exertional hypotension
Chronotropic incompetence
Anginal symptoms during exercise

The predictors of disease severity, listed in Table 5.18, include not only ECG parameters of ischemia but also hemodynamic parameters that better characterize the functional consequences of disease. Global ST-segment abnormalities are characterized by the simultaneous occurrence of ST-segment depression in both anterior and inferior ECG leads. Blumenthal et al. (98) found that almost 60% of their patients with global ischemia had left main coronary artery disease. Marked ST-segment depression occurring early in exercise and persisting long after exercise ended was also predictive of severe disease. Ribisl et al. (102) found that the amount of ST depression during exercise testing was the most powerful indicator of disease severity, with ≥2 mm depression having a sensitivity of 55% and specificity of 80% for triple-vessel plus left main disease.

Morrow et al. (103) have developed a statistical model for identifying high- and low-risk patients for subsequent cardiovascular events using clinical and exercise test data. A score was computed from only four variables as follows: 5 × (congestive heart failure *or* digoxin use [yes = 1, no = 0]) + exercise-induced ST-segment depression (in mm) + change in systolic blood pressure score − METs. The exercise-associated changes in systolic blood pressure score were defined as follows: 0 points = increase >40 mm Hg; 1 point = 31 to 40 mm Hg; 2 points = 21 to 30 mm Hg; 3 points = 11 to 20 mm Hg; 4 points = 0 to 11 mm Hg; and 5 points = decrease below standing systolic blood pressure taken before testing. From this prediction equation three risk groups were categorized: low risk = <−2; moderate risk = −2 to +2; high risk = > +2. Of 2546 male veterans evaluated,

77% were categorized as low risk with an annual cardiac mortality rate <2%; 18% were defined as moderate risk with an annual mortality of 7%; and 6% were identified as high risk with an annual mortality of 15%.

Okin et al. (104), using a simplified version of the maximal ST/HR slope limited to leads V_5, V_6, and aVF, found that a peak slope of more than 6.0 mV/bpm identified three-vessel coronary disease (predictive value, 93%) better than standard ST-segment criteria (predictive value, 50%). These data support the use of more sophisticated exercise ECG analyses to identify severe CHD.

Exercise-induced ST-segment elevation in the absence of infarct Q waves on the baseline ECG not only indicates severe transmural ischemia but also predicts the location of the ischemic process more accurately than ST-segment depression (105). The reason for better localization relates to the proximity of the epicardium to the body surface ECG electrodes. ST-segment elevation confined to leads II, III, and a VF strongly suggests right coronary artery lesions; ST elevation in leads V_{1-3} is predictive of left anterior descending disease. It should be remembered, however, that coronary artery spasm also can cause transmural ischemia and ST elevation in the absence of severe coronary atherosclerosis. Exercise-induced ST elevation in leads with pathologic Q waves in a post-MI patient is usually not an ischemic finding but a reflection of underlying myocardial-wall motion abnormality (106).

Exercise test parameters of severe myocardial dysfunction include low maximal workload (≤4 METs), inadequate blood pressure rise, and exertional hypotension. Although not specific for coronary disease, these parameters are often associated with severe ischemic abnormalities and are predictive of increased morbidity and mortality. Exertional hypotension has recently been redefined as a fall in systolic blood pressure during exercise below the standing preexercise value (106). This abnormality in conjunction with exercise-induced ischemia was associated with a threefold increased risk for new cardiac events (except in recent post-MI patients). Failure of the systolic blood pressure to rise above 130 to 140 mm Hg during exercise may also be prognostically important. Bruce et al. (95) found this to be an important predictor of sudden death in the Seattle Heart Watch study.

An inadequate heart rate response to exercise, called *chronotropic incompetence* by Ellestad and Wan (107), may also be indicative of severe coronary disease, although patients with idiopathic sinus node dysfunction also have this response in the absence of coronary disease. In a study by McNeer et al. (77) patients with maximal heart rates below 120 bpm had a much greater mortality than those whose heart rates exceeded 160 bpm. Unfortunately, it may be that anginal symptoms or myocardial dysfunction was the limiting factor in many patients rather than intrinsic sinus node disease, as suggested by Hammond et al. (109).

Finally, anginal symptoms occurring at low workloads have been correlated with severe CHD and increased morbidity (109). Weiner et al. (79) found that exercise test angina was as sensitive a predictor of cardiac mortality and multivessel disease as ST-segment depression alone. This is an important observation, since many patients may be limited by anginal symptoms during exercise testing before diagnostic ECG changes have occurred. These patients should not be pushed beyond symptoms of moderate severity.

Risk Stratification After Acute MI

Exercise testing soon after acute MI is now routine except in patients who are unstable or who have severe left ventricular dysfunction. The testing protocols and procedures vary considerably, however, depending on physician preference and the clinical characteristics of the patient. In many situations the thallium stress test has replaced ECG stress testing because of improved accuracy, especially in the presence of baseline ECG abnormalities. This section reviews current recommendations for predischarge (or early postdischarge) risk stratification after acute MI. An excellent and comprehensive review of post-MI risk stratification beginning with the CCU admission and including early post-MI care (days 1 to 5), as well as predischarge recommendations, has been published by Krone (110).

The prognosis after acute MI is directly related to three factors (110): (a) the amount of left ventricular dysfunction; (b) the presence and extent of residual myocardial ischemia; (c) and the degree of electrical instability of the myocardium. The purpose of predischarge testing is to identify two subsets of patients. At one extreme, testing is carried out to identify patients at high risk for death or reinfarction who need aggressive management strategies, including revascularization procedures, complex antiarrhythmic therapies, and other costly interventions (including possible heart transplantation). At the other end of the spectrum, testing is used to identify low-risk patients who have an excellent prognosis and who only need standard therapy to modify coronary risk factors and reduce the long-term risk of recurrent coronary disease events. Testing for electrical instability and risk for sudden arrhythmic death usually involves the identification of patients who have severe left ventricular dysfunction and malignant or potentially malignant ventricular arrhythmias. Left ventricular dysfunction is detected by various imaging techniques to quantitate ejection fractions and regional wall motion abnormalities. The potential for malignant ventricular arrhythmias is evaluated by one or more of the following techniques: signal-averaged electrocardiography, ambulatory ECG monitoring, and occasionally invasive electrophysiologic studies (see Chapter 3). Testing for "myocardium at risk" or jeopardized myocardium (which indicates risk for recurrent myocardial infarction or other unstable coronary disease events) involves stress testing to detect myocardial ischemia.

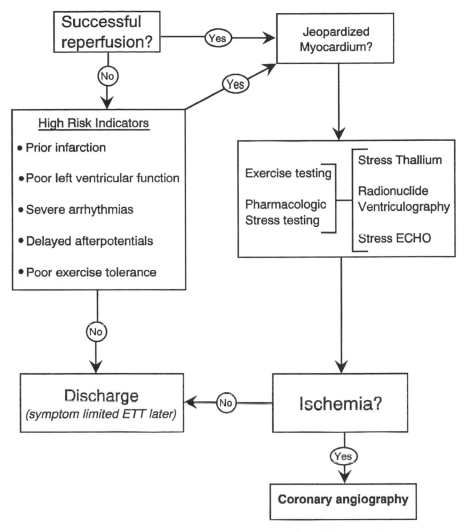

FIGURE 5.20. Predischarge post-MI risk stratification. (Modified from Krone RJ. Ann Intern Med 1992;116:223–237.)

Figure 5.20 illustrates the predischarge risk stratification algorithm proposed by Krone (110), which is based on American College of Cardiology/American Heart Association Joint Task Force recommendations (111). The first decision point asks whether the patient has been successfully reperfused. Essentially all patients treated with thrombolytic agents should undergo predischarge assessment for jeopardized myocardium. Various imaging techniques looking at regional wall motion, ejection fraction, and myocardial perfusion can be used. Provocative maneuvers include exercise, adenosine infusion, and dipyridamole.

227

In the past, when exercise testing was carried out before discharge at 6 to 10 days, many physicians recommended a submaximal protocol that restricted the patient to ≤5 METs work or ≤110 to 120 bpm heart rate. Recent studies have demonstrated the safety and improved detection of high-risk patients using predischarge symptom-limited exercise testing (112). Patients unable to exercise are candidates for pharmacologic stress testing. The same recommendations apply to patients reperfused with angioplasty techniques. If ischemia is found using one of these imaging modalities, then the patient should undergo coronary angiography to assess the potential for coronary revascularization.

Patients who have not been treated with thrombolytic therapy or PTCA should be assessed for clinical indicators of high risk (Fig. 5.20). These include prior myocardial infarction, poor left ventricular function, severe arrhythmias, and poor exercise tolerance. If one or more of these are present or if the patient has a positive signal-averaged ECG, further testing for jeopardized myocardium should be carried out as described above. Coronary angiography is indicated if ischemic abnormalities are detected. If none of these high-risk indicators are present, however, the patient can be discharged with recommendations to undergo symptom-limited exercise testing at a later date. The ideal time for this testing is three weeks post-MI (113). Bad prognostic indicators during symptom-limited exercise testing include (a) inability to achieve a treadmill workload of 4 METs, (b) inability to achieve a peak systolic blood pressure of ≥110 mm Hg, (c) a decrease in systolic blood pressure below baseline, (d) ≥1 mm ST-segment depression, and (e) exercise-induced angina pectoris. Such findings should be followed up with coronary angiography and revascularization if necessary. Thallium stress testing should be substituted for ECG testing if baseline ECG abnormalities preclude adequate recognition of ischemic ST-T-wave changes. Patients with recurrent chest pain or other indicators of ischemia during hospitalization should undergo coronary angiography as soon as possible, preferably before hospital discharge.

In addition to assessing the risk for recurrent coronary disease events, symptom-limited exercise testing carried out after hospital discharge has been shown to have important psychologic benefits to many patients and their families (114). After the physician reviews and discusses the exercise test findings with the patient and family, there is likely to be considerably less anxiety and a restoration of confidence in performing physical activities at home. In this sense the test results have therapeutic value in addition to diagnostic and prognostic value.

FUNCTIONAL EXERCISE TESTING

As discussed earlier in this chapter, the functional assessment of the cardiovascular system is often important in making appropriate diagnostic, prognostic, and treatment decisions. The questions are not so much concerned with the specific etiology of disease but rather the functional consequences of the disease or illness. Such questions are often asked during the workup of patients with dyspnea on exertion, easy fatigability, weakness, and other symptoms of decreased exercise tolerance. The patient's response to exercise testing may be helpful in differentiating cardiovascular impairment from respiratory, skeletal muscle, and other causes of exercise limitations. The rehabilitation of patients with cardiovascular and other disabling diseases requires functional testing to develop safe and effective exercise prescriptions. Finally, there are increasing numbers of patients with end-stage heart disease who are being evaluated for various new heart failure therapies, including better drugs, cardiac assist devices, and heart transplantation. Quantitative measures of functional capacity are important determinants of these therapies and follow-up. This section discusses practical methods for measuring functional capacity in the exercise laboratory. The physiologic concepts of exercise are discussed in Chapter 2.

The term "cardiovascular functional capacity" is, in a sense, a misnomer, since the exercise test response is more an assessment of the patient's total physical work capacity than an isolated test of cardiovascular function. The ability to perform physical work on a treadmill or bicycle requires the coordinated interactions of the respiratory system, central nervous system, hematologic system, skeletal muscles, and cardiovascular system. An impairment within one or more of these organ systems often results in a decreased physical work capacity.

Methods for Functional Exercise Testing

Gas Analysis Techniques

There are several different methods for quantitating ventilation and respiratory gas exchange parameters during exercise testing. Most clinical systems in use today rely on breath-by-breath analysis techniques because they provide the most comprehensive measures of the metabolic response to exercise. The details of these techniques are quite sophisticated and will not be reviewed here. Interested readers are referred to several excellent references on this subject (115, 116).

Three basic parameters are continuously monitored at the mouthpiece during a breath-by-breath exercise study: (a) percent O_2, (b) percent CO_2, and (c) ventilatory air flow. A nonrebreathing valve is connected to the mouthpiece to prevent mixing of inspired and expired air. Oxygen and carbon dioxide gas analyzers are usually incorporated in a "metabolic cart" designed specifically for functional exercise testing. Alternatively, a mass spectrometer can be used to analyze the gas concentrations at the mouthpiece. Respiratory volumes are computed by integrating the air flow signals from a pneumotachometer placed on the expiratory port of the mouthpiece, although some laboratories measure both inspiratory and expiratory volumes. Breath-by-breath volumes of O_2 intake, CO_2 output, and expired ventilation are obtained by integrating the continuous variables over the time course of inspiration (for O_2) and expiration (for CO_2 and $\dot{V}_E$). Average minute volumes are derived from the breath-by-breath data multiplied by the respiratory rate. The gas volumes obtained under ambient conditions are then converted to standard (STPD) conditions using the appropriate conversion equations (116).

Exercise Test Protocols

Exercise protocols were discussed earlier in this chapter. The choice of protocol for functional testing is often determined by the purpose of the test and the exercise tolerance of the person being tested. In evaluating patients with limited exercise tolerance both bicycle and treadmill protocols have been used extensively. The rate of workload progression is somewhat arbitrary, although, as previously discussed, the optimal exercise duration for functional assessment (on the bicycle, at least) is 8 to 17 minutes (22). Bicycle work is quantitated in watts or kpm/min (1 watt ≈ 6 kpm/min). The initial workload is usually 20 to 25 watts (free-wheeling); the workload is then increased by 15 to 25 watts every 2 to 3 minutes until maximal exertion is reached. Alternatively, for electronically braked bicycle ergometers, the workload can be computer controlled, and a ramp protocol (e.g., 10 watts/min) is often utilized. The modified Naughton protocol is recommended for treadmill exercise testing in the heart failure population (27). This protocol is designed to increase the workload by approximately 1 MET (3.5 ml O_2/kg/min) for each 2- or 3-minute stage. Steady-state exercise protocols have also been used in heart failure research studies but have yet to be standardized for clinical testing. More aggressive protocols are used for testing healthy individuals and athletes.

In the heart disease population continuous ECG monitoring and frequent blood pressure measurements are standard requirements during functional testing regardless of the protocol. Hand signals (e.g., 1 to 5 fingers for perceived intensity and thumbs down to stop) are used by the patient during treadmill testing, since verbal communication is usually not possible with the mouthpiece apparatus. Symptoms at maximal exercise that terminate the test include muscle fatigue, exhaustion, extreme dyspnea, and lightheadedness. Cardiac arrhythmias are usually not an indication to stop the test unless sustained tachyarrhythmias develop or the physician monitoring the test feels that further exercise is hazardous. A decrease in systolic blood pressure (below resting pressure) is also a sign of severe left ventricular (LV) dysfunction and an indication to stop the test. Many patients with congestive heart failure, however, fail to significantly increase their systolic blood pressure during exercise because of their LV dysfunction.

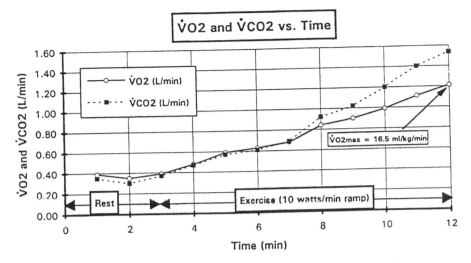

FIGURE 5.21. Minute averages of oxygen uptake ($\dot{V}O_2$) and carbon dioxide output ($\dot{V}CO_2$) as a function of time during a maximal exercise test in a patient with congestive heart failure. A bicycle protocol with a 10-watt/min ramp is used. Carbon dioxide output parallels oxygen uptake until minute 7 when it increased more rapidly because of the added anaerobic component.

A Clinical Example

Figure 5.21 illustrates minute averages of O_2 uptake (L/min) and CO_2 (L/min) output from a patient with chronic congestive cardiomyopathy exercising to maximal exertion on a 10-watt/min ramp bicycle protocol. The patient is sitting at rest for the first three minutes before beginning the ramp protocol. During the first half of exercise (aerobic phase), $\dot{V}O_2$ and $\dot{V}CO_2$ increase in parallel; during the second half, $\dot{V}CO_2$ increases more steeply reflecting the additional CO_2 produced from anaerobic metabolism. The highest $\dot{V}O_2$ at maximal exercise ($\dot{V}O_{2max}$) was 16.5 ml/kg/min (1.2 L/min) and occurred at a workload of 87 watts. Exercise was limited in this patient by generalized exhaustion, including leg muscle fatigue and severe dyspnea. Although some investigators insist that a $\dot{V}O_2$ plateau occur at near maximal exercise before a true $\dot{V}O_{2max}$ is established, this is not always possible, as illustrated by this patient (117). It has been suggested that "peak $\dot{V}O_2$" be used instead of "$\dot{V}O_{2max}$" to define this situation (118).

There are several methods for estimating the ventilatory threshold (V_{at}) from the respiratory gas data (116). In Figure 5.22 the ventilatory equivalents for O_2 and CO_2 (i.e., $\dot{V}_E/\dot{V}O_2$ and $\dot{V}_E/\dot{V}CO_2$) are plotted against $\dot{V}O_2$. From these data the anaerobic threshold (or the $\dot{V}O_2$ at the onset of anaerobic metabolism) is visually identified as the onset of a disproportionate rise in $\dot{V}_E/\dot{V}O_2$ relative to $\dot{V}_E/\dot{V}CO_2$. This occurs because ventilation is being driven by CO_2 production rather than

231

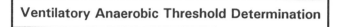

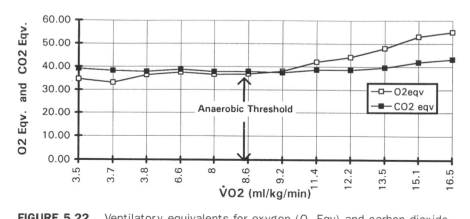

FIGURE 5.22. Ventilatory equivalents for oxygen (O_2 Eqv) and carbon dioxide (CO_2 Eqv) as a function of oxygen uptake ($\dot{V}O_2$). The anaerobic threshold is defined as the onset of a disproportionate rise in O_2 Eqv relative to CO_2 Eqv.

O_2 consumption; the rise in $\dot{V}_E/\dot{V}O_2$ without a change in $\dot{V}_E/\dot{V}CO_2$ indicates that ventilation is increasing in parallel with the increased CO_2 production that occurs with anaerobic metabolism. In the exercise laboratory the anaerobic threshold is usually visually detected from the plotted breath-by-breath exercise data. The anaerobic threshold can also be visually identified as a disproportionate rise of $\dot{V}CO_2$ or $\dot{V}_E$ relative to $\dot{V}O_2$, or a disproportionate rise in end-tidal O_2 relative to end-tidal CO_2 (116).

Unfortunately, there is considerable controversy over the anaerobic threshold concept and its clinical utility (119, 120). One of the problems is related to the interobserver and intraobserver reliability in visually detecting the onset of anaerobic metabolism from the breath-by-breath data (121). To overcome this problem computer detection algorithms have been developed to more objectively measure anaerobic threshold. One successful approach reported by Beaver et al. (122) is called the "V-slope method" and is illustrated in Figure 5.23. In this method the breath-by-breath $\dot{V}CO_2$ data are plotted against $\dot{V}O_2$ and the computer selects the upper and lower slopes by a least-square linear regression technique. The intersection of the two slopes identifies the anaerobic threshold. One can also visually select the breakpoint from the plot of $\dot{V}CO_2$ versus $\dot{V}O_2$ with less ambiguity than using the ventilatory equivalent data.

Clinical Applications—Patients With Disease

The major reasons for ordering a functional $\dot{V}O_2$ exercise test in a patient with disease and/or exercise limitations are (a) to objectively determine the presence

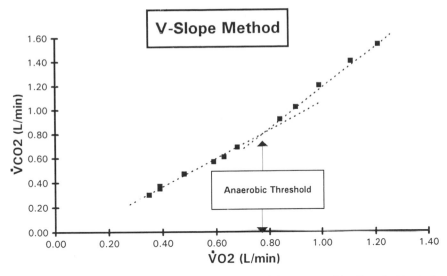

FIGURE 5.23. The V-slope method for determining anaerobic threshold. Carbon dioxide output ($\dot{V}CO_2$) is plotted as a function of oxygen uptake ($\dot{V}O_2$). The anaerobic threshold is defined as the intersection of the two slopes. See text.

and severity of heart and circulatory impairment, (b) to assess the functional consequences of the heart disease, (c) to evaluate the response to various therapeutic interventions, and (d) to assist in making cardiac transplantation decisions. It is well recognized that the traditional New York Heart Association's classification of functional impairment is not always accurate because it is based on a patient's symptoms rather than on objective criteria (123). It is also widely appreciated that *resting* central hemodynamics such as cardiac index, ejection fraction, and pulmonary wedge pressures do not always correlate well with functional impairment measured during exercise testing (124).

The exercise assessment, however, is a global test of a patient's cardiorespiratory functional capacity, since it reflects the entire oxygen transport system beginning with the lungs and pulmonary circulation and including the heart, the oxygen-carrying capacity in the blood, the peripheral circulation, and the skeletal muscles. In patients with heart disease the symptoms of exercise intolerance such as dyspnea on minimal exertion, fatigue, or both result from a complex interplay of mechanisms originating from both central and peripheral components of the oxygen transport system. These symptoms, unfortunately, are nonspecific and may also be medication side effects or caused by other coexisting conditions that may not be related to the underlying heart disease. The exercise test therefore is often helpful in the differential diagnosis of exercise intolerance and symptoms of dyspnea and fatigue (124). Table 5.19 illustrates the various factors that may adversely affect the Fick equation parameters and

TABLE 5.19. Factors Affecting Aerobic Capacity ($\dot{V}O_{2max}$)

Factors That Decrease	Factors That Increase
Aging	Aerobic conditioning
Deconditioning	Increased muscle mass
Acute illness	Genetic factors (heart size, skeletal
Bronchopulmonary disease	muscles, etc.)
Cardiovascular disease	Psychologic factors
Anemia	Increased PO_2 of inspired air
Carbon monoxide exposure	
High altitude	
Skeletal muscle disease	
Drugs that decrease heart rate, stroke volume, etc.	

TABLE 5.20. Functional Classification of Congestive Heart Failure Patients[a]

Class	Severity	$\dot{V}O_{2max}$ (ml/kg/min)	Anaerobic Threshold (ml/kg/min)	Maximal Cardiac Index (L/min/m^2)
A	None to mild	>20	>14	>8
B	Mild to moderate	16–20	11–14	6–8
C	Moderate to severe	10–15	8–11	4–6
D	Severe	6–9	5–8	2–4
E	Very severe	<6	3–4	<2

[a]From Weber KT, Janicki JS. Cardiopulmonary exercise testing. Physiologic principles and clinical applications. Philadelphia: WB Saunders, 1986.

result in a low $\dot{V}O_{2max}$. A knowledge of these factors combined with the results of functional exercise testing and other ancillary tests (e.g., pulmonary function tests) often leads to the correct diagnosis.

Weber and Janicki (115) have proposed an objective grading system, based on values of $\dot{V}O_{2max}$ and anaerobic threshold, that is especially applicable to patients with chronic CHF (Table 5.20). Because of the close relationship between $\dot{V}O_{2max}$ (or anaerobic threshold) and the maximal cardiac index, this grading system provides an excellent measure of disease severity. The classification system has been criticized, however, because it fails to consider age, sex, and weight differences in $\dot{V}O_{2max}$ that occur in normal subjects. Because $\dot{V}O_{2max}$ declines with age and is lower in women than in men, it may be more appropriate to use age- and sex-specific normal values and to classify impairment as a percentage reduction from these normal values. Formulas for predicting $\dot{V}O_{2max}$ in normal sedentary adults have been published for both cycle ergometry and treadmill testing by Wasserman et al. (116), although the database from which they were derived was small.

The direct measurement techniques for quantitating air flow and calculating minute ventilation, oxygen uptake, carbon dioxide output, and anaerobic threshold require on-line computer processing of the signal outputs from gas analyzers and flowmeters. These methods are generally complex, expensive, and demand careful calibrations and equipment maintenance. Commercially available, automated systems have significantly improved the ease with which respiratory data are obtained and analyzed, although these systems also require considerable professional expertise for proper use.

Clinical Applications—Normal Subjects

For many clinical applications the indirect methods of estimating or predicting $\dot{V}O_{2max}$ are reasonable alternatives to the more complex and expensive direct measurement techniques. Submaximal tests for predicting $\dot{V}O_{2max}$ can be used for fitness assessments and exercise prescriptions in the healthy population, although there are many limitations to these tests. The tests can usually be supervised by less experienced and lower salaried personnel than required for maximal testing. Estimations of $\dot{V}O_{2max}$ from maximal treadmill or bicycle tests are more accurate, but they require more careful supervision, take longer to complete, and demand much greater effort from the individual being evaluated.

The oxygen cost during treadmill work can be calculated using the equations presented in Table 5.21, depending on whether the subject is walking (1.9 to 3.7 mph) or running (>5 mph) (1). The total oxygen cost (ml/kg/min) for a given treadmill speed (mph) and elevation (percent grade expressed as a fraction) is the sum of the horizontal and vertical components. It follows that an estimated $\dot{V}O_{2max}$ can be calculated from the maximal speed and elevation achieved during treadmill exercise, provided the subject does not hold on to the side rails. These formulas can also be used for estimating the oxygen costs associated with outdoor activities, but the vertical component for running needs to be multiplied by 2. Estimates of $\dot{V}O_2$ for walking or running speeds from 3.7 to 5.0 mph are less accurate because of individual variations in walking or running patterns during fast walking or slow running.

Montoye et al. (125) compared the equations in Table 5.21 with directly measured exercise $\dot{V}O_2$ in 656 male subjects in all age groups participating in the Tecumseh Community Health Study. The equations were most accurate in estimating $\dot{V}O_2$ in adult males during grade walking, but slightly underestimated $\dot{V}O_2$ during horizontal walking. The formulas also underestimated $\dot{V}O_2$ in subjects under age 18. It should be emphasized, however, that the estimates of $\dot{V}O_2$ using these formulas are for steady-state exercise and may not be as accurate at

TABLE 5.21. Estimations of Oxygen Costs (ml O_2/kg/min) for Treadmill Walking (1.9 to 3.7 mph) or Running (>5 mph)[a]

Walking

Horizontal component: $\dot{V}O_2$ = (speed × 2.68) + 3.5

Vertical component: $\dot{V}O_2$ = (speed × 48.28) × % grade
(as a fraction)

Running

Horizontal component: $\dot{V}O_2$ = (speed × 5.36) + 3.5

Vertical component: $\dot{V}O_2$ = (speed × 24.14) × % grade
(as a fraction)

[a]From American College of Sports Medicine. Guidelines for exercise testing and prescription, 4th ed. Philadelphia: Lea & Febiger, 1991.

TABLE 5.22. Oxygen Requirements for Bicycle Ergometric Workloads[a]

Body Weight		Oxygen Cost								
(lbs)	(kg)	(ml O_2/kg/min)								
88	40	22.5	30.0	37.5	45.0	52.5	60.0	67.5	82.5	97.5
110	50	18.0	24.0	30.0	36.0	42.0	48.0	54.0	66.0	78.0
132	60	15.0	20.0	25.0	30.0	35.0	40.0	45.0	55.0	65.0
154	70	13.0	17.0	21.5	25.5	30.0	34.5	38.5	47.0	55.5
176	80	11.0	15.0	19.0	22.5	26.0	30.0	34.0	41.0	49.0
198	90	10.0	13.3	16.7	20.0	23.3	26.7	30.0	36.7	43.3
220	100	9.0	12.0	15.0	18.0	21.0	24.0	27.0	33.0	39.0
242	110	8.0	11.0	13.5	16.5	19.0	22.0	24.5	30.0	35.5
264	120	7.5	10.0	12.5	15.0	17.5	20.0	22.5	27.5	32.5
Workload										
kpm/min		300	450	600	750	900	1050	1200	1500	1800
watts		50	75	100	125	150	175	200	250	300

[a]From The Committee on Exercise. Exercise testing and training of apparently healthy individuals: a handbook for physicians. Dallas: American Heart Association, 1972.

high treadmill workloads and maximal exercise because the anaerobic component associated with these workloads is not taken into consideration (1).

The standard treadmill protocols described in Table 5.7 have estimated $\dot{V}O_2$ values for each stage of exercise. These values are only applicable if the subject is in a steady state and not holding on to the handrails during exercise. There is a substantial reduction in the $\dot{V}O_2$ and heart rate response to exercise when handrails are used for support (126). This enables the exercising subject to significantly extend the total duration of exercise and falsely elevate the estimated $\dot{V}O_{2max}$. In some individuals who are unable to maintain balance on the treadmill, resting one or two fingers on the rails may still permit a reasonable estimate of $\dot{V}O_{2max}$. The use of handrails for most people can be minimized by the exercise test technician. A careful explanation of the proper techniques for walking on the treadmill followed by a demonstration will usually enable most patients to walk without using the handrails.

Estimates of maximal oxygen uptake can be determined from bicycle ergometric testing (Table 5.22) (127). The following formula can also be used for calculating the oxygen cost for upright bicycle work (1):

$$\dot{V}O_2 \text{ (ml/min)} = \text{(kpm/min} \times 2 \text{ ml/kpm)} + 3.5 \text{ ml/kg/min} \times \text{kg (BW)}$$

The calculation is reasonably accurate for work rates between 300 and 1200 kpm/min. For estimating an individual's maximal aerobic capacity, the maximal workload in kpm/min should be used in the above formula, and the calculated $\dot{V}O_{2max}$ should be divided by the body weight (BW) in kg.

Table 5.23 lists the 5th, 30th, 50th, 70th, and 95th percentile ratings for $\dot{V}O_{2max}$ in healthy adults based on age and sex. These data were collected at The Cooper Clinic and The Institute for Aerobics Research in Dallas, Texas (128). Although the data are derived from a highly motivated group of subjects, they can be used as a standard reference database for aerobic fitness classification. Individuals who are clinically healthy but fall below the 5th percentile are most likely deconditioned as a result of chronic inactivity. These people are ideal candidates for exercise training programs. The extent to which $\dot{V}O_{2max}$ can be improved by physical training is dependent on the initial fitness level, the quality and duration of the exercise training program, and the genetic endowment of the individuals being trained. Values of $\dot{V}O_{2max}$ in the 30th to 70th percentile are found in individuals who may or may not exercise regularly. Some people are physically fit because they engage in physically demanding occupations; others are genetically fortunate to have average or above average exercise tolerance. $\dot{V}O_{2max}$ values above the 95th percentile are primarily observed in highly trained individuals and athletes. These values are likely to be caused by the combination of intense training regimens coupled with an exceptional genetic endowment.

TABLE 5.23. Physical Fitness Standards For Men and Women[a]

| Age (yrs) | $\dot{V}O_{2max}$ (ml O_2/kg/min) | | | | |
	5th Percentile	30th Percentile	50th Percentile	70th Percentile	95th Percentile
Men					
20-29	25.1	38.5	42.4	45.7	54.4
30-39	29.4	37.4	41.0	45.3	52.8
40-49	22.2	35.2	38.7	42.9	51.1
50-59	22.4	31.6	35.2	38.1	46.8
60-69	20.0	28.0	31.1	35.2	43.9
70-79	18.1	23.9	28.0	32.3	39.5
Women					
20-29	23.7	31.6	35.2	39.5	45.3
30-39	24.3	30.2	33.8	36.7	43.9
40-49	22.2	28.0	30.9	33.8	42.4
50-59	18.3	25.1	28.0	30.9	36.7
60-69	18.3	23.7	25.8	28.2	35.2
70-79	18.3	22.2	25.3	29.4	35.4

[a]Data from Cooper Clinic Coronary Risk Factor Profile Charts. Pollock ML, Wilmore JH. Exercise in health and disease. 2nd ed. Philadelphia: WB Saunders, 1990.

Morris et al. (129) have published equations and nomograms for assessing aerobic exercise capacity in men based on maximal treadmill metabolic equivalents (METs) and age. In their study of 1388 male patients, who had a mean age of 57 years (range 21 to 89 years) and who were referred for routine exercise testing, the maximal METs were derived from the final treadmill speed and grade. Exercise capacity was defined as follows:

Exercise capacity = [Observed MET level / Predicted METs] × 100%

Subjects were defined as "active" if they exercised (brisk walking or aerobic sport) for 20 or more minutes three or more times a week. Predicted METs in this subset were derived from regression analyses of METs versus age as follows:

Predicted METs = 18.7 − 0.15(Age)

A similar equation was derived for the "sedentary" subset:

Predicted METs = 16.6 − 0.15(Age)

Exercise capacity values < 100% indicate "below average" exercise capacity relative to one's age group, whereas values > 100% represent a "better than average" exercise performance. The authors suggest that these equations be used to assess exercise tolerance in male patients being evaluated by physicians in an office or hospital-based clinical setting.

CONCLUSIONS

Exercise testing is an important clinical tool for detecting myocardial ischemia, evaluating cardiovascular function and physical working capacity, assessing prognosis and risk for future cardiac disease events, and determining optimal treatment strategies for patients with cardiovascular diseases. The successful use of this tool, however, requires a broad knowledge of cardiovascular structure and function, electrocardiography, clinical characteristics of heart diseases, basic and advanced cardiac life-support techniques, and the principles of clinical judgment. Personnel working in exercise-testing laboratories, moreover, need to keep up with rapidly advancing changes in exercise-testing methodology and applications. Finally, the cost:benefit ratio must always be considered when determining the need for clinical exercise testing to avoid the inappropriate and, at times, potentially harmful use of this procedure. The test is only as good as the cognitive processes and technical expertise of the professional staff using it.

REFERENCES

1. American College of Sports Medicine. Guidelines for exercise testing and prescription. 4th ed. Philadelphia; Lea & Febiger, 1991.
2. Froelicher VF, Myers J, Follansbee WP, Labovitz A. Exercise and the heart, 3rd St Louis; Mosby-Year Book, 1993.
3. Weber KT, Janicki JS. Cardiopulmonary exercise testing. Physiologic principles and clinical applications. Philadelphia; WB Saunders 1986.
4. Wasserman K, Hansen JE, Sue DY, Whipp BJ. Principles of exercise testing and interpretation. Philadelphia; Lea & Febiger, 1987.
5. Subcommitte on Exercise Testing. Guidelines for exercise testing. A report of the American College of Cardiology/American Heart Association Task Force on Assessment of Cardiovascular Procedures. J Am Coll Cardiol 1986;8:725–738.
6. American Heart Association. 1992 heart and stroke facts. AHA Publication 55-0386 (COM). National Center, 7272 Greenville Avenue, Dallas, TX 75231–4596.
7. Kannel WB, Gordon T, eds. The Framingham study: an epidemiological investigation of cardiovascular disease. Vol 12. Bethesda, MD: National Heart, Lung, and Blood Institute, 1968.
8. Weiner DA. Prognostic value of exercise testing early after myocardial infarction. J Cardiac Rehab 1983;3:114–120.
9. Epstein SE, Palmeri ST, Patterson RE. Evaluation of patients after acute myocardial infarction. Indications for cardiac catheterization and surgical intervention. N Engl J Med 1982; 307:1487–1492.
10. Krone RJ. The role of risk stratification in the early management of a myocardial infarction. Ann Intern Med 1992;116:223–237.
11. Young DZ, Lampert S, Graboys TB, Lown B. Safety of maximal exercise testing in patients at high risk for ventricular arrhythmia. Circulation 1984;70:184–191.
12. Ewart CK, Taylor CB, Reese LB, Debusk RF. Effects of early postmyocardial infarction

239

exercise testing on self-perception and subsequent physical activity. Am J Cardiol 1983; 51: 1076–1086.

13. Fletcher GF, Froelicher VF, Hartley et al. Exercise standards. A statement for health professionals from the American Heart Association. Circulation 1990;82:2286–2322.

14. Schlant R, Friesinger GC, Leonard JJ et al. Clinical competence in exercise testing: a statement for physicians from the ACP/ACC/AHA task force on clinical privileges in cardiology. J Am Coll Cardiol 1990;16:1061–1065.

15. Franklin BA. Exercise testing, training and arm ergometry. Sports Medicine 1985;2:100–119.

16. Mellerowicz H, Smodalaka VN. Ergometry: basics of medical exercise testing. Baltimore: Urban & Schwarzenberg, 1981.

17. Mason RE, Likar I. A new system of multiple-lead exercise electrocardiography. Am Heart J 1966;71:196–204.

18. Gamble P, McManus H, Jensen D, Froelicher VF. A comparison of the standard 12–lead electrocardiogram to exercise electrode placements. Chest 1984;85:616–622.

19. Kligfield P, Okin PM, Ameisen O, Borer JS. Evaluation of coronary artery disease by an improved method of exercise electrocardiography: the ST/HR slope. Am Heart J 1986; 112: 589–599.

20. Tam HW, Webster JG. Minimizing electrode motion artifact by skin abrasion. IEEE Trans Biomed Eng 1977;24:134–138.

21. Garber CE, Carleton RA, Camaione DN, Heller GV. The threshold for myocardial ischemia varies in patients with coronary artery disease depending on the exercise protocol. J Am Coll Cardiol 1991;17:1256–1262.

22. Buchfuhrer MJ, Hansen JE, Robinson TE et al. Optimizing the exercise protocol for cardiopulmonary assessment. J Appl Physiol 1983;55:1558–1564.

23. Bruce RA, Kusumi F, Hosmer D. Maximal oxygen intake and nomographic assessment of functional aerobic impairment in cardiovascular disease. Am Heart J 1973;85:346–358.

24. Balke B, Ware RW. An experimental study of "physical fitness" of Air Force personnel. US Armed Forces Med J 1959;10:675–688.

25. Wolthuis RA, Froelicher VF, Fischer J et al. New practical treadmill protocol for clinical use. Am J Cardiol 1977;39:697–702.

26. Ellestad MH, Allen WA, Wan MLK, Kemp GL. Maximal treadmill stress testing for cardiovascular evaluation. Circulation 1969;39:517–522.

27. Naughton J, Sevellus G, Balke B. Physiological responses of normal and pathologic subjects to a modified work capacity test. J Sports Med 1963;31:201–212.

28. Okin PM, Ameisen O, Kligfield P. A modified treadmill exercise protocol for computer-assisted analysis of the ST segment/heart rate slope: methods and reproducibility. J Electrocardiol 1986; 19:311–319.

29. Ellestad MB, Blomqvist CG, Naughton J. Standards for adult exercise testing laboratories. Circulation 1979;59:421A.

30. Glasser SP, Ramsey MR. An automated system for blood pressure determination during exercise. Circulation 1981;63:348–356.

31. Lachterman B, Lehmann KG, Abrahamson D, Froelicher VF. "Recovery only" ST-segment depression and the predictive accuracy of the exercise test. Ann Intern Med 1990;112:11–20.

32. Koppes G, McKiernan D, Bassan M, Froelicher VF. Treadmill exercise testing. I. Curr Probl Cardiol 1977;7:1–69.

33. Stuart RJ, Ellestad MH. National survey of exercise testing. Chest 1980;77:94–100.

34. Cohn PF. Silent myocardial ischemia. Ann Intern Med 1988;109:312–317.

35. Surawicz B. ST-T abnormalities. In: Macfarlane PW, Lawrie TDV, eds. Comprehensive electrocardiology. New York: Pergamon Press, 1989.

36. Vincent GM, Abildskov JA, Burgess MJ. Mechanisms of ST-segment displacement: evaluation by direct current recordings. Circulation 1977;56:559–571.

37. Holland RP, Brooks H. Precordial and epicardial surface potentials during myocardial ischemia in the pig. Circ Res 1975;35:471–480.

38. Elharrar V, Zipes DP. Cardiac electrophysiologic alternans during myocardial ischemia. Am J Physiol 1977;233:H329.

39. Holland RP, Arnsdorf MF. Solid angle theory and the electrocardiogram: physiologic and quantitative interpretations. Prog Cardiovasc Dis 1977;19:431–457.

40. Blackburn H, Katigbak R. What electrocardiographic leads to take after exercise? Am Heart J 1964;67:184–192.

41. Miranda CP, Liu J, Kadar A et al. Usefulness of exercise-induced ST-segment depression in the inferior leads during exercise testing as a marker for coronary artery disease. Am J Cardiol 1992; 69:303–307.

42. Chaitman BR, Waters DD, Theroux P, Hanson JS. S-T segment elevation and coronary spasm in response to exercise. Am J Cardiol 1981;47:1350–1357.

43. Prinzmetal M, Kennamer R, Merliss R et al. Angina pectoris: a variant form of angina pectoris. Am J Med 1959;27:375–381.

44. Lahiri A, Subramanian B, Millar-Craig M et al. Exercise-induced ST-segment elevation in variant angina. Am J Cardiol 1980;45:887–892.

45. Mark DB, Hlatky MA, Lee KL et al. Localizing coronary artery obstructions with the exercise treadmill test. Ann Intern Med 1987;106:53–55.

46. Stiles GL, Tosati RA, Wallace AG. Clinical relevance of exercise-induced ST-segment elevation. Am J Cardiol 1980;46:931–937.

47. Gerson MC, Phillips JF, Morris SN, McHenry PL. Exercise-induced U-wave inversion as a marker of stenosis of the left anterior descending coronary artery. Circulation 1979; 60: 1014–1020.

48. Yano H, Hiasa Y, Aihara T et al. Negative U wave during percutaneous transluminal coronary angioplasty. Clin Cardiol 1991;14:232–236.

49. Vasey C, O'Donnell J, Morris S et al. Exercise-induced left bundle branch block and its relation to coronary artery disease. Am J Cardiol 1985;56:892–895.

50. Whinnery JE, Froelicher VF, Stuart AJ. The electrocardiographic response to maximal exercise testing in asymptomatic men with left bundle branch block. Am Heart J 1977;94:316–322.

51. Smith WM. Mechanisms of cardiac arrhythmias and conduction disturbances. In: Hurst JW, ed. The heart, 7th ed. New York: McGraw-Hill, 1990.

52. Akhtar M. Clinical spectrum of ventricular tachycardia. Circulation 1990;82:1561–1573.

53. Woelfel A, Foster JR, Mcallister RG et al. Efficacy of verapamil in exercise-induced ventricular tachycardia. Am J Cardiol 1985;56:292–297.

54. Rankin AC, Rae AP, Oldroyd KG, Cobble SM. Verapamil or adenosine for the immediate treatment of supraventricular tachycardia. Q J Med 1990;74:203–208.

55. Pritchett ELC. Management of atrial fibrillation. N Engl J Med 1992;326:1264–1271.

56. Busby MJ, Shefrin EA, Fleg JL. Prevalence and long-term significance of exercise-induced frequent or repetitive ventricular ectopic beats in apparently healthy volunteers. J Am Coll Cardiol 1989;14:1659–1665.

57. Sami M, Chaitman B, Fisher L et al. Significance of exercise-induced ventricular arrhythmia in stable coronary artery disease: a coronary artery surgery study project. Am J Cardiol 1984; 54: 1182–1190.

58. Weiner DA, Levin SR, Klein MD, Ryan TJ. Ventricular arrhythmias during exercise testing: mechanism, response to coronary bypass surgery and prognostic significance. Am J Cardiol 1984; 53:1553–1559.

59. Fleg JL, Lakatta EG. Prevalence and prognosis of exercise-induced nonsustained ventricular tachycardia in apparently healthy volunteers. Am J Cardiol 1984;54:572–579.

60. Yang JC, Wesley RC, Froelicher VF. Ventricular tachycardia during routine treadmill testing: risk and prognosis. Arch Intern Med 1991;151:349–353.

61. Wilson RF, Marcus ML, Christensen BV et al. Accuracy of exercise electrocardiography in detecting physiologically significant coronary artery lesions. Circulation 1991:83:412–421.

62. Gianrossi R, Detrano R, Mulvihill D et al. Exercise-induced ST depression in the diagnosis of coronary artery disease: a meta-analysis. Circulation 1989;80:87–98.

241

63. Philbrick JT, Horwitz RI, Feinstein AR. Methodological problems of exercise testing for coronary artery disease: groups, analysis and bias. Am J Cardiol 1980;46:807–814.

64. Detrano R, Lyons KP, Marcondes G et al. Methodological problems in exercise testing research. Are we solving them? Arch Intern Med 1988;148:1289–1295.

65. Fox KM, Selwyn A, Oakley D, Shillingford JP. Relation between the precordial projection of S-T segment changes after exercise and coronary angiographic findings. Am J Cardiol 1979; 44: 1068–1076.

66. Yanowitz FG, Vincent GM, Lux RL et al. Application of body surface mapping to exercise testing: S-T80 isoarea maps in patients with coronary artery disease. Am J Cardiol 1982;50: 1109–1117.

67. Tonkon MJ, Lee G, DeMaria AN et al. Effects of digitalis on the exercise electrocardiogram in normal adult subjects. Chest 1977;72:714–718.

68. Devereux RB, Kramer-Fox R, Kligfield P. Mitral valve prolapse: causes, clinical manifestations, and management. Ann Intern Med 1989;111:305–317.

69. Ellestad MH. Stress testing: principles and practice, 2nd ed. Philadelphia: FA Davis, 1980.

70. Friesinger GC, Biern RO, Likar I, Mason RE. Exercise electrocardiography and vasoregulatory abnormalities. Am J Cardiol 1972;30:733–738.

71. Diamond GA, Forrester JS. Analysis of probability as an aid in the clinical diagnosis of coronary artery disease. N Engl J Med 1979;300:1350–1358.

72. Anderson KM, Wilson PWF, Odell PM et al. An updated coronary risk profile: AHA medical scientific statement. Circulation 1991;83:356–362.

73. Diamond GA, Hirsch M, Forrester JS et al. Application of information theory to clinical diagnostic testing. The electrocardiographic stress test. Circulation 1981;63:915–921.

74. Rifkin RD, Hood WB. Bayesian analysis of electrocardiographic exercise stress testing. N Engl J Med 1977;297:681–686.

75. Patterson RE, Eng C, Horowitz SF. Practical diagnosis of coronary artery disease: a Bayes' theorem nomogram to correlate clinical data with noninvasive exercise tests. Am J Cardiol 1984;53:252–260.

76. Sox HC, Littenberg B, Garber AM. The role of exercise testing in screening for coronary artery disease. Ann Intern Med 1989;110:456–469.

77. McNeer JF, Margolis JR, Lee KL et al. The role of the exercise test in evaluating patients for ischemic heart disease. Circulation 1978;57:64–70.

78. Califf RM, Harrel EF Jr, Lee KL et al. The evolution of medical and surgical therapy for coronary artery disease. A 15–year perspective. JAMA 1989;261:2077–2086.

79. Weiner DA et al. The predictive value of anginal chest pain as an indicator of coronary artery disease during exercise testing. Am Heart J 1978;96:458–463.

80. Elamin MS, Boyle R, Kardash MM et al. Accurate detection of coronary artery disease by a new exercise test. Br Heart J 1982;48:311–317.

81. Quyyumi AA, Raphael MJ, Wright C et al. Inability of the ST segment/heart rate slope to predict accurately the severity of coronary artery disease. Br Heart J 1984;51:395–398.

82. Lachterman B, Lehmann KG, Detrano R et al. Comparsion of ST segment/heart rate index to standard ST criteria for analysis of exercise electrocardiogram. Circulation 1990;83:44–50.

83. Kligfield P, Okin PM, Ameisen O, Borer JS. Evaluation of coronary artery disease by an improved method of exercise electrocardiography: the ST/HR slope. Am Heart J 1986; 112:589–598.

84. Kligfield P, Ameisen O, Okin PM. Heart rate adjustment of ST segment depression for improved detection of coronary artery disease. Circulation 1989;79:245–255.

85. Bobbio M, Detrano R, Schmid J et al. Exercise-induced ST depression and ST/HR rate index to predict triple-vessel or left main coronary disease: a multicenter analysis. J Am Coll Cardiol 1992;19:11–18.

86. Kligfield P, Okin PM. Heart rate adjustment of ST segment depression: is the glass half empty or half full? J Am Coll Cardiol 1992;19:19–20.

87. Kotler TS, Diamond GA. Exercise thallium-201 scintigraphy in the diagnosis and prognosis of coronary artery disease. Ann Intern Med 1990;113:684–702.

88. Beller GA. Pharmacologic stress imaging. JAMA 1991;265:633–638.

89. Verani MS, Mahmarian JJ, Hixson JB et al. Diagnosis of coronary artery disease by controlled coronary vasodilation with adenosine and thallium-201 scintigraphy in patients unable to exercise. Circulation 1990;82:80–87.

90. Limacher MC, Quinones MA, Poliner LR et al. Detection of coronary artery disease with exercise two-dimensional echocardiography. Description of a clinically applicable method and comparison with radionuclide ventriculography. Circulation 1983;67:1211–1218.

91. Picano E. Stress echocardiography. From pathophysiological toy to diagnostic tool. Circulation 1992;85:1604–1612.

92. Pellikka PA. Dobutamine stress echocardiography: methodology and clinical applications. CARDIO January 1994 p.24.

93. Allen WH, Aronow WS, Goodman P, Stinson P. Five-year follow-up of maximal treadmill stress testing in asymptomatic men and women. Circulation 1980;65:522–531.

94. Giagnoni E, Secchi B, Wu SC et al. Prognostic value of exercise stress testing in asymptomatic normotensive subjects. N Engl J Med 1983;309:1085–1089.

95. Bruce RA, Hossack KF, DeRouen T, Hofer V. Enhanced risk assessment for primary coronary heart disease events by maximal exercise testing: 10 years' experience of Seattle Heart Watch. J Am Coll Cardiol 1983;3:565–573.

96. Deedwania PC, Parmley WW. Silent ischemia. In: Parmley WW, Chatterjee K, eds. Cardiology, volume 2, cardiovascular disease. Philadelphia: JB Lippincott 1993.

97. Gordon DL, Ekelund LG, Karon JM et al. Predictive value of the exercise tolerance test for mortality in North American men: the Lipid Research Clinics Mortality Follow-up Study. Circulation 1986;74:252–261.

98. Blumenthal DS, Weiss JL, Mellitis ED, Gerstenblith G. The predictive value of a strongly positive stress test in patients with minimal symptoms. Am J Med 1981;70:1005–1012.

99. Weiner DA, McCabe CH, Ryan TJ. Prognostic assessment of patients with coronary artery disease by exercise testing. Am Heart J 1983;105:749–756.

100. Weiner DA, Ryan T, McCabe CH et al. Prognostic importance of a clinical profile and exercise test in medically treated patients with coronary artery disease. J Am Coll Cardiol 1984; 3: 772–779.

101. Mark DB, Hlatky MA, Harrell FE et al. Exercise treadmill score for predicting prognosis in coronary artery disease. Ann Intern Med 1987;106:793–800.

102. Ribisl PM, Morris CK, Kawaguchi T et al. Angiographic patterns and severe coronary artery disease. Exercise test correlates. Arch Intern Med 1992;152:1618–1624.

103. Morrow K, Morris CK, Froelicher VF et al. Prediction of cardiovascular death in men undergoing noninvasive evaluation for coronary artery disease. Ann Intern Med 1993;118:689–695.

104. Okin PM, Kligfield P. Effect of exercise protocol and lead selection on the accuracy of heart rate-adjusted indices of ST-segment depression for detection of three-vessel coronary artery disease. J Electrocardiology 1989;22:187–194.

105. Mosvatian F, Froelicher VF. ST elevation during exercise testing. Am J Cardiol 1989; 63: 986–988.

106. Dubach P, Froelicher VF, Klein J et al. Exercise-induced hypotension in a male population: criteria, causes, and prognosis. Circulation 1988;78:1380–1387.

107. Ellestad MH, Wan MKC. Predictive implications of stress testing. Circulation 1975;51:363–369.

108. Hammond HK, Kelly TL, Froelicher VF. Radionuclide imaging correlatives of heart rate impairment during maximal exercise testing. J Am Coll Cardiol 1983;2:826–833.

109. Cole JP, Ellestad MH. Significance of chest pain during treadmill testing: correlation with coronary events. Am J Cardiol 1978;41:227–232.

110. Krone RJ. The role of risk stratification in the early management of a myocardial infarction. Ann Intern Med 1992;116:223–237.

111. ACC/AHA Task Force on Assessment of Diagnostic and Therapeutic Cardiovascular Procedures. Guidelines for the early management of patients with acute myocardial infarction. Circulation 1990;82:664–707.

243

112. Jain A, Meyers GH, Sapin PM, O'Rourke RA. Comparison of symptom-limited and low-level exercise tolerance tests early after myocardial infarction. J Am Coll Cardiol 1993;22:1816–1820.
113. Debusk RF, Haskell W. Symptom-limited vs. heart-rated limited exercise testing soon after myocardial infarction. Circulation 1980;61:738–744.
114. Ewart CK, Taylor CB, Reese LB, Debusk RF. Effects of early postmyocardial infarction exer cise testing on self-perception and subsequent physical activity. Am J Cardiol 1983; 51: 1076–1083.
115. Weber KT, Janicki JS. Cardiopulmonary exercise testing. Physiologic principles and clinical applications. Philadelphia; WB Saunders, 1986.
116. Wasserman K, Hansen JE, Sue DY, Whipp BJ. Principles of exercise testing and interpretation. Philadelphia; Lea & Febiger, 1987.
117. Myers J, Walsh D, Buchanan N, Froelicher VF. Can maximal cardiopulmonary capacity be recognized by a plateau in oxygen uptake? Chest 1989;96:1312–1316.
118. Neuberg GW, Friedman SH, Weiss MB, Herman MV. Cardiopulmonary exercise testing. The clinical value of gas exchange data. Arch Intern Med 1988;148:2221–2226.
119. Brooks GA. Anaerobic threshold: review of the concept and directions for future research. Med Sci Sports Exerc 1985;17:22–31.
120. Davis JA. Anaerobic threshold: review of the concept and directions for future research. Med Sci Sports Exerc 1985;17:6–18.
121. Yeh MP, Gardner RM, Adams TD et al. "Anaerobic threshold": problems of determination and validation. J Appl Physiol 1983;55:1178–1186.
122. Beaver WL, Wasserman K, Whipp BJ. A new method for detecting the anaerobic threshold by gas exchange. J Appl Physiol 1986;60:2020–2027.
123. Neuberg GW, Friedman SH, Weiss MB, Herman MV. Cardiopulmonary exercise testing. The clinical value of gas exchange data. Arch Intern Med 1988; 148:2221–2226.
124. Jennings GL, Esler MD. Circulatory regulation at rest and exercise and the functional assessment of patients with congestive heart failure. Circulation 1990; 81(Suppl II):II-5–II-13.
125. Montoye HJ, Ayen T, Nagle F, Howley E. The oxygen requirement for horizontal and grade walking on a motor driven treadmill. Med Sci Sports Exerc 1985;17:640–646.
126. Ragg KE, Murray TF, Karbonit LM, Jump DA. Errors in predicting functional capacity from a treadmill exercise test. Am Heart J 1980;100:581–585.
127. The Committee on Exercise. Exercise testing and training of apparently healthy individuals: a handbook for physicians. Dallas: American Heart Association, 1972.
128. Pollock ML, Wilmore JH: Exercise in health and disease. 2nd ed. Philadelphia: WB Saunders, 1990.
129. Morris CK, Myers J, Froelicher VF et al. Nomogram based on metabolic equivalents and age for assessing aerobic exercise capacity in men. J Am Coll Cardiol 1993;22:175–182.

6

THE EXERCISE PRESCRIPTION

THE EXERCISE PRESCRIPTION represents the carefully regulated dosage of physical activity of a long-term training program. The dosage consists of a coalescence of intensity, duration, and frequency of effort that is undertaken in an exercise mode to achieve specific program objectives. The prescription should be developed in a manner similar to that of prescribing medication, that is, administered in specified amounts based on individual needs. When designed for cardiac rehabilitation and adult fitness, the exercise modes are usually selected for the purpose of enhancing cardiovascular function and lessening the risk of coronary heart disease. Other training objectives such as strength and flexibility have very different prescriptions and are addressed briefly in this chapter, although the reader is referred elsewhere for more in-depth information (1–3). The purposes of this chapter are to present the rationale for an exercise prescription that promotes cardiovascular function; to present the physiologic basis and design of the prescription, the factors that affect the prescription; and to apply the prescription formula to an exercise training program.

PHYSIOLOGIC BASIS OF THE EXERCISE PRESCRIPTION

The physiologic basis of the exercise prescription is the overload principle and the relationship between training stimuli (dosage) and adaptation (response).

Overload Principle

Overload by definition means that the training stimulus must surpass normal daily physical exertion to be beneficial (4). The training stimulus, however, should not provoke undue fatigue, musculoskeletal strain, or mental or emotional burnout. Optimal benefit necessitates regular updating of the overload threshold.

Dose Response

Adaptation is related to the amount of physical exertion, although the relationship is not consistently linear. Dose-response curves depicted in Figure 6.1 (5) represent a relationship illustrating that adaptation does not occur until some minimal effort is expended, that is, overload. The curves do not represent physiologic measures, but rather represent a conceptual comparison of effort versus gain under different circumstances. Training adaptation is modest or nonexistent for most persons until effort approximates 50 to 60% of maximum intensity. Thereafter, gains are rapid until they plateau at the top of the curves, between 85 and 90% of maximal effort, indicating that exercise is too intense or that there is insufficient time for recovery, or both. The dose-response curves shift to the right as physical condition improves. The rate of adaptation varies

FIGURE 6.1. Improvement anticipated from effort expended: A conceptual diagram illustrating training curves in various populations. Note that the trained athlete is required to exercise at a greater intensity to make gains similar to those of normal persons or cardiac patients. Also note that age at onset of training affects the maximal physiologic gain. (Redrawn from Fardy PS. Train for aerobic power. In: Burke EJ, ed. Toward an understanding of human performance. Ithaca, NY: Movement Publications, 1977.)

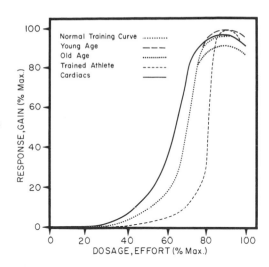

among individuals (4), although improvements are generally similar at different ages and for males and females (6).

COMPONENTS OF THE PRESCRIPTION

The prescription dosage consists of intensity, duration, frequency, and mode of exercise.

Intensity

The single most important factor of the exercise prescription is intensity of effort, usually expressed as a percentage of functional aerobic capacity or maximal heart rate (MHR) (7). There is a strong and consistent correlation between oxygen uptake and heart rate as a percentage of maximum (Fig. 6.2), regardless of the level of physical condition, gender, or muscle groups being compared (8–10).

Several approaches may be used to prescribe training intensity. In any case maximal exercise testing is recommended for best results. The ACSM Guidelines provide clear recommendations for testing (11). Heart rate prescriptions based on submaximal testing or age-estimated maximal heart rates have the potential for considerable error (11) and, as a result, may be too strenuous and pose the risk of injury or too easy and, hence, ineffective.

The target heart rate (THR) is ordinarily established between 70 and 90% MHR, approximately 60 to 80% $\dot{V}O_{2max}$. Those who are poorly conditioned as well as patients with cardiopulmonary disease can benefit from training at heart rates less than 70% MHR, while competitive athletes may require greater than 90% MHR for training adaptation. The THR illustrated in Figure 6.3 (12)

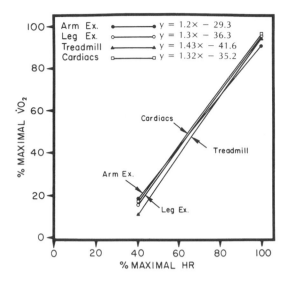

FIGURE 6.2. The regression lines of two groups of normal persons and one group of coronary artery disease subjects show similar relationships between submaximal oxygen intake expressed as percentage of maximum and heart rates as percentage of maximal heart rate. In the formulas, Y = percentage of maximal oxygen intake, X = percentage of maximal heart rate. (Redrawn from Fardy PS et al. Cardiac rehabilitation, adult fitness, and exercise testing. Philadelphia: Lea & Febiger, 1988. Data from Hellerstein HK et al. Principles of exercise prescription for normals and cardiac subjects. In: Naughton JP, Hellerstein HK, Mohler IC, eds. Exercise testing and exercise training in coronary heart disease. Orlando, FL: Academic Press, 1973; and Fardy PS, Webb DP, Hellerstein HK. Benefits of arm exercise in cardiac rehabilitation. Phys Sports Med 1977;5:33.)

provides a training range of 30 to 40 beats from which the specific heart rate is determined by carefully considering age, physical fitness, clinical status, and physical limitations. Trained individuals must exercise at a higher target heart rate than untrained persons because they require a greater intensity of effort to achieve the same benefit (Fig. 6.1). Individuals in poor physical condition experience equal or greater training adaptation at a lower target heart rate compared to highly trained subjects (5).

Submaximal aerobic exercise is recommended to improve muscle endurance and cardiovascular fitness (11). Maximal or near maximal activity, that is, mostly anaerobic exercise, is not necessary for beneficial cardiovascular results and may even compromise the safety of cardiac patients and poorly conditioned individuals. A modest level of activity, such as walking at a brisk pace, may be sufficient for beneficial results. If the intensity of training is excessive, there may be undue cardiovascular and musculoskeletal stress (13–15), including heart

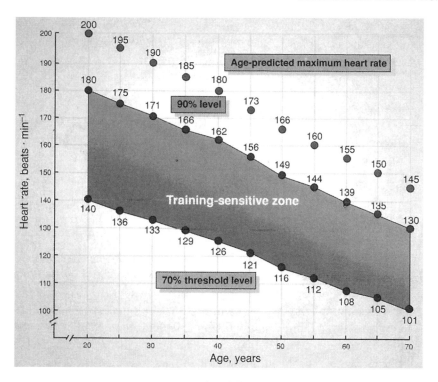

FIGURE 6.3. Maximal heart rates and training-sensitive zones for use in aerobic training programs for people of different ages. (Redrawn from McArdle WD, Katch FI, Katch VL. Exercise physiology: energy, nutrition, and human performance. 3rd ed. Philadelphia: Lea & Febiger, 1991.)

arrhythmias, muscle injury or soreness, and decreased adherence. Modest intensity of exercise is particularly appropriate for persons who were previously active and who tend toward overexertion based on past accomplishments. As a rule of thumb, one should not become excessively out of breath while exercising. This can be assured reasonably well by close adherence to the training heart rate. This level of exertion usually produces perspiration, an increase in breathing, and a not unpleasant sense of fatigue (16).

The simplest method for prescribing training intensity that will accommodate the needs of most individuals is to use the target heart rate range of 70 to 90% MHR attained on the most recent exercise test (Fig. 6.3). Another frequently used method is the Karvonen formula or heart rate reserve method (17). This technique incorporates maximal and resting heart rates; the difference between them is added to the resting rate. The Karvonen formula assumes that training intensity should take into account a percentage of the increase from rest to maximum, not just a percentage of the maximal rate as in the first method. The assertion is that a target rate of 150 would be of greater intensity with a resting rate of 50 and a maximum rate of 200 when compared with a resting heart rate of 100 and a maximal rate of 200. Following are examples of the two methods:

% of Maximal Heart Rate	Karvonen Formula
Maximal heart rate = 200	MHR = 200
	Resting heart rate (RHR) = 80
Training intensity = 70%	Training intensity = 70%
Target heart rate = 140	Target heart rate = 164

Normally the lower limit of intensity using the Karvonen formula is between 50 and 60% of the difference between MHR and RHR, whereas a comparable intensity when taking a straight percentage of MHR is 65 to 70%. The Karvonen formula is a more aggressive approach at a given % MHR. Consequently, training intensity is suggested to be lower when using the Karvonen method.

Another method used to prescribe exercise intensity is with the use of metabolic equivalents, or METs, which represent multiples of resting metabolic rate (one MET is approximately 3.5 ml/kg/min of oxygen uptake) (11). Two METs, therefore, equal twice the resting metabolic rate, and so on. The MET method uses whole numbers, which are simple to understand and are easily available for a variety of activities. From the results of the exercise test, a list of safe and effective activities can be provided. For example, if one attains 10 METs on a maximal exercise test and the training intensity is 70% $\dot{V}O_{2max}$, then activities of 7 METs or less are prescribed as safe and suitable. Tables 6.1 and 6.2 list sample activities and their MET equivalents. METs also can be easily related to other units of work as illustrated in Table 6.3.

The MET method is a simple way to prescribe exercise intensity, although frequently it is used incorrectly. Common errors include the following:

1. *Using published values as precise measurements.* METs are only an estimate of energy expenditure unless resting and exercise oxygen uptake are actually measured. Since resting metabolic rate varies among individuals and is influenced by factors such as physical condition and body size, actual METs may also vary from published values and should be used conservatively.

2. *Failure to allow for effects of skill and competition.* Activities involving skill may have widely varying MET values, whereas activities requiring minimal skill such as walking, jogging, and bicycling are more accurate and vary because of differences in resting $\dot{V}O_2$. The stability of MET values will also be reduced with competition.

3. *Using established values in a nonneutral environment.* Oxygen uptake and METs can be altered by environmental conditions such as wind, temperature, hilly terrain, and texture of the running surface.

TABLE 6.1. Leisure Activities: Sports, Exercise Classes, Games, Dancing—Approximate Range in Energy Cost (METs)[a]

Archery (target or field)	3–4	Horseshoe pitching	2–3
Backpacking	5–11	Hunting (bow or gun)	3–7
Badminton	4–9	Small game (walking, carrying light load)	3–7
Basketball		Hunting (bow or gun)	
Nongame	3–9	Big game (dragging carcass, walking)	3–14
Game play	7–12		
Bed exercise		Jogging (running)	7–15
(arm movement, supine or sitting)	1–2	Mountain climbing	5–10
Bicycling		Paddleball	
(pleasure or to work)	3–8	(or racquetball)	8–12
Bowling	2–4	Sailing	2–5
Canoeing, rowing, and kayaking	3–8	Scuba diving	5–10
Conditioning exercises		Shuffleboard	2–3
(calisthenics)	3–8	Skating, ice and roller	5–8
Dancing		Skiing, snow	
(social and square)	3–7	Downhill	5–8
Fencing	6–10	Cross-country	6–12
Fishing		Sledding	
From bank, boat, or ice	2–4	(and tobogganing)	4–8
Stream (wading)	5–6	Snowshoeing	7–14
Football, touch	6–10	Squash	8–12
Golf		Soccer	5–12
Using power cart	2–3	Softball	3–6
Walking (carrying bag or pulling cart)	4–7	Stair climbing	4–8
		Swimming	4–8
Handball	8–12	Table tennis	3–5
Hiking, cross-country	3–7	Tennis	4–9
Horseback riding	3–8	Volleyball	3–6

[a]Adapted from Fox SM, Naughton JP, Gorman PA. Physical activity and cardiovascular health. III. The exercise prescription: frequency and type of activity. Mod Concepts Cardiovasc Dis 1972;41:25.

4. *Incorrectly determining METs during the exercise test.* Accurate MET values assume a steady state at each work increment. If this assumption is not met, as often happens with certain test protocols, then the published MET values are not valid.

METs are easy to use in prescribing exercise intensity. No monitoring equipment is required, and one does not have to worry about counting the pulse.

TABLE 6.2. Leisure Activities: Nonsports Approximate Range in Energy Cost (METs)[a]

Activity	METs
Carpentry	2–7
Electric vibrator	2
Gardening	
Hoeing	4–8
Digging, shoveling, and pushing	4–8
Wheelbarrow	4–10
Weeding	3–5
Raking	3–6
Home improvement (painting, plumbing)	3–8
Heavy housework (scrubbing floors, making beds)	3–6
Light housework (sweeping, polishing, ironing)	2–4
Mowing lawn	
On cart	2
Power mower	4–5
Hand mower	4–6
Splitting and sawing wood or cutting trees	
Hand	5–10
Power	2–4
Snow shoveling	
Wet snow	8–15
Powder snow	6–9
Walking	
Horizontal or slight grade	3–5
Steep grade	6–8
Upstairs	6–8
Downstairs	4–5

[a]Adapted from Fox SM, Naughton JP, Gorman PA. Physical activity and cardiovascular health. III. The exercise prescription: frequency and type of activity. Mod Concepts Cardiovasc Dis 1972;41:25.

However, the method has limitations and, when a precise exercise intensity is needed (e.g., with cardiac patients), it is better to rely on physiologic data.

Exercise intensity can also be prescribed from ratings of perceived exertion (RPE). The concept of perceived exertion was originally devised by Borg (18, 19) and has been reviewed extensively (18). The RPE scale (Table 6.4) was developed to help quantify perceived exertion and to test its reliability and validity for use in exercise prescription and evaluating the stress of physical activity. The Borg scale ranges from 6 to 20 (1 to 10 in the modified version) and

TABLE 6.3. Comparison of Work Output During Bicycle Ergometry and Treadmill Work[a]

METs	Bicycle Ergometer External Work Output		Energy Expenditure of an Average Individual (70-kg body weight)			Treadmill Work Loads[e]		
	(kpm/min)[b]	(Watts)[c]	O2 Uptake (L/min)	O2 Uptake (ml/kg × min)	Calories[d] (per min)	Speed (mph)		Grade (%)
2.4	150	25	0.6	8.5	3.0	2.0		0.0
3.7	300	50	0.9	13.0	4.5	3.0		0.0
5.0	450	75	1.2	17.0	6.0	3.0		5.0
6.0	600	100	1.5	21.0	7.5	3.0		7.5
7.0	750	125	1.8	26.0	9.0	3.0		10.0
8.5	900	150	2.1	30.0	10.5	3.0		15.0
						4.0		10.0
10.0	1050	175	2.4	36.0	12.0	4.0		14.0
11.0	1200	200	2.7	39.0	14.0	7.0	(running)	0.0
						3.5		16.0
12.0	1350	225	3.0	43.0	15.0	4.0		18.0
						3.5		20.0
13.5	1500	250	3.3	47.0	17.0	8.0	(running)	0.0
						4.2		16.0
14.5	1650	275	3.8	51.0	18.0	3.5		26.0
						4.0		22.0
16.0	1800	300	3.9	56.0	20.0	10.0	(running)	0.0
						5.0		18.0

[a]Adapted from Exercise testing and training of apparently healthy individuals: a handbook for physicians. New York, American Heart Association, 1972.
[b]Kilopond-meter: Energy necessary to lift a 1-kg mass 1 m against the normal gravitational force.
[c]Watt: A unit of power equal to 6.12 kpm/min.
[d]Calorie: A unit of energy based on heat production. One calorie equals 200 ml of O_2 consumed.
[e]Steady state required.

253

TABLE 6.4. RPE Scales[a]

Category RPE Scale (Original)		Category-Ratio RPE Scale (Revised)	
6		0	Nothing at all
7	Very, very light	0.5	Very, very weak
8		1	Very weak
9	Very light	2	Weak
10		3	Moderate
11	Fairly light	4	Somewhat strong
12		5	Strong
13	Somewhat hard	6	
14		7	Very strong
15	Hard	8	
16		9	
17	Very hard	10	Very, very strong
18		•	Maximal
19	Very, very hard		
20			

[a]From Borg GA. Med Sci Sports Exerc 1982;14:377–387.

assigns subjective estimates of effort to numeric scores. The original numeric scale was devised to represent approximately 10% of the heart rate range in healthy young and middle-aged men (18). RPE has also become popularized as a method for determining level of effort in functional and diagnostic exercise stress testing.

Research shows that RPE correlates well with several physiologic functions (e.g., heart rate, oxygen uptake, ventilation, respiratory rate, body temperature, and lactate levels) and is useful and accurate for prescribing exercise both in healthy individuals and in cardiac patients (19–22). Because RPE is sensitive to changes in physiologic data, an individual can be taught to associate a perception-of-effort score with a given heart rate. Although the use of RPE is straightforward in prescribing exercise, considerable practice is recommended for valid results (23). In particular, RPE should be used carefully and sparingly for cardiac patients—more as a reflection of how the patient feels than as an indication of a target heart rate. Careful instructions are needed along with a diagnostic exercise test for cardiac patients. The exercise test is necessary to assure patient safety, because contraindicating signs may occur without symptoms at modest levels of effort and RPE values (24). RPE are especially helpful for patients who are taking heart rate-altering medications such as beta-blockers. Under these circumstances it may be impossible to determine the onset of fatigue from physiologic information. This precaution is seldom important in young, healthy people, although it reinforces the necessity of an exercise test for persons with known or suspected atherosclerotic heart disease.

Duration

Duration, intensity, and frequency interact in such a way that modifications in any one component affects the other two. The exercise session lasts for at least 20 to 30 minutes (11), although highly conditioned individuals often train continuously for an hour or longer. While significant physiologic gains have been reported from 5 to 10 minutes of exercise per day (25), little is known about the effectiveness of exercising several times per day for short durations. The duration of training is sometimes increased while intensity is decreased early in the training program to prepare the musculoskeletal system for vigorous exercise and to reduce the chance of injury.

Frequency

Regular exercise should be performed at least 3 or 4 days a week to be beneficial (11), although fewer sessions may be sufficient for some (4). Less than two days a week will not be beneficial for most persons, although little information is available for the severely deconditioned. It has also been shown that exercising three or four days a week has the same effect as five or more, although athletes and those in superior physical condition typically train 5 to 7 days a week.

The exercise stimulus must be sufficient to provoke a training effect, but excessive exercise should be avoided. Overtraining can be avoided by carefully monitoring physiologic, psychologic, and performance indicators. Guidelines for intensity, frequency, and duration of exercise are summarized in Table 6.5.

The length of the program is another important factor of program design. Most monitored cardiac rehabilitation programs last for eight to twelve weeks, a constraint of reimbursement. Changes in heart rate response to exercise have been documented in as few as two weeks (7), while other changes, (e. g., body composition) many require several months (7, 26). The rate and magnitude of

TABLE 6.5. Exercise Requirements for Achieving Cardiovascular Changes in Highly Trained Persons, Sedentary Individuals, and Cardiac Patients[a]

	Intensity	Frequency	Duration
Highly trained	85–90% max HR	5–7 days	1–2 hours
Sedentary and cardiac	60–85% max HR	3–5 days	15–45 min

[a]From Fardy PS. Training for aerobic power. *In*: Burke EJ, ed. Toward an understanding of human performance. Ithaca, New York: Movement Publications, 1977.

change can vary considerably among individuals and is affected by the intensity of exercise and initial level of fitness.

Modes of Exercise

The exercise mode should reflect the purpose of the program, the interest and ability of the participant, and physical limitations. If the goal is general improvement of physical fitness, then a variety of activities are included. A comprehensive physical assessment should be made to identify musculoskeletal weaknesses, and specific exercises are designed to address those needs. Aerobic exercise is emphasized if the primary objective is to improve cardiovascular endurance.

When an athlete trains for a sport, the exercise training mode is most often task related. Specificity of training is the guiding principle. Adaptation occurs primarily in those muscle groups and even in specific muscle fibers that are overloaded. Few training changes take place in other muscles. Therefore athletes train with activities that resemble the sport, if not the actual activity; for example, a sport that utilizes arm and shoulder exercise requires upper body training.

Cardiovascular function and physical work capacity are best improved through continuous rhythmic exercises that incorporate large muscle groups and are designed to overload the oxygen transport system. Brisk walking, running, jogging, swimming, bicycling, rowing, and cross-country skiing are all excellent. While there is no "best" type of exercise, each of these examples has distinct advantages and disadvantages. Swimming and bicycling are especially good for sedentary individuals and those in poor physical condition, because there is less musculoskeletal trauma compared with weight-bearing activities. However, one must possess specific skills for bicycling and swimming and must meet the facility and equipment requirements. An exercise prescription for swimming is best devised from a swimming test, or at least an evaluation of upper extremity muscles. Swimming prescriptions based on treadmill test results could overload the cardiovascular system and compromise patient safety (27).

One advantage of walking and running is that minimal equipment and facilities are needed. A level surface with resiliency is recommended. Good shoes are important and an orthopedic assessment may prove useful to identify potential podiatric problems. The technology of footwear and orthotics has improved dramatically; shoes and inserts can be designed to meet individual needs, musculoskeletal structures, and orthopedic limitations.

Heavy-resistance and isometric exercises have limited value in enhancing cardiovascular function, especially in elderly, cardiac and coronary-prone populations. Such activities impose a pressure overload as opposed to the volume overload on the left ventricle that is normally observed from continuous aerobic activities, which increase cardiac output and reduce peripheral resistance. Other potential problems include dangerous Valsalva maneuvers, arrhythmias, and increased pressor responses (28, 29). Anatomic changes of the ventricle can occur with both types of exercise, but only training with a volume overload improves ventricular function. Although there is some evidence to suggest that modest cardiovascular benefits are possible from heavy-resistance or isometric activities, especially in those with normal ventricular function (30), they are most effective in developing strength and increasing muscle size. In contrast, low-resistance weight training has been shown to be safe with physical, physiologic, and psychologic benefits for cardiac and high-risk coronary patients (31–33).

Isokinetic exercise is a popular type of resistance training. Many schools, fitness centers, and health clubs are equipped with isokinetic exercise devices. They are fun to use, provide a variety of activities, and are especially beneficial for muscle strength and endurance since specific muscle groups and even muscle fibers can be isolated and trained. Isokinetic exercise enhances strength and cardiovascular function (4, 34). The different types of exercise training programs are discussed later in this chapter.

SPECIAL CONSIDERATIONS

Environmental Factors

Ideal temperatures for exercise are between 40 and 70°F (4 and 24°C) with a relative humidity below 65% (35). Ambient temperatures that approach the shell and core temperature (i.e., above 90°F), especially when combined with high humidity, impose increased thermal regulatory and cardiovascular demands. Evaporation and cooling are impeded when the air is saturated with water vapor. Cardiovascular efficiency and physical work capacity decrease, heart rates rise sharply, and stroke volumes fall because of peripheral vasodilation and decreased venous return. The dosage of effort has to be decreased to maintain the THR. Patients with mild congestive heart failure need to take special precautions in hot and humid weather because heat-related injuries can increase cardiovascular demand. The reader is referred elsewhere for more information about heat-related illnesses (36).

The exercise prescription is affected less by cold. An individual who is healthy and properly clothed generally will have few difficulties adjusting to low temperatures. To avoid frostbite the skin should not be exposed to extremely low temperatures. Cold and dry air may aggravate the respiratory tract temporarily, but this is seldom clinically significant. Wearing a face mask may help to alleviate the discomfort, although the temperature of inspired air rises quickly and is generally above freezing as it reaches the trachea. The elderly, those with known atherosclerotic heart disease, and patients with compromised

Wind Speed (mph)	Thermometer Reading (°F)										
	50	40	30	20	10	0	−10	−20	−30	−40	−50
	(Equivalent temperature [°F])										
5	48	37	27	16	6	−5	−15	−26	−36	−47	−57
10	40	28	16	4	−9	−24	−33	−46	−58	−70	−83
15	36	22	9	−5	−18	−32	−45	−58	−72	−85	−99
20	32	18	4	−10	−25	−39	−53	−67	−82	−96	−110
25	30	16	0	−15	−29	−44	−59	−74	−88	−104	−118
30	28	13	−2	−18	−33	−48	−63	−79	−94	−109	−125
35	27	11	−4	−20	−35	−51	−67	−82	−98	−113	−129
40	26	10	−6	−21	−37	−53	−69	−85	−100	−115	−132
	Minimal Risk				Increasing Risk			Great Risk			

FIGURE 6.4. Wind chill index. (Modified from McArdle WD, Katch FI, Katch VL. Exercise physiology: Energy, nutrition, and human performance. 3rd ed. Philadelphia: Lea & Febiger, 1991.)

left ventricular function must be particularly cautious in cold weather when performing heavy-resistance or isometric exercise, for example, shoveling snow. Cold temperature can cause peripheral vasoconstriction and precipitate left ventricular pressure overload and increased vascular resistance, thereby increasing myocardial oxygen demand and potential ischemia. Vasodilation can also result from vigorous activity when the person is overly dressed. This can lead to venous pooling and decreased venous return, especially with upright exercise and little muscle movement. Wind velocity is an additional important consideration (Fig. 6.4).

The exercise prescription will also be influenced by changes in altitude. Arterial oxygen saturation decreases at high altitudes and causes a chemoreceptor response that increases both the depth and rate of pulmonary ventilation. Arterial blood is approximately 95 to 98% saturated with oxygen at sea level. At altitudes above 5000 feet arterial oxygen saturation decreases, reaching approximately 50% saturation at 15,000 feet. $\dot{V}O_{2max}$ is reduced, although maximal heart rate and stroke volume may not be affected. Diminished arterial saturation and decreased peripheral extraction cause heart rate and cardiac output to increase at submaximal efforts to compensate for decreased oxygenation. Physical work has to be reduced compared to that at low altitudes, although the heart rate prescription generally remains unchanged. Because the physiologic effects can increase cardiovascular risk, a conservative exercise prescription is recommended at high altitudes for cardiac patients and those in poor physical condition. Because of the physiologic advantage of going from high altitudes to sea level, the dosage of exercise can usually be increased.

Acclimatization takes place in two to four weeks, following which the prescription usually can be upgraded.

At attitudes above 5000 feet physical activity should be closely monitored in cardiac patients who normally live at sea level. Myocardial hypoxia can be induced at high altitudes, which, when combined with physical exertion, can precipitate ischemia and possible myocardial infarction. Altitude acclimatization results in increased hemoglobin, growth of new capillaries in organs, and increased myoglobin concentration of the heart and skeletal muscles. These alternatives improve the capacity for transport and utilization of oxygen and increase aerobic capacity toward the normal sea-level value (4).

Air pollution can also affect the exercise prescription and cause specific health-related problems in patients with cardiorespiratory illness. Carbon monoxide causes a negative hemodynamic response to exercise by combining with hemoglobin, for which it has a greater affinity than oxygen, and by forming carboxyhemoglobin. Elevated levels of carboxyhemoglobin can precipitate angina at a reduced rate × pressure product (37, 38), increase myocardial ischemia as evidenced by greater ST-segment displacement (39, 40), and increase mortality from cardiovascular diseases (41). Ozone can also adversely affect exercise. High concentrations are associated with asthma, as well as chronic heart and lung diseases. Patients with cardiorespiratory illness are especially susceptible and may require several hours to recover from ozone attacks. Exercise in high-ozone levels may also have significant short-term effects on healthy individuals by aggravating the respiratory tract, which results in coughing, nausea, and other forms of distress. Considering the health implications associated with physical exertion when air pollutants are elevated, program directors need to be familiar with acceptable air quality standards. Air pollution standards are presented in Tables 6.6 and 6.7.

Cardiac Transplantation

Cardiac transplantation has become a viable surgical procedure with approximately 2500 operations performed in 1989 (42). To date there are no standard guidelines, although several references are available that have nicely summarized experiences in cardiac rehabilitation with these patients (43–45).

The denervated heart has no autonomic nervous system control of heart rate response. Instead circulating catecholamines are primarily responsible for heart rate adaptation to exertion. Heart rate at rest is elevated as a consequence of parasympathetic denervation. At the same time heart rate during submaximal and maximal physical exertion is suppressed because sympathetic stimuli are absent. The heart rate response to activity rises slowly throughout exercise, plateaus in recovery, and slowly returns to a preexercise rate (42, 44).

Because the heart rate response is blunted, the exercise prescription is often based on Borg scale ratings of perceived exertion, generally between 11 and 14,

259

TABLE 6.6. Primary and Secondary Pollutants: Mechanism of Effect, Effect on Exercise Performance, and Factors That Enhance the Effect[a]

Pollutant	Mechanism of Effect	Submaximal Exercise	Maximal Exercise ($\dot{V}O_{2max}$)	Factors Enhancing the Effect	
				Environmental Conditions	Conditions and/or Disease
Primary pollutants:					
Carbon monoxide (CO)	Decreased Hb saturation with oxygen; Decreased ability to deliver O_2 to cells	Little impairment unless levels of COHb greater than 20%	Inversely related to concentration of CO; Significant effect when levels >4.3%	Altitude; Cigarette smokers; Time of day with heaviest traffic patterns; Midwinter (peak values)	Impaired exercise tolerance with CV disease; People with CV may have effect at submaximal exercise with levels as low as 2.5–3%
Sulfur oxides (SO_2, sulfuric acid, sulfate)	Upper respiratory irritant; Bronchoconstriction; Increased airway resistance	Threshold level of effect: 1.0 to 3.0 ppm in healthy individuals	Unknown	Burning of fossil fuels; High humidity; Oral breathing	Asthmatics (threshold levels between 0.2 and 0.5 pm); Respiratory illness; Elderly
Nitrogen oxides (Primary NO_2)	Constriction of small airways and alveoli; Increased airway resistance	Does not appear to have adverse effects in healthy people	Unknown	Peak values with heavy motor vehicle traffic; Increase with smoke (cigarette or fire); Oral breathing; Midwinter (peak values)	Possibly those with chronic bronchitis, COPD, and other respiratory disorders
Primary particles (TSP) (dust, soot, smoke)	Bronchoconstriction; Increased airway resistance; Possible inflammation congestion	Unknown	Unknown	Soot: incomplete combustion of fossil fuels; Dust storms, forest fires, wind storms; Volcanoes	Asthma; Chronic lung disease; Aggravation of CR disease symptoms

260

TABLE 6.6. Cont.

Pollutant	Mechanism of Effect	Submaximal Exercise	Maximal Exercise ($\dot{V}O_{2max}$)	Factors Enhancing the Effect		
				Environmental Conditions	Conditions and/or Disease	
Secondary pollutants:						
Ozone (O_3)	Bronchoconstriction of small airways and proximal alveoli	No effect at light to moderate exercise (increased respiratory discomfort)	Unknown (performance potentially limited at high levels of O_3)	Peak values in afternoon (related to hours of sunlight) Early autumn/summer Heat stress	Asthma Respiratory diseases	
Peroxyacetyl nitrate (PAN)	Minor pulmonary function alterations Eye irritant	No effect	No effect	Ozone		
Aerosols, sulfate, nitrate, sulfuric acid	Particles <3 microns reach alveoli Airway irritation with possible airway constriction	Minimal	Minimal			

*a*Adapted with permission from Pandolf KB: Air quality and human performance. In Pandolf KB, Sawka MN, Gonzalez RR, eds. Human performance physiology and environmental medicine at terrestrial extremes. Indianapolis: Benchmark Press, 1988.

TABLE 6.7. Comparison of the Pollution Standard Index Values With Pollutant Concentrations and Descriptor Words[a]

Index Value	Air Quality Level	TSP (24-hr) $\mu g/m^3$	SO$_2$ (24-hr) $\mu g/m^3$	CO (8-hr) $\mu g/m^3$	O$_3$ (1-hr) $\mu g/m^3$	NO$_2$ (1-hr) $\mu g/m^3$	Health Effect Descriptor
500	Significant harm	600	2620	57.5	1200	3750	
400	Emergency	500	2100	46.0	1000	3000	Hazardous
300	Warning	420	1600	34.0	800	2260	Very unhealthful
200	Alert	350	800	17.0	400	1130	Very unhealthful
100	NAAQS[c]	150	365	10.0	235	[b]	Moderate
50	50% of NAAQS	50	80	5.0	118	[b]	Good
0		0	0	0.0	0	[b]	

[a]Data with permission from Pandolf KB: Air quality and human performance. In: Pandolf KB, Sawka MN, Gonzalez RR, eds. Human performance physiology and environmental medicine at terrestrial extremes. Indianapolis: Benchmark Press, 1988. TSP, total suspended particulates, SO$_2$, sulfur dioxide, CO, carbon monoxide; O$_3$, ozone; NO$_2$, nitrogen dioxide; $\mu g/m^3$=ppm × molecular weight/0.024.

[b]No index values reported at concentration levels below those specified by "alert level" criteria.

[c]NAAQS = National Average Air Quality Standards.

or on oxygen uptake, between 60 to 70% of maximum (42–44). The heart rate reserve method might also be applicable for determining the target heart rate range while taking resting heart rate into consideration (45). Further studies are needed to verify heart rate and metabolic relationships in transplant patients. Exercise sessions are generally stuctured similar to those for postinfarct or CABGS patients, that is, 3 times a week and 30 minutes per session. The prescription is based on the results of maximal exercise testing administered within 1 to 2 months following surgery (42) and incorporating measurement of $\dot{V}O_2$. The benefits of exercise for these patients are outlined in Table 6.8 (42).

Cardiovascular Health

The design of the exercise prescription is significantly influenced by the objectives of the program. If the primary objective is to reduce the risk of coronary disease, as opposed to improving cardiovascular fitness, then adherence to a target heart rate of 70 to 85% MHR is not critical. Little information is available on the dose of exercise required to improve cardiovascular health, although studies have shown that modest dosages reduce the risk of coronary disease (46–48). Furthermore, compliance to a lifetime of regular physical activity is more likely with modest exercise than with more vigorous exercise required to improve aerobic fitness (49).

Weight Control

Intensity of effort is also less important for weight loss. Therefore strict adherence to a target heart rate is usually not required. Instead the prescription focuses on exercise for creating a negative caloric balance, possibly combined with reduced caloric intake. The intensity of exercise is of most interest as it impacts on program duration and the total energy expenditure. Exercise of lower intensity is advisable at the outset to reduce injuries and enhance compliance. Markedly obese persons are more likely to have a successful exercise outcome if the level of intensity is not overly taxing. Another advantage of low intensity exercise is that weight loss can be achieved over time with little or no diet alteration.

Elderly and High-Risk Patients

The exercise prescription will be different in many respects for elderly and high-risk patients compared to young, healthy subjects (50). Habitual physical activity, physical limitations, musculoskeletal condition, age, and body weight are factors that need special consideration in this population. The intensity of effort is usually lower than for the younger subjects, perhaps as low as 30 to 40% $\dot{V}O_{2max}$ or 50 to 70% MHR. When the target heart rate is low, it may be necessary to increase the duration of exercise to provide an overload stimulus. In some instances it may be necessary to reduce intensity and duration.

263

TABLE 6.8. Benefits of Exercise Training for Cardiac Transplant Recipients[a]

Increased maximal oxygen uptake
Increased peak power output
Increased maximal heart rate
Decreased resting heart rate
Decreased submaximal exercise heart rate
Increased maximal systolic blood pressure
Increased anaerobic threshold
Increased lean body mass
Improvement in steroid myopathy
Increased maximal minute ventilation
Decreased submaximal exercise minute ventilation
Reduced exercise ventilatory equivalent for oxygen
Reduced rest and submaximal exercise systolic and diastolic blood pressure
Decreased maximal exercise diastolic blood pressure
Reduced submaximal exercise perceived exertion
Reduced body fat stores[b]
Improved psychosocial function[b]
Improved blood lipid profile[b]

---

[a]From Squires RW. Rehabilitation after cardiac transplantation: 1980–1990. J Cardiopulmonary Rehabil 1991;11:8–92.
[b]Potential benefits.

At times the intensity of effort may be reduced for musculoskeletal considerations. The frequency of activity may also have to be adjusted in light of changes in intensity and duration. The number of exercise sessions per day or week may be increased in response to lowered intensity and shortened duration. Rest intervals may be interspersed between bouts of exercise.

More complete personal history and lifestyle information is recommended for elderly and high-risk patients before prescribing exercise. The prescription will likely be progressed more slowly, and additional modifications may be required based on individual needs. For example, the duration of warm-up and cooldown may be increased. A longer warm-up will enhance flexibility and prepare the musculoskeletal system for increased effort. A prolonged cooldown will be necessary if the heart rate requires a longer time to return to preexercise levels. Exercises that may be stressful for the joints, particularly activities that are weight bearing, should be undertaken cautiously and possibly delayed until the patient is adequately prepared. Shoes with high shock absorbency are recommended for walking and jogging. Resistance exercise is recommended to increase strength and reduce musculoskeletal problems that result from age-induced bone mineral loss (50, 51). Added caution should be taken with high temperature and humidity since heat dissipation through evaporation diminishes with age (51, 52). Exercise intensity may be prescribed by Borg scale ratings of perceived exertion for those who have a difficult time in locating the pulse and accurately counting heart rates.

THE EXERCISE PROGRAM

The exercise program consists of a series of exercise sessions at the designated prescription. A description of the exercise session is discussed thoroughly in Chapters 9 and 10.

Counting the Pulse

The benefits of exercise and compliance are enhanced when the exercise prescription is closely maintained. Exercise heart rates are best measured with pulse monitoring equipment, although the cost and possible discomfort of such equipment may be prohibitive. More likely the THR will be monitored by palpating the heart or pulse, counting the number of beats for a given period, and extrapolating to a full minute. Counting the pulse is relatively simple but must be practiced in advance for accuracy and reliability. Palpating the heart beat through clothing can be difficult in obese persons and in those with a faint pulse. It is generally easier to palpate a pulse following exercise. The carotid and radial pulses are particularly good sites. Patients who have coronary heart disease may be sensitive to carotid sinus reflex (53) and should be careful when palpating at this site.

The best procedure for counting the heart rate manually is to obtain the number of beats in a specified period and convert the count to a minute rate. A more accurate technique requires a stopwatch, taking the time for a designated number of beats, and converting to a minute pulse. Tables 6.9 and 6.10 are suggested for quickly converting time to rate. The stopwatch method is as follows:

1. The stopwatch is started at the first detectable beat, which is counted as zero.
2. The watch is stopped on the last beat, either 10 or 30.
3. Convert to a minute heart rate.

Because the heart rate decelerates rapidly after exercise, especially in well-trained persons, it is important to locate the pulse quickly. The exercise heart rate will be underestimated if it takes too long to locate and count the pulse. Even after 20 to 30 seconds the pulse will begin to slow. Five sources of potential error may affect results:

TABLE 6.9. Conversion of Pulse Beats for 10 Seconds Into Minute Heart Rate

10-Second Rate	Minute Rate	10-Second Rate	Minute Rate
10	60	23	138
11	66	24	144
12	72	25	150
13	78	26	156
14	84	27	162
15	90	28	168
16	96	29	174
17	102	30	180
18	108	31	186
19	114	32	192
20	120	33	198
21	126	34	204
22	132	35	210

TABLE 6.10. Conversion Table for Time of 10 Pulse Beats to Pulse Rate Per Minute[a]

Time (sec)	Heart Rate (bpm)	Time (sec)	Heart Rate (bpm)	Time (sec)	Heart Rate (bpm)
6.0	100	4.8	125	3.6	167
5.9	102	4.7	128	3.5	171
5.8	103	4.6	130	3.4	176
5.7	105	4.5	133	3.3	182
5.6	107	4.4	136	3.2	188
5.5	109	4.3	140	3.1	194
5.4	111	4.2	143	3.0	200
5.3	113	4.1	146	2.9	207
5.2	115	4.0	150	2.8	214
5.1	118	3.9	154	2.7	222
5.0	120	3.8	158	2.6	230
4.9	122	3.7	162	2.5	240

[a]Based on technique of Saltin et al. Scand J Clin Lab Invest 1969;24:323.

1. It takes too long to locate the pulse.
2. Counting may not be accurate, especially at rapid rates.
3. Inaccurate timing.
4. Heart rates taken after exercise do not always reflect the rates during activity.
5. Arrhythmias make pulse counting difficult and less accurate.

Continuous Versus Intermittent Exercise

The choice of either continuous or intermittent (interval) training is going to be influenced by the purpose of the program. There are advantages in each of these training methods, and the best prescription probably contains elements of both. Intermittent training is advantageous for high-intensity exercise. More physical work can be completed in the same length of time with fewer by-products of anaerobic metabolism. Continuous training for at least 4- to 6-minute periods, but usually 10 to 20, is recommended early in the program, especially for those in poor condition, to get the musculoskeletal system prepared for vigorous exercise.

Beginning an exercise program with high-intensity, intermittent training can invite unnecessary muscle soreness, fatigue, and injury. However, intermittent training is particularly beneficial because it is flexible and easily applied in carefully regulated doses and can incorporate a variety of activities.

Types of Training Programs

Various training programs are available from which to choose. Some definitions are appropriate: *Aerobic exercise* consists of low to moderate level activity where the oxygen supply is sufficient to meet the demand. *Anaerobic exercise* is more vigorous, high-intensity activity whereby the oxygen supply to the muscles is inadequate to meet the demands. *Isotonic resistance exercise* describes muscle contraction accompanied by joint movement and resulting in work being accomplished, that is, work = force (resistance) × distance (movement). Resistance may change throughout the range of motion as with weight training, or it may be constant as with certain exercise machines. *Isometric exercise* describes muscle contraction that results in increased muscle fiber tension but no joint movement, that is, no work is being accomplished. *Isokinetic exercise* describes muscle contraction at a constant speed throughout the range of motion. *Continuous exercise* consists of activity that is usually prolonged and aerobic. Generally the target heart rate is achieved and maintained in a steady state throughout the duration of the activity. *Interval or intermittent exercise* consists of short bouts of higher-intensity exercise interspersed with periods of rest. Classic interval training consists of an established pattern of time and distance of work, number of repetitions, and time interval for rest.

Motivation

A measure of program success is the participant's adherence and compliance. Long-term adherence data are discouraging, indicating dropout rates up to 50% during the early months of activity (54). Few individuals are disciplined sufficiently to focus on long-range goals. Many are discouraged by the discomfort of physical exertion, sore muscles and injury, and by benefits that are intangible and difficult to perceive. Because of this the following 10 motivational suggestions are offered.

1. Establish realistic short-term and long-range goals. A system of daily, weekly, or monthly points can help goal attainment.
2. Try to exercise in a group or with a partner. Peer support, group dynamics, and encouragement are extremely valuable.
3. Be sure that the prescription is safe and beneficial.
4. Vary the training program to increase interest.
5. Incorporate professional supervision when possible.
6. Clothing, equipment, and facilities should create a pleasant atmosphere and a safe background for exercise.
7. Utilize positive feedback and demonstrable results that are rewarding and encouraging.
8. Employ tangible rewards such as pins and articles of clothing.
9. Keep a careful record of activity at each session.
10. HAVE FUN!

Prescribing Exercise at the Work Site

Exercise programs at the work site can benefit employers and employees. The size of work-site programs varies according to the resources available, accommodating as few as a handful to as many as the entire workforce of a company. Guidelines for training are the same as those previously discussed. Most work-site programs incorporate a variety of aerobic and resistance type equipment.

While exercise programs at the work site are common, many companies have limited resources. Success often relies on a creative staff who can develop modest yet effective programs (55). An example of creative planning was a stair-climbing exercise program that was developed for employees of a high-rise building in an urban setting. The program was undertaken in the stairwells of the building, and demonstrated excellent compliance, improved cardiovascular function, reduced body fat, and enhanced work efficiency (25, 56). The program showed that regular exercise could be provided without traditional gymnasium facilities at a very modest cost and could be easily scheduled into the regular workday.

School-Based Programs

School-based programs offer another opportunity for a significant impact in health promotion. The focus of programs for children and adolescents should be on primary prevention and the development of lifestyle habits that will continue into adulthood. The onset of atherosclerosis and coronary risk factors in childhood has been well demonstrated (57–60), emphasizing the need for preventive programs at an early age. Risk factors have been shown to track within families (61); therefore school-based programs may also benefit parents and siblings. School-based programs have demonstrated success at improving fitness, reducing risk factors, increasing health knowledge, and improving health behavior (62–66), although additional studies are needed to identify needs and methodologies for ethnic and gender differences.

The Training Session

The training session is the culmination of all the factors that comprise and affect the exercise prescription. It is divided into warm-up, conditioning stimulus, and cooldown.

Warm-up

Warm-up consists of general and specific exercises at low intensity for the purpose of increasing respiration, circulation, and muscle temperature in preparation for more vigorous exercise and to lower the risk of musculoskeletal trauma. Specific warm-up exercises are incorporated for the purpose of complementing the conditioning exercises. For example, flexibility exercises are recommended with running programs to increase range of motion, reducing the possibility of muscle injury at joints not emphasized in the conditioning program. Exercises for the lower back are particularly advisable. Warm-up has also been shown to reduce myocardial ischemia, a benefit that is especially significant for cardiac patients (67). A thorough warm-up should last for a minimum of 10 to 15 minutes.

Conditioning Stimulus

The conditioning stimulus is designed to produce training adaptation. The THR should be maintained at a rate above the overload threshold and maintained for at least 20 to 30 minutes, three or four times a week for most persons.

These guidelines are modified for individuals in very poor or very good physical condition, as well as for other physical or clinical reasons. The conditioning stimulus should ensure the benefits of exercise without undue muscle fatigue, stress, or injury.

Cooldown

Cooldown consists of a gradual tapering off of intensity following the conditioning stimulus. A low level of activity should be continued for 10 to 15 minutes or until the heart rate is substantially reduced and approaches resting values. This helps to replenish the supply of energy reserves and to aid in the removal of the by-products of energy metabolism. The muscles that are utilized in the training phase should be kept in motion to help remove lactic acid from those areas. In general, cooldown should incorporate large muscle groups that have a massaging effect on the veins and enhance venous return. Abruptly terminating exercise causes venous pooling in the lower extremities, decreases ventricular filling, and increases myocardial oxygen demand as a result of compensatory heart rate increase.

Adaptation to Training

Training adaptation occurs centrally and peripherally. Central function consists of cardiac output, that is, heart rate × stroke volume, whereby oxygen is supplied to the muscle cells. Peripheral adaptation involves cellular changes that enable greater oxygen exchange and utilization. Training adaptation in the cardiovascular system is divided into aerobic and anaerobic.

Aerobic Capacity

The most important measurement of aerobic training adaptation is $\dot{V}O_{2max}$. Considered the single best indicator of cardiovascular fitness, $\dot{V}O_{2max}$ (aerobic power) reflects both central and peripheral adaptive mechanisms. The principal central component is cardiac output. Under normal circumstances aerobic training causes heart rates to become lower at rest and in response to a fixed submaximal effort. Maximal heart rates are not appreciably changed and may even decrease slightly. As heart rate decreases, stroke volume increases at rest, at fixed submaximal efforts, and at maximal exertion. Therefore cardiac output remains unchanged at rest and during submaximal work, but at maximal exercise it is increased, thereby providing additional oxygen to the working muscles.

While the delivery system for oxygen and nutrients (i.e., cardiac output) is enhanced through aerobic conditioning, substantial changes also occur in peripheral function. Peripheral adaptation consists of changes that occur within the muscle structure. These changes may be cellular, biochemical, or gross morphologic alterations and may include any of the following (4):

- Increased muscle vascularization
- Increased muscle fiber number
- Increased muscle fiber size
- Increased mitochondria size and number
- Increased oxidative enzymes

- Increased ability to oxidize fatty acids as a source of energy
- Elevated levels of muscle glycogen
- More efficient utilization of muscle glycogen
- Reduced production of lactate

The most important changes are elevated muscle glycogen, increased fat oxidation, increased oxidative enzymes, and increased mitochondria size and number. The magnitude of adaptation varies considerably among individuals and is affected by age and physical condition. Young persons and those initially in poor condition have a greater capacity to improve than older individuals and those who are more highly conditioned. Physical fitness is also affected to a large degree by genetic endowment.

Anaerobic Capacity

Anaerobic capacity is improved by high-intensity training usually performed in short work intervals interspersed with brief periods of rest. Physical effort is usually maximal or near maximal and is generally not more than one or two minutes in duration. Rest intervals between exercise periods must be sufficiently long to spare muscle glycogen depletion and prohibit the buildup of lactic acid. Anaerobic training is often muscle specific, which makes the selection of training exercises extremely important. Because anaerobic training is at a high intensity level, it should be preceded by aerobic conditioning to prepare the musculoskeletal system for the vigorous effort to follow.

Regardless of the training techniques that are employed, physical conditioning should be an ongoing process. Because deconditioning begins soon after training has ceased, a lifetime commitment of regular exercise is necessary. Frequent starting and quitting is ill-advised but is typical of the way that many people approach exercise. As a consequence, potential long-term benefits are not realized and the risk of injury or untoward events is increased.

Untoward Events

The chance of an untoward cardiac event is reduced if exercise is prescribed as a percentage of maximal attained heart rate. Therefore the target heart rate is lower than the peak rate that was attained on the sign-and-symptom–limited exercise stress test. Untoward events may be reduced further by learning to recognize normal and abnormal subjective feelings associated with exercise. Because increases in physical exertion can be perceived accurately, exercise intensity can be estimated subjectively With cardiac patients perceived exertion should be used with objective estimates of intensity because of the possible appearance of abnormalities when effort is perceived as light (24). Untoward signs and symptoms are listed in Table 6.11.

TABLE 6.11. Common Untoward Signs and Symptoms During and Following Exercise[a]

During Exercise	Following Exercise
Angina pectoris	Insomnia
Chest discomfort	Excessive excitement
Skipped beats	Exhilaration
Excessive dyspnea	Weakness
Uncoordination	Fatigue
Lightheadedness	Muscular cramping
Faintness	Skeletal muscular pain
Syncope	Gastrointestinal disturbances
Cold sweat	Nausea
Undue muscle soreness	Vomiting
Fatigue	

[a]Based on Hellerstein HK et al. Principles of exercise prescription: for normals and cardiac subjects. *In*: Naughton JP, Hellerstein HK, Mohler IC, eds. Exercise testing and exercise training in coronary heart disease. Orlando, FL: Academic Press, 1973.

Updating the Prescription

Healthy individuals and cardiac patients with uncompromised or slightly compromised left ventricular function will usually begin to improve after four to six weeks of exercise. Most often the initial rate of improvement is rapid, followed by slower adaptation and eventual plateauing. As adaptation occurs, heart rates are reduced at fixed submaximal levels of effort, thereby requiring more physical work to maintain the THR. Workloads must continue to be increased for training changes.

The exercise staff has the responsibility of updating the exercise prescription when appropriate. This can be done by increasing workloads so that the relative heart rate remains constant and by increasing the target heart rate so that one is exercising at a greater intensity of effort. For example, after a few weeks of exercise, a workload on the bicycle ergometer might be increased from 300 to 450 kpm/min to keep the person at the training target heart rate. After a few more weeks, the target heart rate might be increased from 70 to 75% maximum, which would again result in increased workloads. Increases in heart rate prescription are often in increments of 5% although this guideline doesn't apply for everyone. Over a 12-week cardiac rehabilitation program, the target heart rate is usually increased to 80 or even 85% MHR. Before relative heart rate is increased, the cardiac rehabilitation staff should assess the progress of the patient to assure the most prudent course of action.

Exercise Prescription Form

An exercise prescription form should be developed that includes all of the information necessary for a safe and beneficial exercise training session. The form should include results of the most recent exercise test, medications, comments and recommendations, and the exercise prescription. The prescription form should be signed by the program physician in the case of cardiac patients and should be accessible to supervising staff during training sessions. Information must be updated at subsequent evaluations.

CONCLUSIONS

The exercise prescription is based on the results of an individual evaluation, preferably a sign-or-symptom–limited exercise test, and takes into consideration age, medical history, level of physical condition, physical limitations, and personal interests. Intensity, frequency, duration, and mode of exercise are developed to meet individual needs. Hopefully the exercise regimen will become part of a lifelong plan to foster better health and fitness. Sedentary normal subjects and low-risk cardiac patients should generally train a minimum of 3 times a week, for 20 to 30 minutes per session, at 70 to 85% of the maximal heart rate. The exercise prescription needs to be individualized and must be adjusted as cardiovascular fitness and physical work capacity improve. Training adaptation usually requires a minimum of 4 to 6 weeks. The most appropriate modes of exercise for those interested in cardiovascular function are continuous aerobic activities that utilize upper and lower extremities. Good facilities and equipment are important in well-designed programs, although staff creativity is probably the most important factor of a successful program. High-risk patients, the elderly, and extremely poorly conditioned persons will exercise at a prescription appropriate for them. Additional references are suggested (68, 69).

REFERENCES

1. DiNubile NA. Strength training. Clin Sports Med 1991;10:33–61.
2. Liehman W. Flexibility/range of motion In: American College of Sports Medicine, ed. Resource manual for guidelines for exercise testing and prescription. Philadelphia: Lea & Febiger, 1993.
3. Moffatt RJ, Cucuzzo N. Strength considerations for exercise prescription. In: American College of Sports Medicine, ed. Resource manual for guidelines for exercise testing and prescription. Philadelphia: Lea & Febiger, 1993.
4. McArdle WD, Katch FI, Katch VL. Exercise physiology: energy, nutrition and human performance. 3rd ed. Philadelphia: Lea & Febiger, 1990.
5. Fardy PS. Training for aerobic power. In: Burke EJ, ed. Toward an understanding of human performance. Ithaca, NY: Mouvement Publications, 1977.
6. Astrand I. Aerobic work capacity in men and women with reference to age. Acta Physiol Scand 1960;49(Suppl 169):45.
7. Pollock ML. The quantification of endurance training programs. In: Wilmore JH, ed. Exercise and sport sciences reviews. Vol 1. Orlando, FL: Academic Press, 1973.

8. Fardy PS, Webb DP, Hellerstein HK. Benefits of arm exercise in cardiac rehabilitation. Phys Sports Med 1977;5:33.
9. Franklin B, Hodgson J, Buskirk ER. Relationship between percent maximal O_2 uptake and percent maximal heart rate in women. Res Q Exerc Sport 1980;51:616.
10. Vander LB, Franklin BA, Wrisley D, Rubenfire M. Cardiorespiratory responses to arm and leg ergometry in women. Phys Sports Med 1984;12:101.
11. American College of Sports Medicine: Guidelines for exercise testing and prescription. 4th ed. Philadelphia: Lea & Febiger, 1991.
12. Lester M, Sheffield LT, Trammell P, Reeves TJ. The effect of age and athletic training on the maximal heart rate during muscular exercise. Am Heart J 1968;76:370.
13. Pollock ML et al. Effects of frequency and duration of training on attrition and incidence of injury. Med Sci Sports 1977;9:31.
14. Meytes I. Wenckebach A-V block: A frequent feature following heavy physical training. Am Heart J 1975;90:126.
15. Killip T. Time, place, event of sudden death. Circulation 1975;52 (Suppl 3):160.
16. Wilmore JH. Prescribing exercise for healthy adults. In: Wilson PK, ed. Adult fitness and cardiac rehabilitation. Baltimore: University Park Press, 1975.
17. Karvonen MJ, Kentala E, Mustala O. The effects of training on heart rate. A "longitudinal" study. Ann Med Exp Biol Fenn 1957;35:307.
18. Borg GA. The perceived exertion: a note on "history" and methods. Med Sci Sports 1973;5:90.
19. Borg GA. Psychophysical bases of perceived exertion. Med Sci Sports 1982;14:377.
20. Williams JG, Eston RG. Determination of the intensity dimension in vigorous exercise program with particular reference to the use of the rating of perceived exertion. Sports Med 1989;8: 177–189.
21. Skinner JS, Buskirk ER. The validity and reliability of a rating scale of perceived exertion. Med Sci Sports 1973;5:94.
22. Noble BJ. Clinical applications of perceived exertion. Med Sci Sports Exerc 1982;14:406.
23. Bayles CM et al. Perceptual regulation of prescribed exercise. J Cardiopulmonary Rehabil 1990; 10:25–31.
24. Williams MA, Fardy PS. Limitations in prescribing exercise. J Cardiovasc Pulmon Tech 1980; 3:33.
25. Fardy PS, Ilmarinen J. Evaluating the effects and feasibility of an at-work stairclimbing intervention program for men. Med Sci Sports 1975;7:91.
26. Fardy PS, et al. Effects of two years' exercise training in patients with diagnosed coronary artery disease. Med Sci Sports 1980;12:100.
27. Ribisl PM, Miller HS. Errors in exercise prescription for cardiac patients in aquatic programs using treadmill data. Circulation 1976;54(Suppl 2):226.
28. Atkins JM, Matthews OA, Blomqvist CG, Mullins CB. Incidence of arrhythmias induced by isometric and dynamic exercise. Br Heart J 1976;38:465.
29. Flessas AP et al. Effects of isometric exercise on the end-diastolic pressure, volumes, and function of left ventricle. Circulation 1976;53:839.
30. Fardy PS. Isometric exercise and the cardiovascular system. Phys Sports Med 1981;9:43.
31. Stewart KJ. Introduction to the symposium. Resistive weight training: a new approach to exercise for cardiac and coronary disease prone populations. Med Sci Sports Exerc, 1989;21: 667–668.
32. Goldberg AP. Aerobic and resistive exercises modify risk factors for coronary heart disease. Med Sci Sports Exerc 1989;21:669–674.
33. Ewart CK. Psychological effects of resistive weight training: implications for cardiac patients. Med Sci Sports Exerc 1989;21:683–688.
34. Gettman LR, Culter LA, Strathman TA. Physiologic changes after 20 weeks of isotonic vs. isokinetic circuit training. J Sports Med Phys Fitness 1980;20:265.
35. Yaglou CP. Temperature, humidity, and air movement in industries: the effective temperature index. Am J Physiol 1927;58:439.

36. Vogel JA, Rock PB, Jones BH, Haventith G. Environmental considerations in exercise testing and training In: American College of Sports Medicine, ed. Resource manual for guidelines for exercise testing and prescription. Philadelphia: Lea & Febiger, 1993.

37. Aronow WS, Isbell MW. Carbon monoxide effect on exercise-induced angina pectoris. Ann Intern Med 1973;79:392.

38. Anderson EW et al. Effect of low level carbon monoxide exposure on onset and duration of angina pectoris. A study of 10 patients with ischemic heart disease. Ann Intern Med 1973;79:46.

39. Aronow WS Effect of cigarette smoking and of carbon monoxide on coronary heart disease. Chest 1976;70:514.

40. Aronow WS. Effect of freeway travel on angina pectoris. Ann Intern Med 1972;77:669.

41. Cohen SI, Diane M, Goldsmith JT. Carbon monoxide and survival from myocardial infarction. Arch Environ Health 1969;19:510.

42. Squires RW. Rehabilitation after cardiac transplantation: 1980–1990. J Cardiopulmonary Rehabil 1991;11:84–92.

43. Kavanagh T et al. Exercise rehabilitation after heterotopic cardiac transplantation. J Cardiopulmonary Rehabil 1989;9:303–310.

44. Squires RW. Cardiac rehabilitation issues for heart transplantation patients. J Cardiopulmonary Rehabil 1990;10:159–168.

45. Keteyian S, Ehrman J, Fedel F, Rhoads K. Heart rate-perceived exertion relationship during exercise in orthotopic heart transplant patients. J Cardiopulmonary Rehabil 1990;8:287–293.

46. Morris JN et al. Early exercise training in patients over age 65 years compared to that in younger patients following acute myocardial infarction or coronary artery bypass grafting. Am J Cardiol 1985;55:263–266.

47. Paffenbarger RS Jr et al. Physical activity, all-cause mortality, and longevity of college alumni. N Engl J Med 1986;314:605.

48. Morris JN et al. Vigorous exercise in leisure-time and the incidence of coronary heart disease. Lancet 1973;1:333.

49. Blair S. Rigidity or adaptability in exercise science and clinical practice. Sports Med Bull 1991; 26;5.

50. Williams MA. Exercise testing and training in the elderly cardiac patient. Fardy PS, series editor. Champaign, IL: Human Kinetics, 1993.

51. Wolfel EE, Hossacle JF. Guidelines for the exercise training of elderly healthy individuals and elderly patients with cardiac disease. J Cardiopulmonary Rehabil 1989;9:40–45.

52. Wenger NK. Exercise for the elderly: highlights of preventive and therapeutic aspects. J Cardiopulmonary Rehabil 1989;9:9–11.

53. White JR. EKG changes using carotid artery for heart rate monitoring. Med Sci Sports 1977;9:88.

54. Oldridge NB. Compliance with exercise programs. In: Pollock ML, Schmidt DH, ed. Heart disease and rehabilitation. 2nd ed. New York: John Wiley, 1986.

55. Fardy PS. Prevention is good business: Fitness in Business 1987;1:220–226.

56. Ilmarinen J et al. Training effects of stair-climbing during office hours on female employees. Ergonomics 1979;22:507–516.

57. Berenson GS et al. Review: atherosclerosis and its evolution in childhood. Am J Med Sci 1987;294:429–440.

58. Newman WP et al. Relation of serum lipoprotein levels and systolic blood pressure to early atherosclerosis: the Bogalusa heart study. N Engl J Med 1986;314:138–144.

59. Lauer RM et al. Coronary heart disease risk factors in school children: the Muscatine study. J Pediatr 1975;86:697–706.

60. Fardy PS et al. Coronary risk factors and health behaviors in a diverse ethnic and cultural population of adolescents: a gender comparision. J Cardiopulmonary Rehabil 1994;14:52–60.

61. Perusse L et al. Familial aggregation in physical fitness, coronary heart disease risk factors, and pulmonary function measurements. Prev Med 1987;16:607–615.

62. Walter HJ, Hofman A, Vaughan RD, Wynder EL. Modification of risk factors for coronary heart disease. Five-year results of a school-based intervention trial. N Engl J Med 1988;318: 1093–1100.

275

63. Killen JD et al. The Stanford adolescent heart health program. Health Educ Quart 1989;16:263–283.

64. Wilmore JH, McNamara JJ. Prevalence of coronary heart disease risk factors in boys 8–12 years of age. Pediatrics 1974;84:527–533.

65. Nader PR et al. A family approach to cardiovascular risk reduction: results from the San Diego family health project. Health Educ Quart 1989;16:229–244.

66. Fardy PS et al. Health promotion in minority adolescents: a Healthy People 2000 pilot study. J Cardiopulmonary Rehabil 1995;15:65–72.

67. Barnard RJ et al. Ischemic response to sudden strenuous exercise in healthy man. Circulation 1973;5:936.

68. Yanowitz FG, ed. Coronary heart disease prevention. New York: Marcel Dekker, 1992.

69. American Association of Cardiovascular and Pulmonary Rehabilitation, ed. Guidelines for cardiac rehabilitation programs. Champaign, IL: Human Kinetics, 1991.

III. ADMINISTRATIVE CONCERNS

7

INTRODUCTION TO PROGRAM ADMINISTRATION

THIS CHAPTER CONSIDERS PLANNING, implementation, development, and management of cardiac rehabilitation and adult fitness programs. The material covered is offered as a general introduction to program administration. Greater detail is provided in subsequent chapters. Additional resources on administration are also suggested (1–3).

PLANNING

The initial consideration in administering a program involves a series of steps that pertain to planning. A scheme of these steps is illustrated in Figure 7.1.

The first step in planning for cardiac rehabilitation is to assess the need for and feasibility of a program. The annual data on the prevalence of coronary artery disease and the number of cardiovascular procedures (4), in conjunction with studies of adherence (5, 6), show that approximately 2% of the total population within 20 to 30 minutes of a cardiac rehabilitation center provides a rough estimate of eligible candidates. Approximately 2000 of every 100,000 persons

STEPS IN PLANNING CARDIAC REHABILITATION

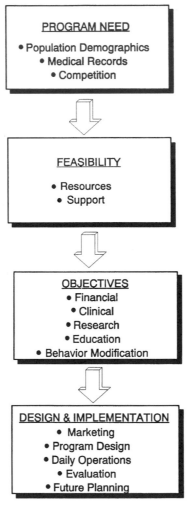

FIGURE 7.1. Steps in planning cardiac rehabilitation.

TABLE 7.1. Sources of Information for Needs and Feasibility Assessment

1.	Population demographics, e.g., age, socioeconomic status
2.	Hospital admissions
3.	Competition
4.	Enthusiasm of medical community
5.	Community needs and interest

would meet the eligibility criteria for cardiac rehabilitation as established by Medicare and most third-party private insurance carriers. Patients meeting the criteria include those recovering from (a) acute myocardial infarction (MI), (b) coronary artery bypass surgery (CABGS), and (c) angioplasty (PTCA), as well as those with stable angina pectoris and cardiac transplant patients. Of this number, 25% is a reasonable expectation of the eventual size of the program (author's personal observation). The actual number will be affected by several factors of which physician support is the most important.

Age and socioeconomic data of the population must also be considered. A large number of elderly citizens, for example, means that there will be more patients eligible for cardiac rehabilitation and more who will depend on Medicare. An aging population will also be more reluctant to drive long distances and will have different activity needs and interests. Furthermore, studies of blue-collar workers have demonstrated poor adherence in cardiac rehabilitation (5, 6), although this might be influenced by how well the program is managed and the motivation of the patients. Community demographics should be carefully evaluated in the early planning phase.

Medical records are useful for obtaining a more accurate number of potential cardiac rehabilitation patients, as well as the names of referring physicians, and can provide a good estimate of the potential size, cost, and revenues of a program. A survey of competition in the area should be undertaken to assess the viability of a new program and to avoid unnecessary replication of services. Methods used to assess need and feasibility are summarized in Table 7.1.

A comprehensive needs assessment is also recommended in planning adult fitness programs. It is important to determine: (a) the perception of need in the community, (b) specific activity interests, (c) competitive programs in the community, and (d) factors that might influence scheduling.

Program Objectives

After the needs and feasibility have been established, the next planning step is to define the program's objectives to ensure that the program director understands what is expected by the institutional administration. The types of objectives include the following: (a) financial, (b) clinical, (c) research, (d) education, and (e) behavior modification (Fig. 7.1).

Financial

The financial objectives should be clarified to establish a budget and cost/revenue expectations. Two questions need to be answered:

1. Is the program expected to make money, break even, or operate at a loss?
2. If operating at a loss is acceptable, how much deficit spending can be sustained?

Most hospital-based programs are established with the primary intent of providing a service rather than making a profit. A small loss is generally acceptable, especially when offset by good public relations and other indirect benefits. Because deficit-operating programs are scrutinized carefully in today's highly competitive hospital industry, financial goals are a very important early priority.

Freestanding, physician-directed centers provide an important clinical service that has high visibility and can be profitable. Sometimes freestanding programs are established for the purpose of complementing diagnostic services that have greater revenue-producing potential, for example, Holter monitoring, exercise stress testing, and echocardiography. The simplest way to develop a freestanding program is with a group of physicians who have a large cardiovascular practice to establish a facility to meet the needs of their patients. The business plan would not count on patient referrals from physicians outside of the practice. A large cardiology practice has a good chance at being profitable.

In a different business arrangement, one that can be equally successful, independent physicians or businessmen would own the rehabilitation center. In this example there might be a larger referral base, although the greater the number of investors the more difficult the program may be to manage and control. Federal regulations have been clearly written that outline the requirements for such centers (7).

An important aspect of financial objectives is the creation of a business plan, which is a long-term strategic document that estimates revenues and expenses. A clear, concise business plan makes review of a proposal much easier. A good business plan should include projected revenues and expenses for both the short and long term. Business plans are discussed in detail elsewhere (8).

Clinical

The clinical objectives refer to the medical rationale for the program and reflect the philosophy of the institution and the professional staff. In general the clinical objectives are divided into primary, secondary, and tertiary prevention.

Primary prevention. The objective is to prevent or reduce the risk of disease onset through health promotion and physical fitness. The focus is on healthy individuals and those with risk factors for coronary artery disease but no disease pathology. Guidelines for testing and training in this population have been developed by the American College of Sports Medicine (9).

Secondary and Tertiary Prevention. In these programs (see Chapter 1) the individual either has asymptomatic coronary artery disease or has already experienced clinical manifestations of disease. The purpose is to prevent clinical disease onset or further complications. Some patients with risk factors qualify for secondary prevention. A few with multiple risk factors may even qualify for reimbursement under some insurance programs. Detailed documentation is required including a list of goals, projected outcomes, and a reasonable time plan for completion. Patients with chronic obstructive lung disease and those with significant cardiac arrhythmias may also be a part of secondary or tertiary prevention. Monitored exercise classes can be useful and relatively inexpensive for adjusting antiarrhythmic medications and determining the prevalence of ectopic beats with physical activity in patients with frequent arrhythmias. Electrocardiographic monitoring during serial exercise sessions will likely reveal more arrhythmias than a single exercise stress test (10, 11). ECG monitoring can also be done during home exercise with transtelephonic electrocardiography.

Research

As a part of program planning it should be decided whether to include research and, if so, the time that will be allotted. The decision ultimately affects personnel, facility, and equipment selection.

Undertaking research can be labor intensive, time consuming, and have limited visible financial benefit. In most instances conducting research will add to the program cost. The exceptions are usually academic institutions with a serious commitment to pursue outside funding. Incurring an additional cost for an objective that is not well understood may be difficult to justify to non–academically oriented administrators and board members. However, a hospital that is perceived as a leading heart research center can ultimately benefit through increased admissions and procedures. While most serious research is conducted at academic institutions, the professional staff at the community hospital can engage in research if adequate resources are available. If the hospital administration opposes the professional staff being engaged in research, then this must be made clear in job descriptions and during the hiring process.

Even when research is not a part of the total program, systematic data collection and analysis are recommended for program evaluation. Evaluating measurable outcomes is considerably more meaningful than subjective evaluation and, if well done, contributes to the program's success.

Education and Behavior Modification

Patient education and behavior modification are important aspects of prevention and cardiac rehabilitation. Because these programs can be expensive and generally are not reimbursed, a decision is necessary about the extent of the commitment to this objective. Cost-benefit analysis must be carried out and must take into account long-term financial and patient-benefit implications. Patient education and behavior modification require a trained professional staff and the equipment and materials to facilitate learning. The facility should be conducive for learning, and the classes should be informative and should motivate individuals to make difficult lifestyle changes.

Ongoing education is also recommended for the professional staff. Continuing education programs that provide credit should be offered to physicians, nurses, and other staff members. Examples of professional education include grand rounds presentations, seminars, conferences, medical society meetings, and meetings of local and state medical associations, nursing associations, and public health and vocational rehabilitation agencies. It is also advisable to provide regular formal and informal progress reports to the medical and nursing staffs and to allow them an opportunity for input. The sessions should be informative and descriptive. Updated materials and information should be attractively packaged and presented. Community education and service should also be a part of cardiac rehabilitation and adult fitness. While these programs constitute an added expense, they may be justified if they increase public awareness of the institution and its commitment to health, physical fitness, and prevention. Because the modern-day medical center is in an excellent position to affect community health, service programs that are provided free or at low cost to the consumer are an excellent marketing strategy. Examples of community service programs include health seminars, speakers bureau, health fairs, risk factor screening, and school-based preventive programs. The cost of service programs should be estimated in advance and weighed against their benefits.

Health and fitness programs are also recommended for the institution's employees. Introducing employee health and fitness as the first phase of a comprehensive program can be an effective way to demonstrate the quality of the professional staff. The employee program is introduced through staff meetings, announcements, and mail notices. The cost to employees should be kept low, although a small fee is suggested to give the employee some ownership. Care should be taken so that the program is available to everyone. This may be difficult in a hospital because of shift work, but it is important to make every attempt to give all employees opportunity to participate.

PROGRAM IMPLEMENTATION

Once the goals of the program have been established and agreed on, it is time for implementation. The steps to be considered are as follows:

- Marketing
- Program design
- Daily operations
- Evaluation
- Future planning

Marketing

A well-conceived marketing strategy should be in place before the program begins. In a hospital-based program the medical staff must be given an opportunity for input that will provide a sense of ownership and encourage their support. A medical advisory board or committee is suggested for keeping physicians informed and responding to their concerns. The advisory board is good for public relations, helps to defuse problems, and is a good vehicle for disseminating information to the medical staff. Physicians who are not a part of the medical staff but practice nearby should be given information about the program and an opportunity for input.

The marketing needs associated with freestanding, physician-owned and -directed clinics are quite different from those that are hospital-based. In the case of a physician-owned facility the principal source of patient referrals is generally the physician owners. In fact, physicians who are interested in owning a freestanding cardiac rehabilitation program should plan to meet their financial goals solely from their own patient referrals. Other physicians should be marketed, especially if no competitive programs exist, but not counted on for referrals.

Primary care physicians are potentially a large source of referrals and should be a significant part of the marketing scheme. Occasionally, they are reluctant to refer patients. Reasons for their nonsupport include the following:

1. Lack of information about cardiac rehabilitation in general and about the program in particular
2. Lack of enthusiasm about potential benefits
3. Loss of patient control
4. Loss of services and income

The marketing scheme must address these issues so that the primary care physician has a level of comfort with the program. In addition to mailing material to the physicians in the area, it is advisable to personally visit these physicians to familiarize them with the program's objectives, procedures, and results. The primary care physician should also be encouraged to perform normal services that are permitted under Medicare guidelines.

The following are marketing strategies that are recommended for both hospital-based and freestanding programs:

1. The medical community must be informed individually about the prospective program. Announcements should be mailed to all physicians in the community, and an "open house" should be planned at an appropriate time.
2. Physicians who refer patients must be regularly updated about their patient's progress.
3. When marketing to physicians emphasize that the essence of the program is to complement, not to replace their care. Pay particular attention to assure them that the patient-physician relationship will not be compromised. Be certain that the referring physician is notified of any emergency or patient problem as soon as possible.
4. Regularly provide documentation about the efficacy of cardiac rehabilitation and risk factor management.

The general public should also be a part of the marketing scheme. Word of mouth is an excellent source of patient referral and should be encouraged. Media advertising to the public must be careful to include a statement that a referral from the personal physician is required.

An advisory board of influential citizens from the community is also suggested. The advisory board helps to sell the program to the community, provides assistance on special occasions, provides feedback from the community to the program director, and promotes good public relations. It is also advisable to work closely with service organizations, health agencies, educational institutions, and large employers in the community. Use local resources whenever possible. An individual with marketing expertise can be a valuable addition to the professional staff.

Adult fitness centers should utilize news events to attract media coverage. Although the media is unlikely to provide free advertising for profit-based programs, they will cover newsworthy items. Keep the name of the center regularly in the news. Be sure that the marketing plan responds to the socioeconomic level of the community and the clientele of the center. Examples of media news events include health-fitness days, fun runs, health screenings, health-fitness columns in the newspaper, and radio shows. A well-conceived marketing plan is even more necessary in promoting adult fitness programs since competition is so keen.

Facilities, equipment, and personnel are discussed in detail in the following chapters. The information provided here is to serve as a reminder that these topics need to be addressed in program planning.

Facilities

The different phases of cardiac rehabilitation have varying facility requirements. In the case of a new building or renovation the program administrator should become familiar with architectural plans and work closely with the architect. The architect is usually not too familiar with the details of the program, and consequently shortcomings in the facility's plans may be better recognized by the program director. Facilities are also discussed elsewhere (12, 13).

Equipment

Equipment requirements are also different in each phase of the program, and the program administrator has the responsibility of becoming familiar with the various choices. Because there are often so many equipment options, it is recommended that demonstrations and, if possible, short-term loans of equipment be considered before purchasing. The professional staff who will use the equipment should be actively involved in the selection process. Equipment is discussed elsewhere (12, 13).

Personnel

As a general rule, the size and the background of the professional staff are determined by the scope of the program. A comprehensive interdisciplinary and multidisciplinary cardiac rehabilitation program might include physicians, nurses, exercise specialists, educators, nutritionists, psychologists, physical and occupational therapists, administrators, business manager, marketing expert, and support staff. Some staff members may be hired on a part-time basis as consultants or subcontractors. Staff are added as the program expands, resources become available, and patient needs are identified.

Most of the professional personnel in adult fitness have a background in physical education, with a specialty in exercise science, exercise physiology, or corporate fitness. Health classes that complement exercise may require personnel with specific training. Examples are aerobic dance, stress management, nutrition, and selected sport skills. A business manager, marketing person, and support staff are also necessary.

Regular personnel evaluations and reports are needed to enhance job performance and to provide an opportunity for a formal exchange of ideas and feelings between the director and the individual program staff members. The personnel review should include the information listed in Table 7.2. The program administrator should use the review process as a positive experience to motivate individual staff members. Good managerial skills are required to avoid parties becoming intimidated and defensive.

TABLE 7.2. Job Performance Review

- Knowledge of subject
- Enthusiasm
- Organization
- Communication
- Diligence
- Attentiveness to detail
- Punctuality
- Self-starting
- Innovative, creative
- Responsible
- Initiative and resourcefulness
- Sound judgment
- Personal appearance
- Personality
- Professional goals
- Satisfactions and disatisfactions
- Suggestions

TABLE 7.3. Program Costs

- Facility (rent, renovation, construction)
- Equipment (purchase, lease)
- Personnel (salaries, consultants, subcontractors)
- Supplies (reusable, expendable)
- Maintenance
- Service contracts (laundry, cleaning)
- Insurance
- Publications (printing, copying, journal costs, artwork, etc.)
- Professional travel
- Marketing
- Utilities
- Special events
- Miscellaneous

Billing and Reimbursement

Projections of expenses and revenues are a part of all program planning. The cost of a program can be estimated from the items listed in Table 7.3. Revenues are projected from the estimated number of patients and average reimbursement. The amount of reimbursement varies significantly among insurance carriers and individual coverage.

Because of the complexity of billing it is advisable to have a financial administrator who is experienced with these procedures, who understands how to deal with commercial third-party carriers, as well as Medicare and Medicaid, and who is familiar with the diagnosis-related group (DRG) system. In the case of a freestanding facility it may be worthwhile to employ an outside agency for this service. A good billing service is familiar with procedures and possesses the computer technology to do the job efficiently. The cost of this service is typically between 5% and 10% of collections. In addition to understanding the nuances of reimbursement, the person responsible for billing must be familiar with diagnostic and billing codes (14, 15). Since these may change, it is essential to keep abreast of current information and trends.

Referral and Orientation

A patient must have a written physician referral to enter into a cardiac rehabilitation program. The referral includes the patient diagnosis and basic clinical information. A sample referral form is provided (Fig. 7.2). If there is a question of the patient's suitability for rehabilitation, it is the responsibility of the medical director to make the final decision. A program orientation is suggested following the referral to introduce the staff; discuss objectives, procedures, and financial obligations; show the facility and equipment; and provide an opportunity for questions and answers.

Patient Follow-Up

The patient and family have to understand that cardiac rehabilitation is about changing lifestyle and that success depends on a lifetime commitment. Therefore a plan for follow-up is essential to provide ongoing personal contact, updated information, motivation, and reinforcement. The patient must be provided with sufficient information to accept greater personal responsibility for changing living habits. Procedures used in follow-up are discussed further in Chapters 3 and 5. A flowchart of the patient's progress through a program is shown in Figure 7.3. Patient support techniques are an integral part of follow-up programs, particularly at the conclusion of phase II when many patients opt to continue with exercise at home. Heart health clubs, regular social functions, and newsletters are examples that provide an ongoing source of information, group interactive dynamics, and patient motivation. Many of these approaches can quickly be turned over to patient leadership.

REFERRAL FORM
(to be completed by physician)

Patient's Name_____ Date_____
                Last   First   Middle Initial

Address_____ _____
        Street   City   State   Home Telephone

Birth Date_____ Age_____ Spouse's Name_____

Insurance Company_____ Policy No._____

Diagnosis: _____Bypass Surgery   _____Myocardial Infarct
                  _____Cardiac Patient   _____Angioplasty
                  _____Symptomatic Coronary Artery Disease (Angina)
Other:_____ Explain_____

Specific Cardiac Information_____

Other Limitations_____

Date of Most Recent Hospital Admission_____

Medications	Dosage	Frequency	Date Prescribed	Physician Prescribing

Please fill in information below if possible:
Date of Examination_____
1. Urine: sp. gr._____ Alb._____ Glucose_____ Micro._____
2. Complete blood count: Hbg_____ Hct_____ WBC_____ Diff._____
3. ECG, 12 lead (enclose copy)_____
4. Blood pressure: Systolic R_____ L_____ Diastolic R_____ L_____
5. Cholesterol _____mg%; HDL _____mg%; LDL _____mg%; Triglycerides _____ mg%
6. Exercise Stress Test Results (enclose, if available)

Impression of above information_____

Signed _____, M.D.

Type or Print:

Name of Physician_____
Address_____
Phone_____

FIGURE 7.2. Referral form.

Medicolegal Considerations

The risk of fatal or serious complications associated with exercise is relatively small for both healthy adults and patients with diagnosed coronary disease (16–19). However, issues of safety and liability must be given serious attention. It is recommended that the professional staff be familiar with medicolegal and

PROGRESSION THROUGH CARDIAC REHABILITATION

```
┌──────────────────────────────────────────────┐
│           Physician Referral to Phase II       │
└──────────────────────────────────────────────┘
(within days)              ⇩
┌──────────────────────────────────────────────┐
│              Program Orientation               │
└──────────────────────────────────────────────┘
(immediately)              ⇩
┌──────────────────────────────────────────────┐
│              Sign-up for Program               │
└──────────────────────────────────────────────┘
(within days)              ⇩
┌──────────────────────────────────────────────┐
│           Evaluation and Prescription          │
└──────────────────────────────────────────────┘
(within days)              ⇩
┌──────────────────────────────────────────────┐
│                 Enter Phase II                 │
└──────────────────────────────────────────────┘
(4-24 weeks)               ⇩
┌──────────────────────────────────────────────┐
│          Evaluation of Effects of Phase II     │
└──────────────────────────────────────────────┘
(within days)              ⇩
┌──────────────────────────────────────────────┐
│             Enter Long-term Program            │
└──────────────────────────────────────────────┘
(6-12 months)              ⇩
┌──────────────────────────────────────────────┐
│     Regular Follow-up and Updated Prescription │
└──────────────────────────────────────────────┘
```

FIGURE 7.3. Progression through cardiac rehabilitation.

safety factors (20). Adequate liability insurance is required, necessitating that administrators of freestanding programs shop around and negotiate for the best coverage. The program administrator must be familiar with city, state, and federal regulations that affect the conduct of the program. Standards for conduct have been developed and published by the American Medical Association (21), American Heart Association (22), American College of Sports Medicine (9), and the American Association of Cardiovascular and Pulmonary Rehabilitation (1). In addition, a detailed description of policies and procedures should be developed for use in planning and program management. Patient records must be carefully maintained and contingency plans for emergencies need to be

291

TABLE 7.4. Common Areas of Potential Liability and Exposure

In the course of conducting exercise programs, certain common claims seem to be the most likely sources of litigation. A summary follows:

1. Failure to monitor an exercise test properly and/or to stop an exercise test in the application of competent professional judgement.

2. Failure to evaluate the participant's physical capabilities or impairments competently, factors that would proscribe or limit certain types of exercise.

3. Failure to prescribe a safe exercise intensity in terms of cardiovascular, metabolic, and musculoskeletal demands.

4. Failure to instruct participants adequately as to safe performance of the recommended physical activities or the proper use of exercise equipment.

5. Failure to supervise properly the participant's exercise during program sessions or to advise individuals regarding any restrictions or modifications that should be imposed in performing conditioning activities during unsupervised periods.

6. Failure to assign specific participants to an exercise setting with a level of physiologic monitoring, supervision, and emergency medical support commensurate with their health status.

7. Failure to perform or render performance in a negligent manner in a variety of other situations.

8. Rendition of advice to a participant that is later construed to represent diagnosis of a medical condition or is deemed tantamount to medical prescription to relieve a disease condition and that subsequently and/or proximately causes injury and/or deterioration of health and/or death.

9. Failure to refer a participant to a physician or other appropriately licensed professional in response to the appearance of signs or symptoms suggestive of health problems requiring medical or other professional attention.

10. Failure to disclose certain information in the informed consent process or failure to maintain proper and confidential records documenting the informed consent process, the adequacy of participant instructions with regard to performance of program activities, and the adequacy of their physical responses to physical activity regimens.

11. Failure to respond adequately to an untoward event with appropriate emergency care.

developed and practiced regularly. The most common sources of litigation for exercise programs are listed in Table 7.4 (20).

Evaluation

The effectiveness of the program must undergo regular evaluation. The process should include the following information:

- Patient enrollment
- Efficiency of patient flow

- Program benefits
- Cost-benefit analysis
- Program safety
- Personnel assessment

MANAGERIAL SKILLS

Implementing programs also requires day-to-day management skills. An effective administrator possesses:

- Good interpersonal skills
- Well-organized thoughts and actions
- Innovative and creative thinking
- The ability to follow through
- Effective communication skills
- A thorough understanding of program information
- Futuristic thinking
- The ability to delegate responsibility
- Good leadership skills
- Time management
- Insightfulness

One may be an effective administrator without being equally proficient in all of these skills, but should at least possess most of these abilities. Good administrators will recognize their personal shortcomings and constantly strive to improve themselves. Managerial skills are discussed elsewhere (8).

CONCLUSIONS

Although a good administrator is one who can successfully delegate responsibilities, this does not detract from the importance of being a skilled manager. To review, the key factors for an administrator to consider in developing a program are as follows:

1. Establish the need and feasibility.
2. Define the objectives.
3. Have a thorough understanding of the project's financial requirements.
4. Be familiar with all aspects of a comprehensive program.
5. Have a good understanding of marketing techniques.
6. Have an appreciation for planning and developing facilities.
7. Be familiar with equipment.
8. Understand personnel requirements.
9. Have an understanding of the nuances of billing and reimbursement.

10. Know the patient flow through the program.
11. Develop a detailed, clear, and concise policy and procedure manual.
12. Have a knowledge of medicolegal considerations.

REFERENCES

1. American Association of Cardiovascular and Pulmonary Rehabilitation. Guidelines for cardiac rehabilitation programs. Champaign, IL: Human Kinetics, 1991.
2. American College of Sports Medicine, eds. Resource manual for guidelines for exercise testing and prescription. 2nd ed. Philadelphia: Lea & Febiger, 1993.
3. Hall LK, Meyer GC, eds. Cardiac rehabilitation: Exercise testing and prescription. Vol 2. Champaign, IL: Life Enhancement Publications, 1988.
4. Heart facts. Dallas: American Heart Association, 1992.
5. Oldridge NB. Compliance and exercise in primary and secondary prevention of coronary heart disease: a review. Prev Med 1982;11:56.
6. Oldridge NB. Compliance with exercise programs. In: Pollock ML, Schmidt DH, eds. Heart disease and rehabilitation. 2nd ed. New York: John Wiley, 1986.
7. Medicare hospital manual. Department of Health and Human Services, Health Care Financing Administration, Transmittal No. 312, HCFA Pub. No. 10, Sept. 1982.
8. Gettman LR. Management skills. In: American College of Sports Medicine, eds. Resource manual for guidelines for exercise testing and prescription. 2nd ed. Philadelphia: Lea & Febiger, 1993.
9. American College of Sports Medicine, eds. Guidelines for exercise testing and prescription. 4th ed. Philadelphia: Lea & Febiger, 1991.
10. Williams MA, Fardy PS. Limitations in prescribing exercise. Cardiovasc Pulmon Technol 1980; 8:33.
11. Simoons M, Lap C, Pool J. Heart rate levels and ventricular ectopic activity during cardiac rehabilitation. Am Heart J 1980;100:9.
12. Guidelines for cardiac rehabilitation centers. Los Angles: American Heart Association, Greater Los Angeles Affiliate, 1982.
13. Grantham WC, Howley ET. Facility design, equipment selection, and calibration. In American College of Sports Medicine eds. Resource manual for guidelines for exercise testing and prescription. 2nd ed. Philadelphia: Lea & Febiger, 1993.
14. Fanta CM et al. Physicians current procedural terminology. 4th ed. Chicago: American Medical Association, 1985.
15. International classification of diseases. 9th revision. Clinical modification. Vols 1 and 2. Ann Arbor, MI: Commission on Professional and Hospital Activities, March 1980.
16. Haskell WL. Cardiovascular complications during exercise training of cardiac patients. Circulation 1978;57:920.
17. Thompson PD. Cardiovascular hazards of physical activity. In: Terjung RL, ed. Exercise and sport sciences reviews. Philadelphia: Franklin Institute Press, 1982.
18. Rochmis P, Blackburn H. Exercise tests: a survey of procedures, safety, and litigation experience in approximately 170,000 tests. JAMA 1971;217:1061.
19. Thompson PD. The safety of exercise testing and participation. In: American College of Sports Medicine, eds. Resource manual for guidelines for exercise testing and prescription. 2nd ed. Philadelphia: Lea & Febiger, 1993.
20. Herbert WG, Herbert DL. Legal considerations. In: American College of Sports Medicine, eds. Resource manual for guidelines for exercise testing and prescription. 2nd ed. Philadelphia: Lea & Febiger, 1993.
21. American Medical Association. Standards and guidelines for cardiopulmonary resuscitation (CPR) and emergency cardiac care (ECG). JAMA 1980;244:453.
22. American Heart Association. Special report exercise standards, a statement for health professionals. Circulation 1986;82:2286.

IV. REHABILITATION AND DISEASE PREVENTION PROGRAMS

8

Cardiac Rehabilitation: Phase I

THE FOLLOWING CHAPTERS DESCRIBE each of the three phases of cardiac rehabilitation, beginning with phase I.

DEFINITION

Phase I of cardiac rehabilitation is an inpatient program that is designed primarily for those recovering from myocardial infarct or coronary artery bypass graft surgery (CABGS). To a lesser degree phase I includes angioplasty (PTCA), valve surgery, cardiac transplant, stable angina, and coronary artery disease (CAD) risk factor patients. The program combines low-level exercise and patient education, generally lasting from 3 to 6 days. The length of a typical program has decreased significantly in recent years because of shorter hospital stays. Currently, programs are often condensed to only a few days. Phase I is designed as the initial step in preparing the patient for a return to an active and productive lifestyle.

OBJECTIVES

The objectives of phase I are outlined in Table 8.1. In the past the objectives have focused on (a) avoiding problems associated with extended bedrest, and (b) educating the patient about the components and benefits of a healthy life-style. As the length of the hospital stay has become shorter, these objectives may no longer be achievable. Little information is available about the benefits of phase I as it currently exists.

CONDUCT OF THE PROGRAM

When to Start

Entrance to phase I begins with a written order from the attending physician. Generally, this is done once at the beginning of the program and may even be in the form of a "standing order" that applies to all eligible patients. Occasionally, a physician's signature is required on a daily basis for the patient to be advanced. In most instances the inpatient program is the responsibility of the cardiac rehabilitation staff, although other personnel may contribute significantly. Careful coordination is required among program staff, attending physicians, and nursing personnel.

Phase I should be started as soon as the patient's condition has stabilized, usually 24 to 48 hours after infarct or bypass surgery. In the case of surgical patients the program may actually begin with presurgical instructions that prepare the patient for the procedure and follow-up programs. A routine of progressive exercise and ambulation is developed on an individual basis. Education and counseling are introduced when appropriate.

Exercise Program

Inpatient exercise starts with a physician's order. Low-level exercise during the hospital stay has been shown to be safe (1), feasible (2), and beneficial (3), although significant improvement in cardiovascular fitness or other physical measurements should not be expected (4). Early physical activity has been

TABLE 8.1. Objectives of Phase I

1. To assist the patient in becoming ambulatory.
2. To prepare the patient, family and significant others for a healthy life-style, thereby decreasing further risk of coronary artery disease.
3. To reduce psychologic and emotional disorders that frequently accompany myocardial infarction, CABGS, and diagnosed CAD.
4. To facilitate adjustment to the hospital environment and to the acute event.
5. To begin to identify and ultimately modify coronary artery disease risk factors.
6. To create a positive attitude that will motivate the patient to make a long-term commitment.

shown to reduce the risk of thrombi, maintain muscle tone, reduce orthostatic hypotension, and maintain joint mobility (5).

The attending physician is responsible for determining when phase I should begin and writing the order. The nurse and cardiac rehabilitation staff are actively involved in assessing eligibility and recommending suitable candidates. Ambulatory exercise, even low level, may be contraindicated in the event of any of the conditions listed in Table 8.2 (5).

At the beginning of the program background information on medical history and clinical status is obtained from the patient's chart. This is an excellent opportunity for the cardiac rehabilitation staff to interact with the physician and nurses. A meeting is usually scheduled with the patient and family to introduce the program and key personnel and to discuss objectives and procedures. This initial contact between the staff and patient is important for establishing a good working relationship and a positive tone for the program. Much of the program's success will depend on psychologic and attitudinal factors. At the beginning the intensity of exercise is very modest, emphasizes range of motion, and progresses in a stepwise fashion throughout the hospitalization. The patient is advanced through a series of passive, active, and resistance exercises in the supine, sitting, and upright positions (Figs. 8.1 to 8.16). Because the duration of phase I is usually only a few days most patients begin with active exercise. Passive range of motion is occasionally warranted for patients with significant myocardial damage or other compromising complications. While patients are confined to bed, they are encouraged to move their legs and feet to minimize venous stasis (Figs. 8.3 to 8.7).

The exercise program is outlined on Fig. 8.17, with each step described separately on an exercise card. Supervised exercise sessions usually last 10 to 15 minutes and may include informal education and conversation. They are recommended at least twice daily. The exercise sessions are usually led by the cardiac rehabilitation nurse, an exercise specialist, or physical therapist. Most

299

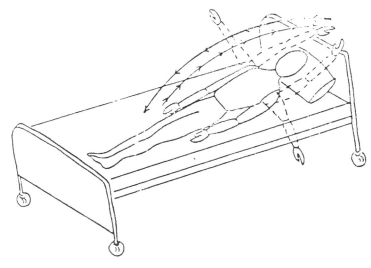

FIGURE 8.1. Phase I shoulder exercises: abduction, adduction, flexion, and extension. (Adapted from Phase I, Peninsula General Hospital and Medical Center, Salisbury, MD.)

TABLE 8.2. Contraindications for Exercise

1. Unstable angina
2. Heart failure (acute, decompensated)
3. Uncontrolled arrhythmias or high-grade A-V block
4. Resting systolic blood pressure >200 mm Hg; resting diastolic blood pressure >100 mm Hg
5. Moderate or severe aortic stenosis
6. Acute systemic illness or fever
7. Active pericarditis or myocarditis
8. Recent embolism
9. Thrombophlebitis
10. Resting ST displacement >3 mm
11. Uncontrolled diabetes
12. Orthopedic problems that would prohibit exercise

exercise sessions are conducted at the bedside, in adjacent corridors, and in stairwells. A few institutions have an exercise room specifically established for phase I exercise. In these instances the program is usually intended for CABGS and other patients who can be exercised aggressively. Electrocardiogram monitoring is usually accomplished with telemetry and may be required for reimbursement. These programs are safe and beneficial (6), although there are no comparative data with traditional phase I programs. For bedside programs a

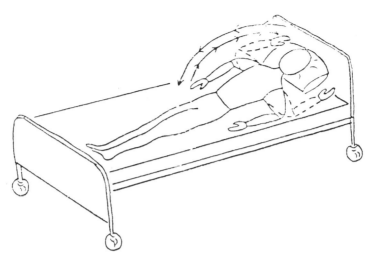

FIGURE 8.2. Phase I shoulder exercises: internal and external rotation. (Adapted from Phase I, Peninsula General Hospital and Medical Center, Salisbury, MD.)

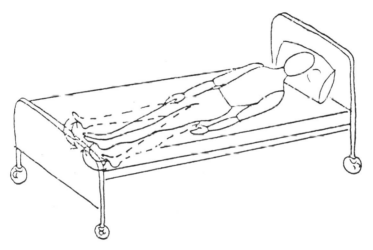

FIGURE 8.3. Phase I hip exercises: abduction and adduction. (Adapted from Phase I, Peninsula General Hospital and Medical Center, Salisbury, MD.)

central monitoring station or portable monitors may be used. Phase I equipment and facilities are also discussed in Chapter 7.

CABGS and PTCA patients are usually exercised more aggressively than myocardial infarct patients since there is little or no permanent damage to the myocardium. Typically, patients are progressed one or two steps each day. Physical exertion at each session increases from <2.0 to 4.0 METS or approximately 1.0 to 5.0 kcal/min. The duration of exercise initially is 5 to 10 minutes per session and is gradually increased to 20 or even 30 minutes per session, two to

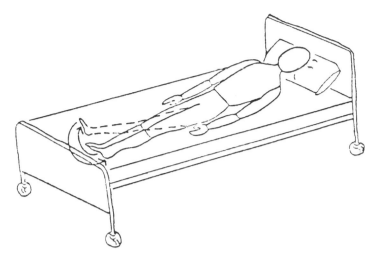

FIGURE 8.4. Phase I hip exercises: flexion and extension. (Adapted from Phase I, Peninsula General Hospital and Medical Center, Salisbury, MD.)

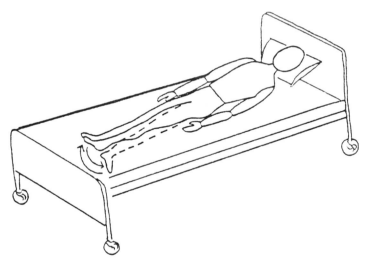

FIGURE 8.5. Phase I hip exercises: internal and external rotation. (Adapted from Phase I, Peninsula General Hospital and Medical Center, Salisbury, MD.)

four times daily (5–7). Walking in the corridors or on a treadmill and bicycle ergometry are the most common modes of exercise. Exercise is terminated if signs or symptoms appear (Table 8.3) (5).

The patient's progress is reviewed daily by the cardiac rehabilitation staff. Prior to exercise the patient is evaluated for pulse, blood pressure, electrocardiogram, muscular and joint limitations, dizziness, general appearance, and symptoms. Activity cards that detail the objectives and procedures for the day are left at the patient's bedside to be reviewed with the cardiac rehabilitation

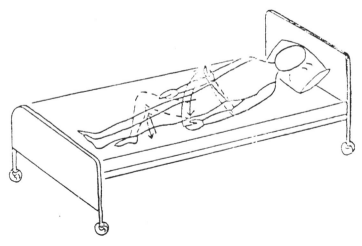

FIGURE 8.6. Phase I knee and elbow exercises: flexion and extension. (Adapted from Phase I, Peninsula General Hospital and Medical Center, Salisbury, MD.)

TABLE 8.3. Criteria for Terminating Exercise

1. Fatigue
2. Light-headedness, confusion, ataxia, pallor, cyanosis, dyspnea, nausea, or peripheral circulatory insufficiency
3. Onset of angina with exercise
4. Symptomatic supraventricular tachycardia
5. ST displacement ≥3 mm from rest
6. Ventricular tachycardia
7. Exercise induced left bundle branch block
8. Onset of 2nd- or 3rd-degree A-V block
9. R on T PVCs
10. Frequent multifocal PVCs (30% of the complexes)
11. Exercise hypotension (>20 mm Hg drop in systolic BP)
12. Excessive blood pressure risk: systolic >220 or diastolic >110 mm Hg
13. Inappropriate bradycardia (drop in heart rate greater than 10 beats/min) with increase or no change in workload

staff. Heart rate and blood pressure are recorded immediately preceding and following each exercise session. Physiologic and clinical responses to exercise are reported to the nurse in charge and are documented in the physician's progress notes.

In cardiac transplant patients passive range of motion exercises are begun at extubation and, as with infarct, and CABGS patients, are performed twice a day. Borg scale ratings in the range of 11 to 13 are used as an indication of exer-

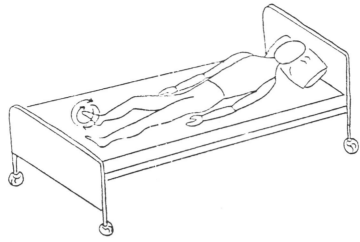

FIGURE 8.7. Phase I exercise: foot circles. (Adapted from Phase I, Peninsula General Hospital and Medical Center, Salisbury, MD.)

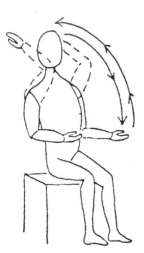

FIGURE 8.8. Phase I shoulder exercises, flexion and extension. (Adapted from Phase I, Peninsula General Hospital and Medical Center, Salisbury, MD.)

cise intensity (5, 8). Ratings of perceived exertion (RPE) are recommended to assess these patients because of denervation of the heart. Exercise, including walking and stationary bicycling, can be performed in the patient's room during isolation. A program for the transplant patient is described in detail in Table 8.4 (8).

The physician has the prerogative to alter Phase I at any time, depending on the patient's clinical status. The rate of advancement depends on the patient's daily progress, which is regularly reviewed by the cardiac rehabilitation staff. Positive feedback to the patient is very encouraging and reinforces the goal of an active and healthier lifestyle.

Some patients are allowed bedside exercise without supervision. Although generally not recommended, such exercise may be appropriate and necessary on occasion. If the patient is monitored from a central station, then unsupervised exercise might be better than canceling the session when supervision is not available. Physician approval is required for unsupervised exercise.

FIGURE 8.9. Phase I shoulder exercises: abduction and adduction. (Adapted from Phase I, Peninsula General Hospital and Medical Center, Salisbury, MD.)

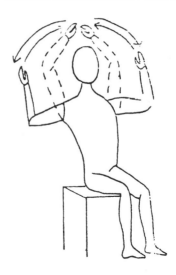

FIGURE 8.10. Phase I shoulder exercises: internal and external rotation. (Adapted from Phase I, Peninsula General Hospital and Medical Center, Salisbury, MD.)

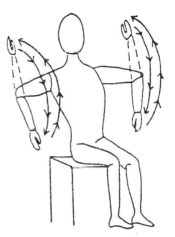

Exercise Testing

A low-level exercise test may be ordered prior to discharge for the purpose of assessing the patient progress, helping determine appropriate home exercise, and to begin assessing patient risk and prognosis.

The low-level exercise test is generally conducted with the following possible end points: 20 to 30 beats above resting heart rate, a maximal heart rate of 120 to 140, 4 to 6 METS, or 70 to 75% age-estimated maximal heart rate (5). For patients on beta-blockers an RPE of "hard" may be suggested as an end point (5). A low-level test may be performed prior to or shortly after discharge, depending on clinical circumstances. Testing from three days to three weeks after an event is usually considered as an early test. The safety and application of early testing has been well documented (9–14). Patients who respond well to early exercise testing and in whom contraindications for exertion do not appear are good candidates for continuation of physical activity at home or in the supervised phase II program. Those who respond poorly to exercise will need to be assessed thoroughly and progressed cautiously. Predischarge and postdischarge exercise testing is discussed further in Chapter 5.

TABLE 8.4. Activity Levels for Inpatient Physical Therapy After Cardiac Transplantation

---

Level 1

   Reeducation of neuromuscular relaxation to counteract muscle tension
   Reeducation of thoracic and diaphragmatic breathing
   Review of posture principles, body mechanics, and transfer techniques
   Exercises (up to 10 repetitions, supine)
      Shoulder flexion
      Shoulder abduction
      Shoulder horizontal abduction
      Hip/knee flexion and extension
      Hip abduction
      Ankle pumps
   Up in chair 20-30 minutes
      Performed with a wand
Level 2
   Breathing and relaxation techniques
   Exercises (up to 10 repetitions, seated)
      Wand exercises per level 1
      Shoulder circling
      Trunk rotation
      Hip/knee flexion (seated marching)
      Knee extension
      Ankle pumps
      Gait: standing pregait activities (dips, weight shifting)
   Up in chair 30-60 minutes
Level 3
   Exercises (up to 10 repetitions, standing)
      Head circles
      Arm circles
      Trunk rotation
      Trunk lateral flexion
      Dips
      Toe raises
      Wand exercises
   Gait: short walks in the room, as tolerated
   Up in chair ad libitum

TABLE 8.4. Cont.

Level 4
  Exercises (up to 10 repetitions, standing)
    Head circles
    Arm circles
    Trunk rotation
    Trunk lateral flexion
    Toe raises
    Wand exercises: progress to wrist weights (begin at 1 pound)
    When patient has full shoulder range of motion,
      elbow flexion/extension with wrist weights
  Gait: walk in room ad libitum
  Stationary cycle: 5 min at minimal resistance
Level 5
  Exercise and walking as per level 4
  Stationary cycle: 10 min at minimal resistance
  Add cooldown stretches for quadriceps and heel cords
Level 6
  Exercise and walking as per level 4
  Stationary cycle: 15 min at minimal resistance
  Cooldown stretches as per level 5 plus hamstring stretch
Level 7
  Exercise and walking as per level 6
  Stationary cycle: 20 minutes at mild resistance (RPE 11-13)
    (include 2-3 minute slower warm-up and cooldown)
  Cooldown stretches as per level 6

Psychosocial Testing

Psychosocial evaluation has been recommended as a significant component of cardiac rehabilitation (15), although it is seldom utilized and little information is available. The psychosocial status of the patient influences learning, compliance, attitude toward intervention, lifestyle modification, and other aspects of cardiac rehabilitation. Identifying appropriate psychosocial test instruments and interventions for phase I requires much more study (15).

PERSONNEL

The most important personnel in phase I include the cardiac rehabilitation nurse, physical therapist, exercise specialist, educator, psychologist, physician, and floor nurses.

307

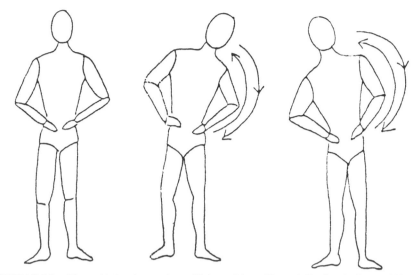

FIGURE 8.11. Phase I lateral exercises. (Adapted from Phase I, Peninsula General Hospital and Medical Center, Salisbury, MD.)

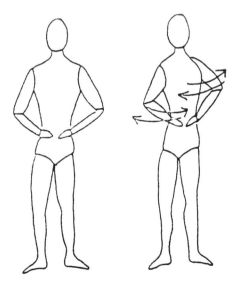

FIGURE 8.12. Phase I exercises: trunk twisting. (Adapted from Phase I, Peninsula General Hospital and Medical Center, Salisbury, MD.)

Cardiac Rehabilitation Nurse

A cardiac rehabilitation nurse is usually the program leader and is responsible for coordinating the rehabilitation team; leading exercises; scheduling meetings with patients, spouses, and significant others; and directing patient education. The role of the cardiac rehabilitation nurse is elaborated on throughout the chapter.

Physical Therapist

In some programs physical therapists are responsible for phase I exercise and may be involved in other aspects of the program. In particular the physical therapist is used to assess musculoskeletal dysfunction and joint mobility. In the case of impaired joint mobility the therapist may prescribe additional exercises to meet specific needs. Sometimes it is necessary to continue with physical therapy following discharge from the hospital. Although the order for therapy is from the attending physician, input from the cardiac rehabilitation staff is often

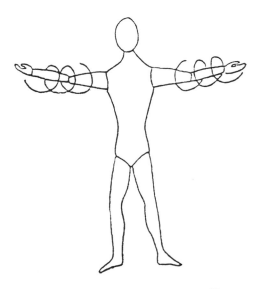

FIGURE 8.13. Phase I shoulder exercise: arm circles. (Adapted from Phase I, Peninsula General Hospital and Medical Center, Salisbury, MD.)

FIGURE 8.14. Phase I shoulder exercise: scapular adduction. (Adapted from Phase I, Peninsula General Hospital and Medical Center, Salisbury, MD.)

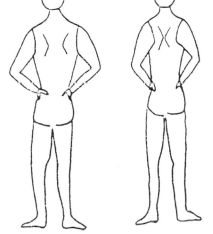

valuable. Physical therapists who work with cardiac patients must be able to recognize adverse cardiovascular signs and symptoms. While the physical therapist may be very useful in cardiac rehabilitation, the reality is that there is a shortage of therapists, which frequently limits their involvement.

Exercise Specialist

An exercise specialist may be used for leading exercises and teaching patients about the value of physical activity, as well as addressing patient questions concerning exercise. The exercise specialist must understand the appropriateness and clinical implications of different types of physical activities.

Psychologist/Psychiatrist

In most instances a psychologist, psychiatrist, or social worker is responsible for psychologic testing and intervention. A professional with training in psychology is important is dealing with the psychosocial aspects of heart disease. Both understanding and addressing the patient's psychologic needs are necessary for the

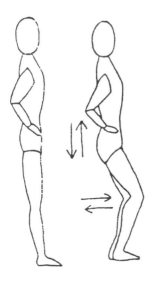

FIGURE 8.15. Phase I exercise: slight knee bends. (Adapted from Phase I, Peninsula General Hospital and Medical Center, Salisbury, MD.)

success of the entire rehabilitation program. The psychology professional is responsible for assessing patient and family needs, psychosocial testing, defining objectives, and patient and family counseling.

Nurses

The floor nurses should be actively involved in cardiac rehabilitation. They can lead exercise and participate in patient education and their activities should be closely coordinated with those of the cardiac rehabilitation team. In hospitals without a full-time cardiac rehabilitation staff a cardiovascular nurse generally assumes a leadership role. An active role by the nursing staff is very important for a successful program. In-service presentations are recommended so that the nursing staff better understands the goals and procedures of the program. In-service education helps to train the nurses in leading exercise, recognizing appropriate and inappropriate responses to exercise, and properly documenting activities. The nursing staff should be actively involved in assessing the readiness to progress exercise and should be familiar with all aspects of the program even though not actively involved. This will help to foster a greater sense of participation and to motivate the floor nurse to be enthusiastic about the program rather than to perceive it as an additional burden.

Educator

An educator, especially one with training in behavioral modification, is a valuable addition for helping to plan short- and long-term educational programs. Educational objectives and benefits probably need to be reevaluated in many programs, especially because of the brevity of hospitalization for many patients.

Physician

In some ways the physician is the key professional in the program. Technically, the physician is responsible for writing patient orders or providing a standing referral order. The referral should be the beginning of an active role in motivating the patient and significant others to adopt a positive attitude about the rehabilitation program. A few words of encouragement can be a powerful motivator for the patient, family and friends.

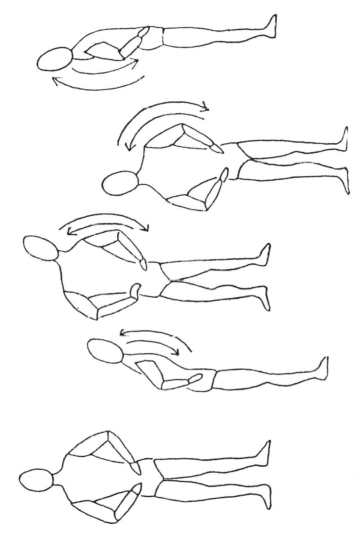

FIGURE 8.16. Phase I exercise: four-way body bends. (Adapted from Phase I, Peninsula General Hospital and Medical Center, Salisbury, MD.)

Five to ten repetitions of each exercise will be performed.

STEP 1

Active Range of Motion to all extremities while lying in bed using proper breathing. <u>Shoulder</u>: abduction, adduction, flexion, extension (Fig. 8.1), internal and external rotation (Fig. 8.2). <u>Hip</u>: abduction, adduction (Fig. 8.3), flexion, extension (Fig. 8.4), internal and external rotation (Fig. 8.5). <u>Knee and elbow</u>: flexion and extension (Fig. 8.6). <u>Active foot</u>: circling at least one time per hour (Fig. 8.7). <u>Surgical patients</u>: up in chair two times daily, ambulation with assitance in room. MET level: 1.0 to 1.5

STEP 2

Repeat all exercises as in Step 1. <u>Surgical patients</u>: with bed at 45° angle. Up in chair ad lib. at least two times daily. Short walks with assistance in room and corridor.
MET level: 1.0 to 1.5

STEP 3

Repeat all exercises as in Step 2 with mild resistance. <u>Surgical patients</u>: exercises done while sitting on bed. Increase walking, chair sitting as in Step 2.
MET level: 1.0 to 2.0

STEP 4

Active Range of Motion to all extremities while sitting using mild resistance and proper breathing. <u>Shoulder</u>: exercise done with flexed elbow (Figs. 8.8 to 8.10). <u>Surgical patients</u>: up ad lib. in room without assistance. Longer walks in hall with assistance at least two times daily.
MET level: 1.5 to 2.0

STEP 5

Repeat exercises of Step 4 with moderate resistance and proper breathing. Walk to tolerance, not more than 50 feet. <u>Surgical patients</u>: exercises in standing position with 1- to 2-pound weights, lateral side bends, trunk twists (Figs. 8.11 and 8.12). Continued walking.
MET level: 1.5 to 2.0

FIGURE 8.17. Cardiac rehabilitation Phase I exercise program.

EDUCATION AND LIFESTYLE MODIFICATION

Patient education and an introduction to lifestyle modification are additional objectives of phase I. Individual or group sessions are used to enable the patient and family to cope with hospitalization, render physical and emotional support that will enhance recovery, and assist in identifying appropriate lifestyle modifications. The classes serve as an introduction to the long-term program following discharge from the hospital. From an educational perspective it is best to identify the most important patient needs and to concentrate on those issues.

STEP 6

Active Range of Motion activities to all extremities with 1- to 2-pound weights while standing. Shoulder: add arm circles (Fig. 8.13), scapular adduction (Fig. 8.14). Walk to tolerance, not more than 100 feet. Surgical patients: walking ad lib. without assistance.
MET level: 1.5 to 2.0

STEP 7

Repeat exercises in Step 6. Walk to tolerance, not more than 200 feet. Surgical patients: repeat Step 6. Add slight knee bends (Fig. 8.15); continue walking, walk down one flight of stairs with assistance (up on elevator).
MET level: 1.5 to 2.5

STEP 8

Repeat exercises in Step 7. Walk to tolerance, not more than 300 feet. Surgical patients: repeat Step 7. Continue walking, walk down two flights of stairs with assistance (up on elevator).
MET level: 1.5 to 2.5

STEP 9

Repeat exercises in Step 8. Add slight knee bends, fourway body bends (Fig. 8.16). Walk to tolerance, walk down one flight of stairs with assistance (up the elevator). Surgical patients: up one flight of stairs, down one.
MET level: 2.0 to 2.5

STEP 10

Repeat exercises in Step 9. Down two flights of stairs with assistance. Surgical patients: Repeat Step 9.
MET level: 2.0 to 2.5

STEP 11

Repeat exercises in Step 10. Down one flight of stairs and up with assistance.
MET level: 2.5 to 3.0

FIGURE 8.17. Cont.

Information and material provided in phase I should be reinforced in subsequent phases as part of an ongoing effort. The most important short-term goal is to create a positive attitude in the patient and significant others. This will carry over into the follow-up programs and strengthen the commitment to a healthier lifestyle.

Although patient education and behavioral changes are usually the responsibility of the cardiac rehabilitation staff, a multidisciplinary and interdisciplinary approach is recommended. The professional staff may conceivably consist of physicians, nurses, social workers, dieticians, psychologists, exercise specialists, occupational and physical therapists, and other professionals.

Patient education should be initiated early during hospitalization (16, 17) and should involve the patient's family and friends when possible and appropriate. In some instances education may precede the start of exercise. For most patients education can start almost immediately, for example, an introduction to the coronary care unit. In the case of CABGS and transplant patients, presurgical teaching prepares the patient and family for the upcoming proce- dure and follow-up program. Educational sessions usually last from 15 to 45 minutes with shorter sessions being held earlier in recuperation. Longer classes may be appropriate for family and friends, although the appropriate moment must be evaluated for teaching effectiveness.

The information and objectives of each educational session should be well documented. The content of educational programs is presented in Figures 8.18 and 8.19. The cardiac rehabilitation staff should utilize assessment skills to identify teachable moments and the appropriateness of the material to be dis- cussed. Tables 8.5 and 8.6 include a list of individual and group sessions.

Education and counseling sessions are also planned for the family and signifi- cant others. Long-term adherence has been shown to be better when the spouse has a favorable attitude toward the program (18). It has also been shown that risk factors for coronary disease are often familial and track into adulthood (19–22), making family educational sessions of even greater significance. Educational classes generally last from 30 to 60 minutes and are informally structured to allow time for questions and answers and to address specific patient needs. Shorter classes may be more appropriate at the very beginning.

As the program continues and the patient's clinical status improves, regularly scheduled group classes are suitable and encouraged if time is available. The classes should be conducted in a pleasant environment to facilitate learning. The patients can ambulate or be transported to a classroom with other patients, family members, and friends. Information and materials that are appropriate at this time are recommended by the cardiac rehabilitation staff according to group needs. Regularly scheduled group classes include topics such as those listed in Table 8.6. Sample class schedules are presented in Figures 8.20 and 8.21. Figure 8.22 summarizes phase I education and exercise, and Figure 8.23 includes bed- side activities and self-care sessions.

A comprehensive program of patient education has been developed by the American Heart Association, *An Active Partnership for the Health of Your Heart* (23). This is an example of an educational program that could be introduced during phase I and extended through phase II. More will be said about this program in Chapter 9. The emphasis of these classes is on introducing information that will be taught later in more detail. Long-term educational objectives and lifestyle modification become part of an ongoing plan for the patient. The brevity of

PENINSULA REGIONAL MEDICAL CENTER

Cardiac Patient Education Documentation

ADDRESSOGRAPH / PATIENT LABEL

PROCEDURE	DATE	COMMENTS	INITIALS
1. Orientation to unit			
2. Orientation to Active Partnership Program			
3. Recovery following a heart attack (AHA book)			
4. Orientation/admission to Cardiac Rehabilitation			
5. Understanding Coronary Artery Disease - Video #1			
6. Risk Factor I.D.- Video #2			
7. Patient's Modifiable Risk Factors:			
A.Nutrition/Diet Changes			
B.Exercise - Video #5			
C.Stress - Video #6			
D.Smoking Cessation - Video #3			
E.Weight Loss			
F.Diabetes			
H.Hypertension			
Patient Preferred Teaching			
1._____ 2._____			
8. Understanding Angina & Medication Management			
9. Spouse Education			
10. Pre-operative Teaching			
11. Discharge Instructions:			
A. MI D/C Summary			
B. Medication Review			
12. Discharge Exercise			
Guidelines:			
A.Cardiac Rehab. Ref.			
B.General Guidelines by Units			
13. Other Teaching Needs/Classes Attended			

Signature	Initials
_____	_____
_____	_____
_____	_____
_____	_____
_____	_____
_____	_____

Comments: _____

_____

_____

_____

_____

_____

_____

253

CR-204 (11/93)

FIGURE 8.18. Cardiac patient education documentation.

phase I only allows for an introduction to these important skills. Subsequent practice, reinforcement, and long-term follow-up are necessary to ensure success. The use of new technologies such as computers and video techniques need to be explored, developed, and used when appropriate.

PENINSULA REGIONAL MEDICAL CENTER

Coronary Artery Bypass Teaching Guide

ADDRESSOGRAPH / PATIENT LABEL

CONTENT	Patient. Responsible Person Instruction [DATE]	Patient/ Responsible Person Demonstrated Understanding [DATE]	CONTENT	Patient. Responsible Person Instruction [DATE]	Patient/ Responsible Person Demonstrated Understanding [DATE]
I. PREOPERATIVE PLAN			6. Stomach and Urinary Tubes		
A. Received Teaching Plan			7. Turning Frequently and Chest P.T.		
B. Orientation to Unit and Staff			8. ICU Environment		
C. "Before and After Your Surgery"			9. Pain Control		
D. Tour of ICU/Visit with Post-operative Heart Patient			10. Visiting Hours, Phone Calls, Communication		
E. Special Skin Preparation			11. Removal of Tubes and Catheters, Dressing Changes		
F. Personal Belongings			B. West Two		
G. Cough and Deep Breathing, No Smoking			1. Activity Progression		
H. Medication Changes			2. Dressing Changes		
I. Pre-Operative Night Routine			3. Condition checks, Less Frequent		
			4. Cough and Deep Breathing		
II. OPERATIVE PROCEDURE			5. Diet [Lo-cholesterol, No Added Salt]		
A. Atherosclerosis and Risk Factors			6. Fluid intake		
B. Normal blood vessel vs. Atherosclerosis			7. Usual Length of Stay		
C. Blood supply to heart					
D. Oxygen deficit and Angina			C. Discharge Instruction		
E. Vein bypass - Purpose, site, Operative Procedure			1. Activity		
F. Incision			2. Diet		
G. Heart-Lung Bypass			3. Follow-Up		
			4. Medications		
III. POST-OPERATIVE CARE			5. Daily weight		
A. ICU			6. Specific Instructions		
1. Purpose of Unit and staffing			A.		
2. Endotracheal Tube, Respirator, Suctioning			B.		
3. Radial Line and I.V.'s					
4. EKG Monitoring, Pacing Wires					
5. Chest Tubes					

Patient or Person Responsible: _____

Nurse: _____   Date: _____

NUR-004 (10/93)

FIGURE 8.19. Coronary artery bypass teaching guide.

FACILITIES

Most of phase I exercise is performed at the patient's bedside and in adjacent corridors and stairwells. Some hospital programs, particularly those with a large cardiovascular surgery commitment, have separate exercise facilities for low-level, monitored physical activity. Coronary artery bypass graft surgery patients and other cardiac patients with less severe disease might benefit from a more vigorous inpatient program than that which is normally conducted at the

TABLE 8.5. Topics for Individual Patient Classes

Preoperative teaching for coronary artery bypass surgery

Orientation to cardiac rehabilitation—phase I

Orientation to cardiac rehabilitation—phase II

Orientation to critical care environment

Anatomy of the heart; disease and the healing process

Home walking and home stationary bicycle program and pulse taking

Angina pectoris

Medications

TABLE 8.6. Topics for Group Classes

Family adjustment

Psychosocial adjustment to coronary artery disease

Inpatient rehabilitation program-nutrition intervention

Coronary disease risk factors

Physical activity and coronary artery disease

Sexual activity and coronary artery disease

---

bedside. Figures 8.23 and 8.24 are examples of separate phase I exercise rooms. A separate room should also be included for individual and group counseling sessions. Sufficient space should be allocated to accommodate at least 5 to 10 persons. The teaching/counseling room should be quiet, well lit, pleasantly decorated, and easily accessible.

EQUIPMENT

Phase I programs require relatively little equipment. The exercise program is usually conducted at the bedside and requires light weights (1 or 2 pounds), blood pressure apparatus, a stopwatch or watch with a sweep second hand, and perhaps some small game balls. In a few phase I programs exercise bikes are used in the patient's room for more vigorous activity. Exercise bicycles and treadmills are used in those programs that have dedicated facilities for their phase I patients.

Audiovisual equipment and supplies are necessary because of the emphasis on patient education and lifestyle modification. A typical list of items includes cameras, audio and video recorders and players, tapes, slides, flip charts, manuals, books, filmstrips, and a variety of handout materials. Computers with self-help software programs might also be considered and definitely have application in phase II and phase III programs. If ECG monitoring is done in phase I,

317

	Monday	Tuesday	Wednesday	Thursday	Friday	Saturday	Sunday
A.M.	Exercise—PT Visit	Exercise—PT Visit	Exercise—PT Visit	Exercise—PT Visit	Exercise—PT Visit	Exercise—PT Visit	Exercise—PT Visit
10:00 to 10:45	Class—Risk Factors	Class—Diet	Class—Discharge	Class—Activity	Class—Emotional Reactions	—	—
P.M.	Exercise—With Nurse	Exercise—With Nurse	Exercise—With Nurse	Exercise—With Nurse	Exercise—With Nurse	Exercise—With Nurse	Exercise—With Nurse
3:45 to 4:30	Class—Activity	Class—Emotional Reactions	Class—Risk Factors	Class—Diet	—	Class—Activity	—
6:30 to 7:15	—	—	—	—	Class—Discharge	—	Class—Discharge

PT, physical therapist

FIGURE 8.20. Cardiovascular center at LDS hospital. Cardiac rehabilitation program. Phase I: classes and exercise schedule.

MONDAY	Cardiac Risk Factors 4:00 P.M.	Discharge Classes Medical Patients 6:15 P.M. Surgical Patients 6:15 P.M.
TUESDAY	Dietary Review 11:00 A.M.	Stress Management 7:00 P.M. The Caregiver 6:00 P.M.
WEDNESDAY	Medication Information 4:00 P.M.	Discharge Classes Medical Patients 6:15 P.M. Surgical Patients 6:15 P.M.
THURSDAY	Dietary Review 4:00 P.M.	_____
FRIDAY	The Caregiver 10:00 A.M. Stress Management 11:00 A.M. Cardiac Risk Factors 4:00 P.M.	Discharge Classes Medical Patients 6:15 P.M. Surgical Patients 6:15 P.M.
SATURDAY	Diet Film 3:00 P.M.	_____

FIGURE 8.21. Cardiac rehabilitation weekly patient class schedule. All patients and family members are encouraged to attend any and all classes. Activity recommendations are made individually with exercise therapists and nurses. (Courtesy of the Cardiovascular Center and LDS Hospital.)

056

PENINSULA REGIONAL MEDICAL CENTER
SALISBURY, MARYLAND 21801

PHASE 1 - CARDIAC REHABILITATION
DOCUMENTATION - PROGRESS REPORT

TEACHING PROGRAM	DATE PRESENTED	EVALUATION
General Admission A & P Packet Given		
Nutrition Class		
Individual Nutrition Instruction		
Risk Factors Class		
Discharge Class		
Home Walking Program		
Spouse Education		
Family/Patient Support Class		
Other Individual Needs		
MI Video Review		
CABG Video Review		

PHASE I - EXERCISE

DATE	STEP NUMBER	WGTS	POSITION	RESTING HR	RESTING BP	EXERCISE HR	EXERCISE BP	EKG	

FIGURE 8.22. Phase I cardiac rehabilitation documentation—progress report.

CR-202 (R 5/93)

IMPRINT PATIENT'S PLATE HERE

	SIGNATURE

Diagnosis: _____

Admission Summary: _____

_____

_____

_____

Additions: _____

_____

_____

_____

* Positions: H - Head of Bed 45°
                S - Sitting
                ST - Standing

COMPONENT

EVALUATION/COMMENTS/SYMPTOMS	SIGNATURE

FIGURE 8.22. Cont.

321

	SELF CARE	BEDSIDE ACTIVITIES	CALISTHENICS/BREATHING	WALKING/BICYCLING/STAIRS	
				MI	SURGERY
			See Additional Notes on Supervised Exercise on the other side of this sheet	See Additional Notes on Supervised Exercise on the other side of this sheet	
1	•Feed self •Use bedside commode •Wash hands/face •Brush teeth	•Sit in bed with firm back support	•Passive ROM, all extremities •Active plantar/dorsiflexion •Ankle circles •Diaphragmatic breathing	none	none
2	•Bathe self at bedside •Wash hands, face, upper body and personal areas (nurse assist with back and legs) •Comb hair •Shave self	•Dangle legs on side of bed •Sit up in chair for 20 minutes (NOT at mealtime or immediately before or after another activity such as bathing) •Light reading	Same as above, plus: •Active assisted ROM, all extremities •Shoulder shrugs	*Met level:* — *Walk in halls:* —	1.5 100-200 ft. (2-5 min)
3	•Bathe self at bedside or sitting in chair in front of sink (nurse assist with back and legs)	•Walk to bathroom in room with assistance •Sit up in chair as tolerated •Sit in bedside chair for meals	Same as above, plus: •In supine position flex knees to 75°	*Met level:* — *Walk in halls:* —	1.5 200-360 ft. (2-5 min)
4	•Take warm shower if appropriate	•Sit in bedside chair as tolerated •Sit in bedside chair for meals •Walk to bathroom with assistance as needed	Same as above, plus 1 minute each of the following: •In supine position flex knees to 75° •Sitting knee extension •Sitting push and pull	*MET level:* 1.5-2.0 *Walk in halls:* 100-200ft (2-5min) *Treadmill/Bike:* —	1.5-2.0 400-600 ft. (5-7 min) 5-7 min

FIGURE 8.23. Cardiovascular center at LDS Hospital. Daily activity levels for patients.

	SELF CARE	BEDSIDE ACTIVITIES	CALISTHENICS/BREATHING	WALKING/BICYCLING/STAIRS MI	WALKING/BICYCLING/STAIRS SURGERY
5	•Take warm shower if desired	•Increased beside chair sitting time as tolerated	Same as above, plus 1.25 min. each, 3× a day of the following; •Sitting knee extension •Sitting with lateral trunk bender •Sitting push and pull	MET level: 1.5-2.0; Walk in halls: ≤500 ft. (5-7 min); Treadmill/Bike: 5 min; Stairs: 3-6	MET level: 1.2-2.5; ≤1000 ft. (5-10 min); 5-10 min; 3-6
6	•Continue as above plus standing self care	•Continue with bedside chair and bathroom privileges	Same as above, 1.5 min each, 3× a day	MET level: 1.5-2.5; Walk in halls: ≤1000 ft. (5-10 min); Treadmill/Bike: 5-10 min; Stairs: 6-12	MET level: 1.2-2.5; ≤2000 ft. (10-15 min); 10-15 min; 6-12
7	•Up ad lib	•Up ad lib	Same as above plus add the following: •Standing one arm overhead •Standing lateral bend	MET level: 1.5-2.5; Walk in halls: ≤2000 ft. (10-15 min); Treadmill/Bike: 10-15 min; Stairs: up to 14	MET level: 2.0-3.0; ≤3000 ft. (15-20 min); 15-20 min; up to 14

Additional Notes on Supervised Exercise

•Blood pressure is recorded before and immediately after each exercise session.
•Heart rate is recorded before, during, and one minute after each exercise session.
•Exercise therapists will supervise calisthenics, treadmill, bicycling, and stairs two times a day, and nursing staff will assist patients once a day.

Specific Learning Objectives

•Patients will be encouraged to attend all scheduled cardiac classes.
•Exercise therapists and nursing staff will review concepts taught in cardiac classes and during exercise sessions and will help patients learn pulse monitoring during each exercise session.
•Home program preparation will begin on level 6.

FIGURE 8.23. Cont.

then a decision must be made concerning the best choice of equipment. If a central monitoring station is used in the patient unit, it can also be used to observe patient responses to exercise. If a central station is not available or is insufficient to monitor all patients, then a portable system should be considered. Portable units are moderately priced and can easily be transported. Since ECG monitoring is often required for reimbursement and its use enhances patient safety, some type of a system is necessary. In phase I programs with a separate exercise room, the exercise equipment needed is similar to that for phase II exercise. The most notable difference between phases I and II is the emphasis on lower body exercise in the former, especially for postsurgical patients because of their inability to do much upper body work following surgery.

BENEFITS

Additional controlled studies that evaluate the effectiveness of phase I programs are needed to determine the following: (a) the extent of knowledge gained, (b) the effect on behavior modification, (c) reliability and validity of self-administered questionnaires, (d) readiness of the patient for intervention, (e) development of instruments that measure effectiveness, and (f) long-term benefits of phase I (24). Intuitively it makes sense to incorporate educational classes as a regular part of phase I. However, there is little information available to substantiate the value of these programs.

CONCLUSION

Phase I consists of a combination of low-level physical activity and patient education. These programs have been shown to be safe and beneficial, although benefit is less well documented at present when programs have been substantially shortened. While physical benefits may be more difficult to observe, there may very well be short- and long-term attitudinal improvements that are escaping evaluation. The most important objective is to prepare the patient for the beginning of a lifetime commitment to a healthier lifestyle.

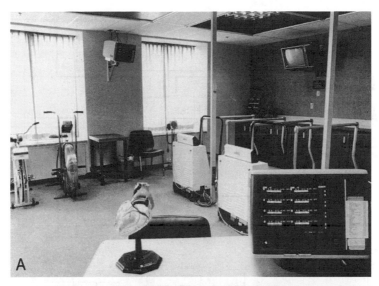

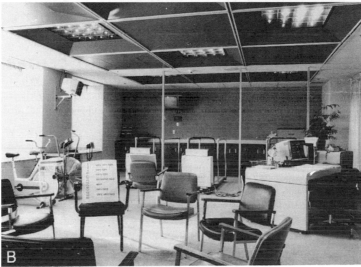

FIGURE 8.24, A and **B.** Phase I exercise area. (Courtesy of MidAmerica Heart Institute: St Luke's Hospital of Kansas City; Patricia Caldwell, Coordinator; David Venner, Photographer.)

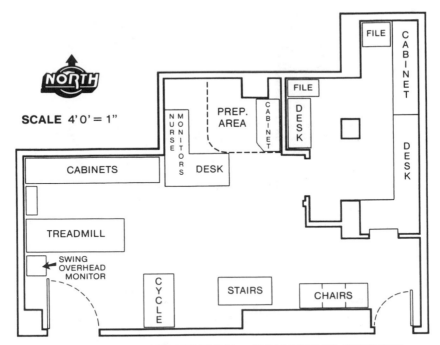

CARDIAC REHABILITATION · INPATIENT CENTER
MOUNT SINAI MEDICAL CENTER, MILWAUKEE, WI.

FIGURE 8.25. Phase I cardiac rehabilitation facility. (Courtesy of Mount Sinai Medical Center, Milwaukee, WI; Neil Oldridge, PhD, Director.)

REFERENCES

1. Wenger NK. Critical evaluation of cardiac rehabilitation. Chest 1977;71:317.
2. Graber AL. Cardiovascular disease prevention programs in a community hospital. J Tenn Med Assoc 1977;70:95.
3. Gilliland MM, Jones WL. A quest for earlier and more organized rehabilitation of the coronary patient. SD J Med 1976;29:7.
4. Sivarajan ES et al. Treadmill test responses to an early exercise program after myocardial infarction: a randomized study. Circulation 1982;65:1420.
5. American College of Sports Medicine. Guidelines for exercise testing and prescription. 4th ed. Philadelphia: Lea & Febiger, 1991.
6. Pollock ML et al. Exercise prescription for rehabilitation of the cardiac patient. In: Pollock ML, Schmidt DH, eds. Heart disease and rehabilitation. New York: John Wiley, 1986.
7. Pollock ML, Ward A, Foster C. Prescription of exercise in a cardiac rehabilitation program. In: Fardy PS, Bennett JL, Reitz NL, Williams MA, eds. Cardiac rehabilitation: implications for the nurse and other health professionals. St. Louis: CV Mosby, 1980.
8. Squires RW. Cardiac rehabilitation issues for heart transplantation patients. J Cardiopulmonary Rehabil 1990;10:159.
9. Ibsen H et al. Routine exercise ECG three weeks after acute myocardial infarction. Acta Med Scand 1975;198:463.
10. DeBusk R, Houston N, Markiewicz W. Prognosis of early postinfarction exercise testing. Circulation 1976;54(Suppl 2):9.

11. Sasterhaug A, Nygaard P. Early discharge and early rehabilitation and return to work after acute myocardial infarction. J Cardiopulmonary Rehabil 1989;7:268.

12. Dubach P, Froelicher VF. Recent advances in exercise testing. J Cardiopulmonary Rehabil 1991;11:29.

13. Leitschuh ML et al. The effect of pre-discharge exercise testing on activity recommendations and patient confidence following PTCA. J Cardiopulmonary Rehabil 1990;10:359.

14. Harper GR et al. Pre-discharge assessment of functional capacity in 94 coronary artery bypass patients. J Cardiopulmonary Rehabil 1990;10:359.

15. Southard DR, Broyden R. Psychosocial services in cardiac rehabilitation. A status report. J Cardiopulmonary Rehabil 1990;10:255.

16. Parmley WW. President's page: position report on cardiac rehabilitation. JACC 1986;7:451.

17. Wenger NK. Rehabilitation of the patient with acute myocardial infarction during hospitalization: early ambulation and patient education. In: Pollock ML, Schmidt DH, eds. Heart disease and rehabilitation. 2nd ed. New York: John Wiley, 1986.

18. Heinzelman F. Social and psychological factors that influence the effectiveness of exercise programs. In: Naughton JP, Hellerstein HK, Mohler IC, eds. Exercise testing and exercise training in coronary heart disease. Orlando, FL: Academic Press, 1973.

19. Webber LS, Cresanta JL, Voors AW, Berenson GS. Tracking of cardiovascular disease risk factor variables in school-age children. J Chronic Dis 1983;36:647.

20. Webber LS, Cresanta JL, Croft JB, Srinivasan SR, Berenson GS. Transition of cardiovascular risk from adolescence to young adulthood—the Bogalusa Heart Study II. Alterations in anthropometric, blood pressure and serum lipid variables. J Chronic Dis 1986;39:91.

21. Khoury P et al. Clustering and interrelationships of coronary heart disease risk factors in school children age 6–19. Am J Epidemiol 1980;112:524.

22. Must A et al. Long-term morbidity and mortality of overweight adolescents: a follow-up of the Harvard Growth Study of 1922 to 1935. N Engl J Med 1992;327:1350.

23. American Heart Association. An active partnership for the health of your heart. Dallas, TX: AHA, 1990.

24. Godin G. The effectiveness of interventions in modifying behavioral risk factors of individuals with coronary heart disease. J Cardiopulmonary Rehabil 1989;9:223.

9

CARDIAC REHABILITATION: PHASE II

Emergency Procedures
Motivation and Adherence
ADAPTATION
SUMMARY AND CONCLUSIONS

PHASE II OF CARDIAC REHABILITATION is a supervised outpatient program of individually prescribed exercise with continuous or intermittent electrocardiogram (ECG) monitoring. It may be operated as a hospital-based or freestanding physician-directed facility. The exercise program is based on an individualized prescription of intensity, duration, frequency, and mode of activity (1–4). Patient education and lifestyle modification are integral parts of phase II that are discussed in detail in Chapter 11.

OBJECTIVES

The objectives of phase II are to do the following:

1. Enhance cardiovascular function, physical work capacity, strength, endurance, and flexibility
2. Detect arrhythmias and other ECG changes during exercise
3. Educate patients on the proper techniques of exercise
4. Work with patients, family, and significant others to establish healthy lifestyles
5. Enhance the psychologic function of patients
6. Prepare patients for a return to work and resumption of normal familial and social roles
7. Provide patients with guidelines for long-term exercise

This chapter discusses the significant issues of program planning, organization, and operation.

ELIGIBILITY

Criteria for Eligibility

Patient eligibility is mostly determined by the diagnoses approved for reimbursement:

1. Documented myocardial infarction
2. Coronary artery bypass surgery or angioplasty
3. Heart transplant surgery
4. Valvular and congenital heart disease surgery
5. Stable angina pectoris

Patients with elevated risk factors and other diagnosed cardiovascular abnormalities can also benefit from cardiac rehabilitation, although they may not be eligible for insurance reimbursement. Medicare has developed the most widely used guidelines for reimbursement (5), although substantial differences exist among insurance carriers. The final decision on individual questions of reimbursement lies with individual insurance companies.

Referral

Medicare guidelines require documented physician referral to precede entrance into phase II. Generally, the referral is provided by the primary care physician, cardiologist, or surgeon. If the referring physician is not responsible for the patient's primary care, then all physicians who participate in therapy decisions should confer on the rehabilitation treatment. Referrals are often prompted by the nursing and cardiac rehabilitation staffs. The attitude of the patient and the success of the program are substantially influenced by physician support (6–8). The referral process should be more than a passive letter. Instead, the referring physician is encouraged to assume a proactive role. Referral is encouraged as soon as the patient's condition is stable since delaying the process may negatively affect adherence.

Orientation

Following the written referral the patient and family or friends are invited to attend an orientation program. The purpose is to enhance the patient's level of comfort about the program as outlined by the objectives in Table 9.1.

The orientation may be planned for individual patients, couples, or small groups of patients and guests. If possible the patient should be given an opportunity to observe an exercise class, to visualize the fun and safety of exercise, and to alleviate potential fear, anxiety, and apprehension. The best time for a patient to observe a class is in conjunction with planning for discharge in the case of a hospital program or shortly following discharge in the case of a freestanding facility. The patient should be encouraged to enroll during the

TABLE 9.1. Objectives of Orientation

1. Introduce staff
2. Show facility
3. Demonstrate equipment
4. Explain procedures for exercise and lifestyle modification
5. Discuss financial obligations and arrangements
6. Establish patient objectives
7. Provide opportunity for questions
8. Sign-up

orientation. Allowing a long time to elapse between the event and entering phase II may result in a loss of interest as the patient begins to feel better but has not undertaken changes in lifestyle to prevent recurring problems.

PROGRAM STRUCTURE

Content

The content or scope of the program should be decided on during early planning. Financial objectives are clarified, revenues and expenses are estimated, and sources of funding are discussed. The benefits of non-income producing programs are weighed against their cost. The contents of a Phase II program are outlined in Table 9.2.

Evaluation

Phase II is preceded and followed by a detailed evaluation that enables the staff to assess eligibility, establish the exercise prescription, and provide baseline data against which progress is measured. The exercise stress test is the most important part of the evaluation and can be a part of phase II or administered separately in the physician's office or at a hospital testing center. If exercise testing is separate from phase II, then a standard test protocol is encouraged for referral purposes. Evaluation procedures can provide a substantial source of revenue, although they also increase the cost of the program through added personnel, equipment, and facilities. When deciding if exercise testing is feasible as a part of the rehabilitation program, one must consider the possibility of a conflict with physicians who have made a personal investment in exercise test equipment and facilities. Cardiac rehabilitation does not want to be perceived as a competitor of physicians who might be a source of referrals. Evaluation procedures are discussed in Chapters 3 to 5.

TABLE 9.2. Program Content

1.	Evaluation
2.	Exercise
3.	Education and lifestyle modification
4.	Research
5.	Community service
6.	Home programs
7.	Other programs

Stratification

In current clinical practice cardiac rehabilitation patients are often stratified based on prognostic risk for the purpose of recommending the appropriate supervision and monitoring required. Guidelines for stratification are provided in Table 9.3 (9). Specific purposes include the following: (a) to determine the appropriateness of an individual patient for exercise training, (b) to assess the adequacy of the current medical regimen, as well as the need for coronary revascularization, and (c) to determine the extent of ECG monitoring during exercise (10).

The shortcoming of this currently popular practice is its failure to consider important patient needs other than clinical risk. For example, some patients are dependent on the security of continuous monitoring until their level of self-

TABLE 9.3. Guidelines for Risk Stratification[a]

Risk level	Characteristics
Low	Uncomplicated clinical course in hospital
	No evidence of myocardial ischemia
	Functional capacity ≥ 7 METs
	Normal left ventricular function (EF ≥50%)
	Absence of significant ventricular ectopy
Intermediate (Moderate)	ST-segment depression ≥ 2 mm flat or downsloping
	Reversible thallium defects
	Moderate to good left ventricular function (EF 35 to 49%)
	Changing pattern of or new development of angina pectoris
High	Prior myocardial infarction or infarct involving ≥ 35% of left ventricle
	EF < 35% at rest
	Fall in exercise systolic blood pressure or failure of systolic blood pressure to rise more than 10 mm Hg on exercise tolerance test
	Persistent or recurrent ischemic pain 24 hours or more after hospital admission
	Functional capacity < 5 METs with hypotensive blood pressure response or ≥ 1 mm ST-segment depression
	Congestive heart failure syndrome in hospital
	≥ 2 mm ST-segment depression at peak heart rate ≤ 135 bpm
	High-grade ventricular ectopy

Note. 1 MET = 3.5 ml O_2/kg/min; EF = ejection fraction.
[a]From AACVPR. Guidelines for cardiac rehabilitation programs. Champaign IL: Human Kinetics, 1991.

confidence is raised. In others, issues of group dynamics, compliance, and long-term adherence are also important. Some individuals respond more favorably with group support than by being on their own, which is the basis of support groups such as Alcoholics Anonymous and Weight Watchers.

It is suggested therefore that patient stratification include psychosocial, as well as clinical, assessment. If a goal of cardiac rehabilitation is a lifetime commitment to healthy behavior, then all factors that can influence adherence must be considered.

Exercise

The focus of Phase II is regular aerobic exercise that is designed primarily to improve muscular endurance and cardiovascular fitness. When planning the exercise program, try to envision its growth to determine equipment, facility, and personnel needs for the future. Socioeconomic background, occupation, leisure activity interests, and possible scheduling problems should be considered.

Education and Lifestyle Modification

Although exercise is the foundation of phase II, patient education and lifestyle modification are also very important. These programs must be planned in advance since they are heavily labor intensive and generate limited revenues. The American Heart Association has developed a comprehensive education program and workbook, *An Active Partnership for the Health of Your Heart (11)*. The contents of the AHA program are outlined in Table 9.4. The use of computers with self-help software programs should also be considered for patients and significant others. More information about patient education and lifestyle modification are presented in Chapter 11. Budgetary considerations, facilities, equipment, and personnel are all affected.

Research

Exercise testing, prescription, and training provide an excellent opportunity for research, which can be stimulating for the staff and provide additional information about the program. However, a significant commitment to research is time consuming and affects the selection of a program director. A research-oriented professional may not be an advisable choice for the position of program director in job situations where research will be discouraged. Nevertheless, a systematic evaluation is very important in measuring outcomes, whether for the purpose of scientific research or not.

Community Service

The services provided in phase II can be a source for community service and favorable public relations for the hospital. The expected payback for service programs that are offered to the public free or at a nominal fee is the increase in

TABLE 9.4. An Active Partnership for the Health of Your Heart

I. Introduction

II. Understanding heart disease

III. Food
  A. Where do you stand?
  B. Making changes
  C. What's good to eat?
  D. A practical guide to shopping, cooking and eating out
  E. Answers to some common questions
  F. Special problems

IV. Exercise
  A. What types of exercise?
  B. Your personal exercise prescription
  C. Making plans
  D. Getting started
  E. Enjoying yourself: exercising comfortably
  F. Increasing your exercise
  G. Making exercise a lifelong habit

V. Stress
  A. What is stress?
  B. What stress does and why
  C. Keeping track of your stress
  D. Four basic ways to cope with stress
  E. Stress management skills
  F. Making your plans change

VI. Smoking
  A. Understanding the urge to smoke
  B. Emergency urge control
  C. Planning for urges
  D. Food and fun
  E. Snuffing out slips
  F. How to quit

hospital referrals. Because community service is labor intensive, requiring staff, equipment, and facilities, the decision to offer these programs should be made during program planning.

Home and Ancillary Programs

The large majority of patients who are eligible for cardiac rehabilitation never participate in a supervised program (12). Home-based programs are developed to provide a reasonable alternative. A good home program requires careful planning, including time and personnel allocation. Frequent follow-up by telephone, written records of activity, staff visits to the home, transtelephonic ECG monitoring, and periodic patient visits to the rehabilitation center are all potential components of a home program. The patients must feel that they are being carefully managed even though they are not regularly supervised. Home programs generate few revenues.

Phase II presents several opportunities for complementary programs. These include psychologic, physical, occupational, and recreational therapy and pulmonary rehabilitation. Other programs that include a significant exercise component can share equipment and facilities at the same time as cardiac rehabilitation if the patients interact well and neither program is disrupted.

Facilities

The size and floor plan of the facility are affected by the program's financial resources. The following features are important to consider in facility planning: location, exercise testing and training, education and lifestyle modification, staff offices, business operations, employee comforts, and ancillary programs.

Location

A good location is one that is easily accessible and not more than 20 to 30 minutes travel distance for the patient (13). Hospital-based programs are usually situated in or near the hospital, whereas a freestanding facility can be located at any site selected by the staff. The best location is one that is near the population center with easy access by automobile and public transportation. The building should have good parking with ease of entrance and exit. The appearance of the building, facility, and surrounding area must be pleasing and provide a sense of safety and comfort. The center can be located on the ground floor or on a higher floor if a good view is provided. Basement space is less expensive and can be a good choice if the design and decor are aesthetically pleasing. All of these features influence the patient's perception of the program.

Before making a final decision, a variety of locations should be visited and thoroughly researched. The location should provide the best chance for the program to succeed. Patient demographics come before personal interest in making the final decision. Figure 9.1 is an outside view of a modern medical building in which the top two floors are dedicated to cardiac rehabilitation.

Budget

Budgetary considerations also need to be carefully analyzed as a part of facility planning. The cost of rent, renovations, or property purchase is especially important in a freestanding facility. It is often prudent to start small and simple and to move into larger and more luxurious accommodations as the program grows.

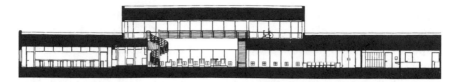

FIGURE 9.1. Building section plan. Cardiovascular Disease Prevention and Rehabilitation Program facilities are within the third floor and mezzanine level floor of the Cardiac Center of Creighton University. (Courtesy of Richard D. Nelson Co., Architecture and Interiors.)

Large facilities with a lot of open area may be aesthetically appealing but have wasted space, are costly to maintain, and compromise safety when patients are not supervised as closely.

Floor Plans

After the site and space have been determined, specific floor plans are prepared. The services of an architect are recommended (14), preferably one with experience in planning exercise facilities. While not required under all circumstances, an architect will generally save the project money and better ensure a functional and pleasant facility. The architect must balance several elements: (a) aesthetics—the appearance of the facility; (b) technology—construction and control of the facility's internal environment; (c) economics—the project budget; and (d) function—the purpose of the facility. Once there is agreement concerning these issues, it is possible to advance to the next stage.

The four distinct stages in the development of a facility are as follows (14):

1. Conceptual design—taking ideas and putting them into a general layout.
2. Development design—developing specific plans for each room.
3. Construction documents and bidding—the final plans and taking bids for construction.
4. Construction—the job of supervising construction, which is the responsibility of the general contractor. The architect, however, can do on-site inspections and serve in the role of liaison to the contractor. Remember that the architect works for the program administration and must set the financial limitations of the construction. Figure 9.2 is the interior floor plan from Figure 9.1. This particular facility includes both phase II and phase III of cardiac rehabilitation. Additional phase II facility floor plans are presented in Figures 9.3 to 9.5.

Space Requirements

The most important factor in allocating space is a realistic estimate of size and future growth. Estimate the number of patients likely to use each part of the

336

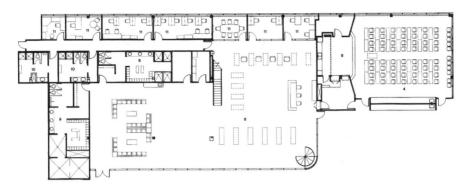

FIGURE 9.2. Third-level floor plan, including those facilities dedicated to the Cardiovascular Disease Prevention and Rehabilitation Program, Cardiac Center of Creighton University. Third-level floor plan also includes mezzanine-level floor plan, which provides for the walk/jog surface that is above and looks down onto the third-floor exercise area. (Courtesy of Richard D. Nelson Co., Architecture and Interiors.)

facility at a given time. A facility may not be functional if the area is not well utilized. The following recommendations are for floor space in a traditional phase II facility:

1. One hundred square feet of the exercise training area is suggested for each patient. For example, if individual classes are planned to accommodate six to eight patients, then 600 to 800 square feet is recommended. The actual area used for exercise will be less when equipment, storage, drinking fountain, sink, counter top, and decorative items are added. If the available space is less than that recommended, mirrors can help to create the appearance of greater size and modifications in the program may be needed. Care should be taken that the facility does not appear "clinical." Colored walls, murals, pictures, hanging plants, mirrors, stereo music, and carpeting are encouraged. An interior designer is well worth considering.

2. The dressing area must be large enough to accommodate the maximum number of patients who will utilize the room at one time. If classes are going to overlap, then the number of patients should include those finishing exercise plus those reporting for the next class. A larger dressing and shower area is usually suggested for males since they constitute a greater percentage of patients, and are more likely to use the shower facilities. The need to accommodate increasing numbers of female patients must be carefully considered. For class sizes of eight or fewer, two shower stalls are usually adequate for men, while one may be sufficient for women. It is suggested that 150

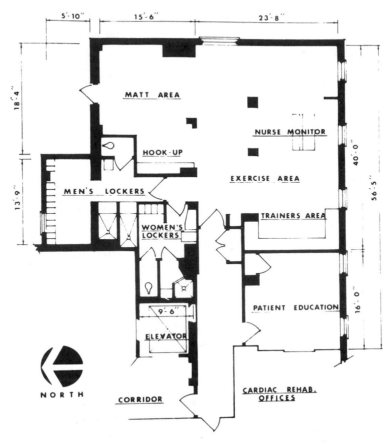

FIGURE 9.3. Phase II cardiac rehabilitation facility. (Courtesy of Mt Sinai Medical Center, Milwaukee, WI.)

to 200 square feet be allotted for each dressing and shower area.

3. One hundred square feet is a minimal area recommended for exercise testing. An additional 75 to 100 square feet per station is recommended if more than one test will be performed simultaneously. One or more adjacent areas of approximately 50 square feet are suggested for patient preparation when a large volume of tests will be the norm. The testing area must be large enough to accommodate personnel, equipment, and supplies. There must also be sufficient room to manage an emergency. Finally, a work area, including desk and telephone, should be provided for the physician to dictate reports and utilize time effectively between tests.

4. Electrical requirements can usually be met by standard 115 voltage. If 220 voltage is projected for future use, it is easier and less expensive to add an electrical line at the beginning. There should be a

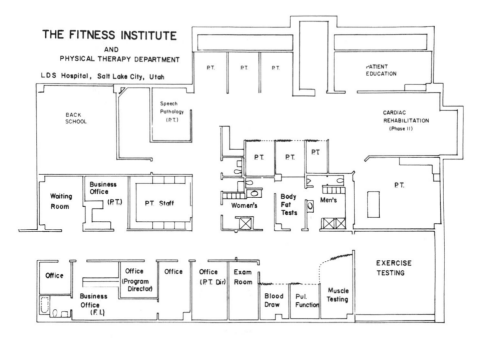

FIGURE 9.4. Cardiac rehabilitation and adult fitness facility. (Courtesy of the Fitness Institute, LDS Hospital, Salt Lake City, UT.)

sufficient number of electrical outlets, including floor and ceiling strip outlets every 6 to 12 feet. The electrical system should be designed with isolated transformers and outlets on separate circuits to avoid electrical overloading, voltage surges, and circuit breaker problems. Separate electrical circuits are suggested with computer equipment that is sensitive to voltage changes. Two and three-phase electrical circuits are important and often require special lines.

5. Space should be planned for patient education and lifestyle modification classes. A conference room large enough to accommodate 10 to 20 persons is suggested. If space is limited, then larger numbers can be accommodated with classroom seating style compared to round table. More space is needed for less structured classes and small group discussions. A minimum of 300 square feet is suggested for a conference room. The room should be quiet, well lit, and comfortable. The conference room should have a wall writing board, screen, and dimmer lights and should be well equipped for audiovisual presentations such as slides, videos, and movies. A separate but smaller room should be available for individual counseling and teaching. The small room has the same requirements for sound, light, comfort, and decor.

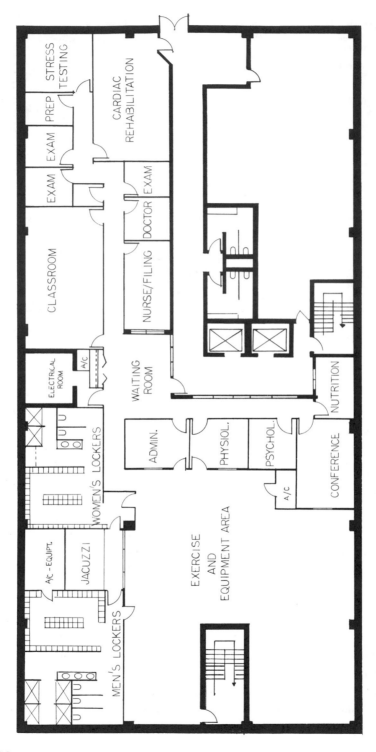

FIGURE 9.5. Floor plan of cardiac rehabilitation and adult fitness facility. (Courtesy of North Arundel Cardiac Rehabilitation/Fitness Center, Glen Burnie, MD; Linda Carlson, Designer.)

6. A waiting area is recommended for patients and guests. The area should be large enough for one visitor per patient, since a spouse, relative, or friend is often present. One hundred square feet is usually sufficient.

7. Adequate office space is required for the staff. Offices should be pleasant and functional, allowing a minimum of 50 to 60 square feet for each person. The program director requires a private office that is large enough to be a small meeting room.

8. A business office is needed for the freestanding facility. It must be large enough for personnel, equipment, and supplies. Filing space should be planned to maintain patient records for at least three years. One hundred to 150 square feet are recommended for a business office. An additional 50 to 100 feet is recommended if the business office also serves as a reception area. Privacy is important in situating the business office. Because conversations are often personal, the area should be quiet, private, and away from classes.

Additional space might be used for a research laboratory, staff lounge, library, media center, large conference room, and special teaching areas such as a kitchen and a quiet room. Two thousand to 3000 square feet is suggested for a program that expects to enroll 200 to 300 patients annually. Less space can be satisfactory if the program is well planned and organized.

Floor Plan

The floor plan should be developed after space requirements have been defined. Traffic patterns, patient privacy, business operations, light, noise, and environmental factors need to be considered. The floor plan should be designed to minimize interference among different aspects of the program. Because some patients are sensitive to interruptions and outside visitors, the number of such visits should be controlled, and patients should be given advance notice whenever possible. The traffic pattern must also be planned for patient safety. In the case of an emergency, the patient must be reached easily for treatment. There should be sufficient room for emergency equipment, personnel, and patient evacuation. There should also be minimal noise from one area to the next. Conference or teaching rooms should not be contiguous to the exercise area. Instead, noisy areas should be situated away from those that demand quiet. All rooms should be adequately lit and should use natural light sources when possible. The location of rooms should also take advantage of the outside environment. If the facility is located in a scenic area, then the design should include expanses of windows so that the view is enjoyed. Outdoor facilities are feasible when temperature and humidity are within acceptable guidelines (15,16). Other outdoor factors to consider are altitude, air pollution, noise, sunlight, wind, and safety. Noise and light distractions should be kept to a minimum.

Equipment

The most substantial equipment used in phase II is for exercise testing, training, patient monitoring, and emergencies. Because there are so many manufacturers, choosing the best equipment can be time consuming. Comparative prices, technology, service, contract agreements, future needs, and possible compatibility with other components and systems need to be considered.

A traditional phase II program incorporates a variety of exercise devices that are used for upper and lower extremity muscle groups. These include arm and leg ergometers, rowing machines, treadmills, wall pulleys, shoulder wheels, light weights, and stepping devices. At least one heavy-duty treadmill is recommended for obese patients. The exercise equipment should be quantitative and calibratable, enabling the patient to observe and measure progress. Examples of phase II exercise equipment are presented in Figures 9.6 to 9.9.

Electrocardiogram monitoring is accomplished with telemetry or hard-wire systems. Although telemetry is used more extensively, hard-wire monitoring is adequate and is much less expensive. Choosing the best monitoring system can be difficult. Cost, reliability, availability of service, simplicity of maintenance, ease of use, and equipment features must all be considered. Those who will regularly use the equipment should play an active role in the selection. Equipment companies are generally cooperative about demonstrations and usage on a trial basis.

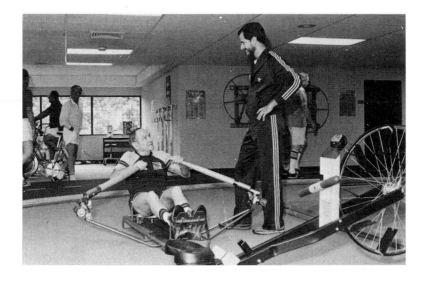

FIGURE 9.6. Exercise area for cardiac rehabilitation and adult fitness. (Courtesy of the Health Institute, St Luke's Hospital, Kansas City, MO; David Venner, photographer.)

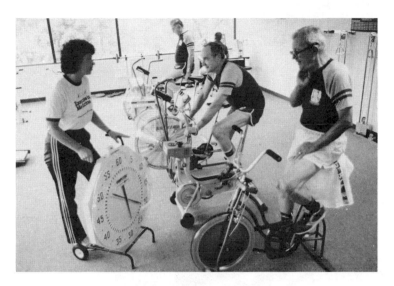

FIGURE 9.7. Supervised exercise on stationary bicycles. (Courtesy of the Health Institute, St Luke's Hospital, Kansas City, MO; David Venner, photographer.)

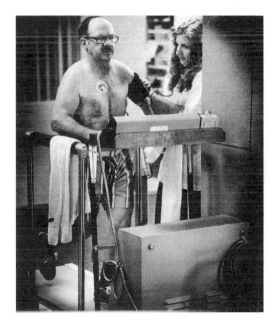

FIGURE 9.8. Phase II exercise, Mt Sinai Medical Center, Milwaukee, WI. (Photograph courtesy of Michael Pollock, PhD.)

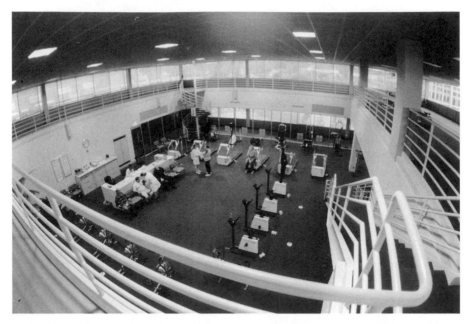

FIGURE 9.9. Overhead view of exercise area. Cardiovascular Disease Prevention and Rehabilitation Program, Cardiac Center of Creighton University. (Photograph courtesy of Michael H. Sketch, Sr., MD.)

Equipment for ECG monitoring is for the purpose of detecting and monitoring arrhythmias and ischemia. Ischemic changes are more difficult to assess because of reduced frequency response in most telemetry systems, lead placement errors, and poor patient preparation. As with exercise testing, careful preparation is vital for obtaining good records. Monitoring systems, electrode placement, and transmitter attachment are shown in Figures 9.10 to 9.12. Newer models of monitoring equipment feature storage of arrhythmias, miniature transmitters, transmitters that can be used underwater, and trending devices that display and later print average heart rates and frequency of arrhythmias. Although these features provide interesting and useful data, they may seldom be used and will not justify the added expense.

Transtelephonic ECG monitoring systems, originally developed for pacemaker checks, are used today in cardiac rehabilitation. The equipment is particularly useful in assessing patients between phases I and II or for home-based programs. Because only a small number of eligible patients participate in supervised cardiac rehabilitation, transtelephonic electrocardiography may be a viable alternative that provides at least short bouts of discontinuous monitoring. Several types of transtelephonic equipment are available. There are significant differences among these systems. Figures 9.13 to 9.15 illustrate the transmitter and receiving units. Figures 9.16 and 9.17 illustrate a

344

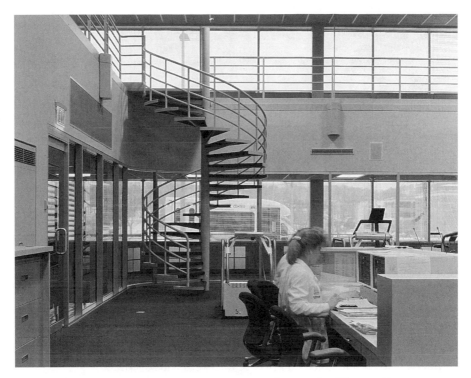

FIGURE 9.10 Exercise area workstation. Cardiovascular Disease Prevention and Rehabilitation Program, Cardiac Center of Creighton University. (Photograph courtesy of Mike Sinclair, Sinclair-Reinsch Photography.)

transtelephonic telemetry system that can monitor real-time ECG responses to exercise.

There are many exercise stress test systems from which to choose. Some are expensive and include sophisticated electronics, information retrieval, and patient information printout. Excellent low-cost systems are also available that provide only the basic components required, that is, a multichannel recorder, scope with non-fade capability, and treadmill. Ultimately, the choice of stress test equipment depends on its use and budget considerations. Excellent guidelines for equipment needs and test procedures have been published (17–19).

Other large purchases required for phase II include equipment for emergencies and for operating a business office. Emergency equipment includes defibrillator, medications, oxygen, suction, and other items required for resuscitation. A business office would use a computer, word processor, copier, and fax machine for preparing forms, data collection, storage and analysis of data, physician reports, accounting and billing, and rapid transmittal and reception of documents.

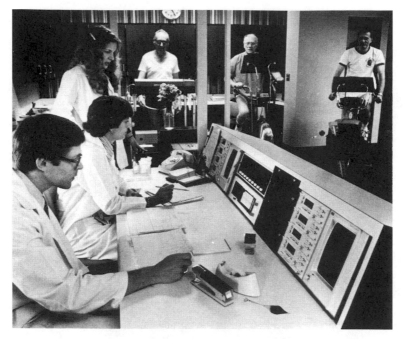

FIGURE 9.11. Phase II ECG monitoring systems, Mt Sinai Medical Center, Milwaukee, WI. (Photograph courtesy of Michael Pollock, PhD.)

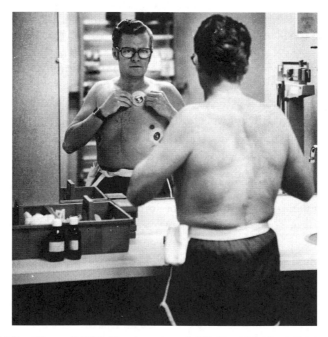

FIGURE 9.12. Phase II ECG "hookup area." Mt Sinai Medical Center, Milwaukee, WI. (Photograph courtesy of Michael Pollock, PhD.)

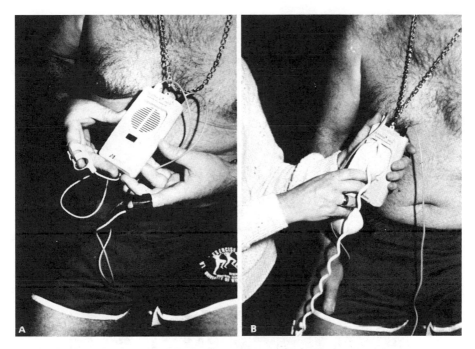

FIGURE 9.13. Telephone ECG. **A.** Finger cups. **B.** Telephone (lead I).

Personnel

Key personnel of phase II include a cardiac rehabilitation nurse (CRN), exercise specialist, and the program director who may or may not be a physician. In the case of a nonphysician director a medical advisor is a key member of the professional staff. A health educator or behaviorist is recommended for programs that emphasize education and lifestyle modification. The referring physician is also an important part of the professional team although seldom present during classes.

In most instances the CRN is the most visible member of the professional staff and is responsible for much of the program operation, patient care, reading and interpreting ECGs, and providing emergency care. In some instances these responsibilities are assumed by other professional staff. The nurse or supervisor will have certification in cardiac rehabilitation and advanced cardiac life support (ACLS) and should be able to communicate effectively with physicians. As a general rule one cardiac rehabilitation specialist is responsible for monitoring up to four patients per exercise class.

The exercise leader is in charge of leading activity classes, teaching lifestyle classes, and possibly serving as an exercise test technician. The exercise leader is usually trained in physical education, exercise physiology, or exercise science, although occasionally professionals trained in nursing or physical therapy

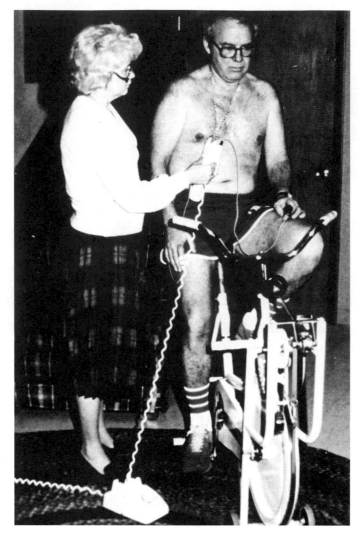

FIGURE 9.14. Patient telephoning in ECG.

assume this role. The exercise leader should be American College of Sports Medicine (ACSM) certified (19), knowledgeable with clinical factors that affect physical activity, and be able to assist with risk factor modification and lifestyle management classes. A background in exercise testing, prescription, and training is suggested.

A health educator is suggested to help plan and manage patient education and behavior modification programs that complement exercise training and provide a multidisciplinary approach to prevention. Education sessions are most effective in small groups or individually. In most instances the health educator will be part-time, although a large program may require a full-time position.

348

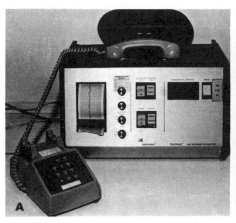
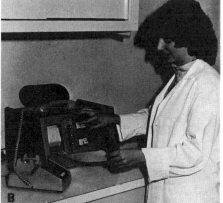

FIGURE 9.15. Telephone ECG being received at medical facility (**A** and **B**).

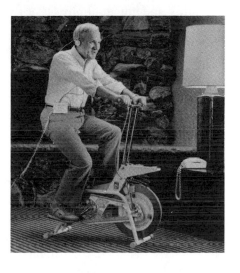

FIGURE 9.16. Transtelephonic telemetry system: patient monitoring. (Courtesy of FutureCare Systems, Minneapolis, MN.)

The physician director or advisor is often minimally involved with the daily operation but is responsible for determining the exercise prescription, evaluating clinical problems, and managing medical emergencies. Medicare guidelines require that the physician be in the vicinity of the exercise area when classes are in session. An active role by the physician is a source of motivation and emotional support for the patient. Most physician directors are board certified in cardiology or internal medicine. They should have a reasonable understanding of exercise physiology. ACLS certification is also required (9).

The referring physician is not likely to be a member of the professional staff but nevertheless has an important role in cardiac rehabilitation and must be provided with regular patient reports. The information will help to assure continuity of care and will be useful in making appropriate therapeutic decisions. If the attitude of the referring physician is positive and supportive, then the patient is more likely to experience success (6–8). It is suggested that all personnel, including support staff, be certified in basic cardiopulmonary resuscitation (CPR) and that regular training sessions in managing emergencies be scheduled.

349

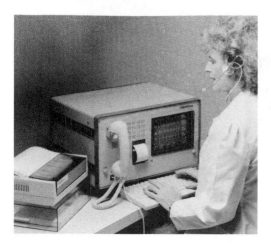

FIGURE 9.17. Transtelephonic telemetry system: receiving monitor and printout. (Courtesy of FutureCare Systems, Minneapolis, MN.)

CONDUCT OF THE PROGRAM

The patient enters phase II after a physician referral and orientation. Individual meetings with new patients are advisable for establishing short- and long-range objectives. It is made clear that phase II is just the beginning of a lifetime commitment of physical activity and positive health behavior. The orientation meeting can also be used for this purpose.

A comprehensive evaluation is administered prior to training and includes medical and lifestyle history, physical examination, laboratory and blood tests, physical fitness assessment, and the exercise stress test (19). Many of these tests can be performed by the referring physician. Psychologic screening is also recommended to help design a program that will best meet the patient's needs.

A typical exercise class consists of patient preparation, warm-up, exercise training, cooldown, and relaxation.

Patient Preparation

A list of preexercise instructions is provided to the patient prior to the first class (Table 9.5). Skin preparation, electrode placement (Fig. 9.18), and the use of monitoring equipment are taught at the initial exercise class. After the electrodes are self-applied, the patient answers questions from the staff concerning medications and any recent adverse symptoms. Body weight should be taken before each class along with resting heart rate, blood pressure, and an ECG rhythm strip. The patient is then ready for warm-up.

Warm-up

A warm-up is performed at the beginning of each exercise session. The benefits of warm-up have been well studied and reviewed (20–23). The procedures are illustrated in Figure 9.19.

Training Stimulus

The goal of exercise training is to achieve a target heart rate (THR) that reaches the training adaptation threshold. Individual THRs, exercise workloads, and the sequence of exercise modes are provided on an exercise prescription card

TABLE 9.5. Patient Instructions Before Exercise

1. Do not eat a large meal for at least 2 hours prior to the exercise session. A small snack is fine.
2. Alcohol should not be consumed before exercise.
3. Do not drink beverages with caffeine, i.e., coffee, tea, cola, etc., for at least 2 hours prior to exercise.
4. Do not smoke at least 1 hour prior to exercise.
5. Wear comfortable clothing to exercise, i.e., gym shorts, loose-fitting slacks, sneakers, socks, loose-fitting blouse or shirt, etc.
6. Please be prompt! Try to arrive 10 to 15 minutes prior to the scheduled time of the exercise class to get ready.
7. If you experience any unaccustomed symptoms of pain, discomfort, or soreness, let the nurse know before starting to exercise.
8. Inform the nurse of any changes in medications before exercising.
9. Bring a lock to the class to secure your valuables.

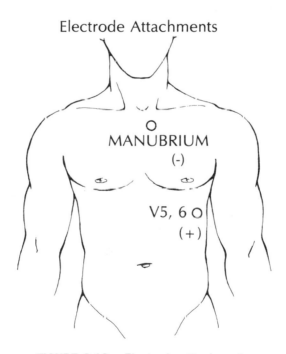

FIGURE 9.18. Electrode attachments.

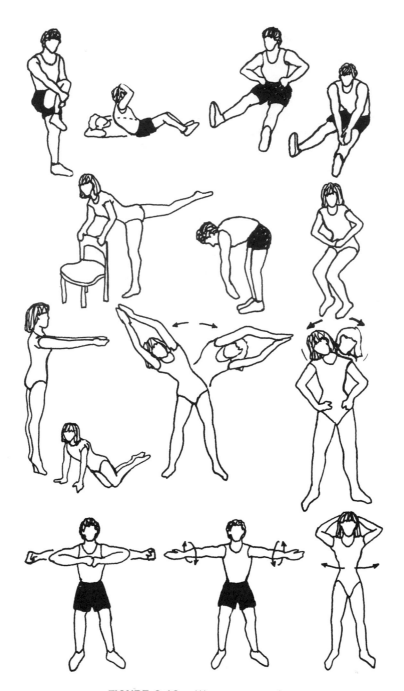

FIGURE 9.19. Warm-up exercises.

Name_____
            Last   First

Target Heart Rate_____

Device and Order	Work Load	Adjusted Work Load

FIGURE 9.20. Exercise prescription card.

(Fig. 9.20), which is given to the patient at the beginning and collected at the end of each session. The intensity of effort is increased gradually until the THR is attained and maintained at that level for the duration of the session with continuous training, or interspersed with brief periods of rest with intermittent training. More work can be completed in the same amount of time, exercise intensity can attain higher heart rates, and a greater variety of activities are feasible with intermittent training.

Dynamic-rhythmic and aerobic activities are emphasized. Isometric, isotonic resistive and isokinetic resistive exercises have become increasingly popular, although generally are not included until after completion of phase II. The traditional exercise program is designed to improve upper and lower extremity muscle groups, and may incorporate the following types of equipment: bicycle ergometer, arm ergometer, treadmill, wall-pulley, steps, arm crank, rowing machine, and light weights. The patient usually exercises 5 to 10 minutes on each of several modalities with approximately 1 minute between bouts. Exercise classes, including time for dressing and showering, take about one hour and are generally held three times a week. Arm training is especially important as there is little crossover adaptation from leg exercise. Arm ergometers, bicycle ergometers modified for arm use, light weights, vertical climbing devices, and cross-country ski simulators can be used. Increased muscle fatigue is associated with some modes of arm exercise as a consequence of a greater amount of isometric activity and localized metabolic demands.

Exercise programs are sometimes modified for patients with specific needs or limitations. These changes may be slight or substantial depending on the individual. Many of these modifications reflect the "art" used in prescribing exercise. High-risk patients are discussed later in the chapter.

Cooldown

The level of effort is gradually reduced following exercise to maintain systemic blood flow at a level that doesn't increase myocardial oxygen demand. This is accomplished by the massaging effect of contracting and relaxing muscles on veins, thereby enhancing venous return. Ventricular filling is increased and stroke volume augmented in accordance with the Frank-Starling mechanism (24). Vigorous exercise that is stopped suddenly is associated with venous blood pooling in the lower extremities, reduced return to the heart, and compensatory increase in heart rate. Hypotension, decreased blood flow to the brain, light-headedness, dizziness, and fainting are possible. Maintaining adequate circulation also enhances removal of metabolic by-products, especially lactic acid, hastens recovery, and reduces the possibility of muscle soreness following exercise (24). Although lactic acid buildup is seldom significant in cardiac rehabilitation, continuing light activity in the muscle groups that have been active is a good training principle.

Upgrading the Prescription

The exercise prescription is upgraded in response to training adaptations. As heart rates decrease in response to exercise, the exercise workloads are increased to maintain the THR. Initial reductions in heart rate response to exercise are often a result of decreased anxiety and familiarization with equipment and the environment, whereas later changes are more likely attributed to training. In either case the same adjustments have to be made. Target heart rates may be increased after initial changes in workloads are made. Typically, the THR is increased by 5% every 4 to 6 weeks. The rate of progression is very individualized and is affected by age, level of fitness, clinical prognosis, and the rate of adaptation.

Relaxation

Relaxation exercises are recommended for the end of cooldown and can be effective for reducing heart rate, blood pressure, and cardiac arrhythmias (25–27). Sufficient time for cooldown needs to be allotted prior to relaxation. Lying down quickly after vigorous activity may increase myocardial oxygen demand (MVO_2) by creating a left ventricular volume overload.

Relaxation techniques are useful for patients who are hyperactive. Too often the hectic pace of the day extends into the training session as these patients rush into the exercise session, often late, try to hurry through the class, rush to shower, and on to the next appointment. Benefits from exercise are likely to be negated by this behavior. Relaxation exercises ensure a brief respite from frantic activity, and might be helpful to relieve stress and improve sleep. A sample of relaxation exercises is provided in Table 9.6. The basic technique incorporates

TABLE 9.6. Instructions for Relaxation Exercises

1. Close eyes and relax (in a supine position)
2. Take a deep breath. . . . . .and relax.
   Concentrate on your breathing. Allow 10 to 15 sec between commands.
3. Again, a deep breath. . . . . .and relax.
4. Now, contract the muscles in one arm (either one). . . . . .and relax.
5. Repeat with opposite arm.
6. Contract the muscle in one leg. . . . . . . .and relax.
7. Repeat with opposite leg.
8. Now contract the muscles of an arm and the leg of the opposite side. . .
   . . . . . .and relax.
9. Repeat with other arm and leg.[a]

[a]Initially, an assistant might check that the muscles are being completely relaxed. If they are, one should be able to lift the designated limb with no muscular resistance.

controlled breathing with alternating muscle contraction and relaxation. It is important that these techniques be regularly practiced.

Electrocardiogram Monitoring

Electrocardiogram monitoring is an issue of considerable debate that has implications for safety, program effectiveness, and cost containment. The following questions need to be addressed: (a) Is ECG monitoring necessary? (b) Do all patients need to be monitored? (c) How much monitoring is appropriate? (d) Is ECG monitoring needed more with certain types of exercise? (e) Is self-monitoring an acceptable alternative?

Although there are no universally accepted guidelines governing the use of ECG monitoring, several recommendations have been made (28–30). The most obvious use is for identifying and counting arrhythmias, which are more likely to be detected with continuous patient monitoring than exercise testing (30–32). Long-term data on the clinical significance of arrhythmias in patients with adequate left ventricular function and no ischemic changes are inconclusive. What is known is that patients with poor left ventricular function and complex and frequent arrhythmias and other patients who are at high risk require careful supervision and continuous ECG monitoring. The rationale for continuous monitoring is that patients adhere better to the exercise prescription, are less anxious about exercise, and can exercise safely. Nonmonitored exercise has been shown to be safe and beneficial for low-risk patients (33), although factors other than clinical need to be considered. For low-risk patients the argument is that continuous monitoring is costly, of questionable benefit, may become a crutch for some, and is not feasible for everyone. DeBusk and others (33) have shown that home-based and infrequently monitored programs can be safe and beneficial, perhaps lessening the

TABLE 9.7. Frequency of Significant Arrhythmias During 12-Week. Phase II, Monitored Exercise[a]

Week of Program	Total Patients With Significant Arrhythmias	New Patients With Significant Arrhythmias
1	14	14
2	15	8
3	15	5
4	14	8
5	18	6
6	18	2
7	18	5
8	13	1
9	10	1
10	18	3
11	12	1
12	13	1

[a]Data from Fardy PS, Doll N, Williams M. Monitoring cardiac patients: how much is enough? Phys Sports Med 1982;10:146.

need for monitoring in certain patients. Additional studies are needed before a definitive policy can be established.

Table 9.7 illustrates the frequency of significant arrhythmias throughout a 12–week phase II program (30). In this instance significant arrhythmias were defined as ventricular tachycardia, ventricular bigeminy or trigeminy, PVC couplets, and more that five PVCs per minute. Significant arrhythmias were detected in 50% of patients during the 12–week program compared to 12% during stress testing. These data are similar to findings reported elsewhere (31, 32). Although the frequency of significant arrhythmias decreased in weeks 8 to 12, 13% of the total population experienced new events. It is noteworthy that at least one new patient each week exhibited a significant event for the first time. Based on these results continuous ECG monitoring is recommended for at least 7 weeks and could be justified for as long as 12 weeks. Data beyond 12 weeks are lacking. Electrocardiogram monitoring is also recommended whenever the prescription is changed. From the results of Table 9.7 it can be concluded that monitoring exercise, even for only a few sessions, is likely to enhance patient safety.

A few sessions of ECG monitoring can also help to provide guidelines for safe home exercise. Home programs require careful self-heart rate monitoring because asymptomatic contraindications to exercise can occur frequently (34).

Electrocardiogram monitoring can also be useful for arrhythmia detection in patients with a history of frequent, complex multiform ventricular arrhythmias, with or without coronary disease. Having these patients monitored as a part of phase II, or as in an arrhythmia detection clinic, is an effective and relatively inexpensive way to assess medication therapy compared to serial exercise testing or Holter monitoring. ECG monitoring can help to determine if the occurrence of arrhythmias is heart rate or exercise mode related. Additional evidence in support of patient monitoring is that significant untoward events rarely occur in monitored programs (35, 36).

Other forms of monitoring are important as well. For example, there is a greater need for monitoring adverse signs or symptoms as the number of high-risk patients in cardiac rehabilitation is increased. Cardiac transplant patients need to be monitored by ratings of perceived exertion as heart rate response to exercise has been impaired by sympathetic denervation. Chronic obstructive lung disease (COPD) patients and cardiac patients with pulmonary complications should be monitored for oxygen desaturation, in addition to heart rate, ECG, and other adverse signs or symptoms. Other cardiac patients who may have special monitoring needs include those with severe physical limitations, those on negative or positive chronotropic medications, and patients with other pathology requiring additional supervision.

Length of Phase II

A traditional phase II program lasts for 12 weeks or 36 sessions. Patients who fail to demonstrate progress and continue to display contraindicating signs and symptoms can be continued for an additional 12 weeks, although it is not usual that Medicare will reimburse for this service. Reimbursement is more likely with careful clinical documentation especially in conjunction with the occurrence of a clinical event such as angina, bypass surgery, and reinfarction that requires rehospitalization. Private insurance carriers may reimburse the extended program on a case-by-case basis. Definitive exit criteria from phase II would help to clarify this problem. Some guidelines have been published (19), although they are quite general. Exit criteria have to be individualized. Five METs work capacity may be an acceptable criterion for daily home activities, but may be unacceptable for returning to work. Some factors that need to be considered in evaluating a patient's progress include the amount of adaptation, appearance of contraindicating signs or symptoms, and the presence of coronary risk factors.

Exit from phase II should signal the beginning of a lifetime commitment to healthy behavior. Physician approval is required before advancing to more strenuous exercise. The uncomplicated myocardial infarct or coronary artery bypass graft surgery patient needs reassurance that return to a normal lifestyle is within reach.

Untoward Events

The risk of life-threatening events in phase II is small (35, 36). Proper medical supervision, continuous patient monitoring, individualized exercise prescription, complying with the guidelines for exercise, and having the necessary equipment to handle untoward events help to promote safety. Potential untoward events following phase II may be reduced by teaching patients to monitor themselves. Studies show that subjective indications of exercise intensity can be perceived accurately (37, 38), thereby making it possible to self-regulate the prescription. To do this well requires considerable practice.

Emergency Procedures

Emergency planning is needed that considers procedures for cardiorespiratory care, personnel assignments and responsibilities, patient transfer and hospitalization, and other factors that affect patient safety. It is recommended that the entire staff responsible for patient care be certified in basic cardiac life support and that all nonphysician staff who are medically responsible for patient care be certified in advanced cardiac life support (ACLS) as established by the American Heart Association (9). In a freestanding facility, at least one staff person certified in ACLS must be available at all times. The program director is generally responsible for developing an action plan to direct emergency procedures until a physician is present.

If an emergency occurs, it is important to monitor the electrocardiogram, document the time of the event, and to notify the medical director and referring physician at an opportune time. Patients are directed to a nearby location where they are supervised by a member of the professional staff to lessen anxiety and explain what has transpired. The emergency team leader is responsible to direct the following: CPR, defibrillation, setting up intravenous infusion, inserting an airway if needed, providing oxygen, and preparing medications until the physician arrives. The patient is transferred to the emergency room at the discretion of the attending physician. The medical director or program supervisor is responsible for scheduling periodic reviews of emergency procedures, including mock calls for the staff. Emergency procedures are outlined by the American Association of Cardiopulmonary Rehabilitation (9).

Motivation and Adherence

One of the most powerful motivators for persons with a recent cardiac event is the fear of death or being a cardiac cripple (39, 40). As the patient recuperates, the advantages of the rehabilitation program assume greater importance, that is, the quality of leadership, social aspects of group participation, and the recognition of improvement (41, 42). Feedback to the patient is important and group interaction is encouraged. The latter should be enhanced with occasional social events. Keep in mind that exercise is not easy. Few are disciplined well enough to exercise by themselves. Most persons find it easier to be in a group where they can share the joy and hard work of becoming fit (41, 42).

TABLE 9.8. Effects of Habitual Physical Activity[a]

Increase in maximal oxygen uptake, cardiac output, and stroke volume

Reduced heart rate at given oxygen uptake

? Reduced blood pressure

Reduced heart rate × blood pressure product

Improved efficiency of heart muscle

? Improved myocardial vascularization

Favorable trend in incidences of cardiac morbidity and mortality

Increased capillary density in skeletal muscle

Increased activity of "aerobic" enzymes in skeletal muscles

Reduced lactate production at given percentage of maximal oxygen uptake

Enhanced ability to utilize free fatty acid as substrate during exercise: glycogen
  saving

Improved endurance during exercise

Increased metabolism: advantageous from a nutritional viewpoint

Counteracts obesity

Increase in the HDL/LDL ratio

Improved structure and function of ligaments, tendons, and joints

Increased muscular strength

Reduced perceived exertion at given work rate

Increased release of endorphins

?Enhanced fiber sprouting

Enhanced tolerance to hot environment: increased rate of sweating

Reduced platelet aggregation?

Counteracts osteoporosis

Can normalize glucose tolerance

? = There are not general agreements about these effects.
[a]Compiled by P.-O. Astrand, from Adams TD, Edgington CE. The physician's role in promoting physical activity. In: Yanowitz FG, ed. Coronary heart disease prevention. New York: Marcel Dekker, 1992, with permission.

Adherence is better if the patients derive enjoyment and benefit from the program. The program will be enjoyable if activities are diversified and the staff is pleasant, enthusiastic, and attentive to the needs of the patients. The program's benefit is determined from objective evaluation and subjective feelings of improvements, both of which are important. Attendance should be carefully documented as another measure of the program's success. A certificate of completion or "graduation" is inexpensive yet very meaningful for some.

Name_____ Date _____ Target Heart Rate_____
　　　　Last　　　　　　　First

Have you had any health problems since your last exercise session?

Have you taken your medication today? Yes_____ No_____

Have there been any medication changes? Yes_____ No_____

Resting Heart Rate_____　　　　　　　　　　　　　DEVICES: A = Arm Ergometer
Resting Blood Pressure_____/_____　　　　　　　　　　　　　　　　B = Bicycle
Recovery Blood Pressure_____/_____　　　　　　　　　　　　　　　R = Rowing Machine
　　　　　　　　　　　　　　　　　　　　　　　　　　　　　　　　　S = Step
　　　　　　　　　　　　　　　　　　　　　　　　　　　　　　　　　T = Treadmill

EXERCISE DATA

Order	Exercise Device	Work Load	ECG Changes	Signs and Symptoms	Exercise Heart Rate	Recovery Heart Rate
0.	Warm-Up					
1.						
2.						
3.						
4.						
5.						
6.						
7.	Relax					

Average Exercise Heart Rate_____

Comments:_____

FIGURE 9.21. Exercise training session.

ADAPTATION

Patients at low risk generally exhibit normal, acute responses to exercise. Increased sympathetic adrenergic drive results in elevated heart rate, blood pressure, respiratory frequency, and volume. Variations from normal adaptation are mostly a result of myocardial dysfunction and pharmacologic agents. Special populations of patients exhibit other different responses to exercise. For example, heart rate and blood pressure changes are blunted in transplant patients because of denervation and reliance on circulating catecholamines. Patients with ventricular dysfunction have faster heart rates than normal as a compensatory mechanism for decreased contractility and ejection fraction. In the appearance of COPD expect a rapid heart rate, perhaps as high as 100% age-estimated values with very low levels of effort as a result of oxygen desaturation.

Long-term benefits of exercise are summarized in Table 9.8 (43). Some of these changes are more likely to occur in phase III, the long-term program. Training adaptation may begin in as few as 4 to 6 weeks, although it may take as long as 6 months for significant changes in body fat (44). Some patients have a more rapid rate of adaptation than others, a function of myocardial damage and left ventricular asynergy. Adaptation in myocardial infarct and CABG patients is similar (45), although surgical patients are often exercised more aggressively.

The results of each training session together with ECG rhythm strips are documented and become a part of the patient's personal file (Fig. 9.21). Long-term adaptation is the basis of exercise prescription changes and feedback to the patient.

SUMMARY AND CONCLUSIONS

The purpose of phase II is to enhance physical work capacity and prepare the patient for a lifetime commitment to healthy behavior. The focus of traditional phase II is aerobic exercise, three times a week for at least 30 minutes per session. Lifestyle modification classes should be included. Structure and conduct of the program are discussed, as well as adaptation to exercise. On completion the patient is eligible for phase III, long-term cardiac rehabilitation.

REFERENCES

1. Pollock ML, Pels AE III, Foster C, Ward A. Exercise prescription for rehabilitation of the cardiac patient. In: Pollock ML, Schmidt DH, eds. Heart disease and rehabilitation. 2nd ed. New York: John Wiley, 1986.
2. Pollock ML, Wilmore JH, Fox SM. Exercise in health and disease: evaluation and prescription and rehabilitation. Philadelphia: WB Saunders, 1984.
3. Franklin BA, Hellerstein HK, Gordon S, Timmis G. Exercise prescription for the myocardial infarction patient. J Cardiopulmonary Rehabil 1986;6:62.
4. Metier, CP, Pollock ML, Graves JE. Exercise prescription for the coronary artery bypass graft surgery patient. J Cardiopulmonary Rehabil 1986;6:85.
5. Department of Health and Human Services. Medicare and Medicaid guide. Health Care Financing Administration, Chicago: Commerce Clearing House, 1984.
6. Dismuke SE, Miller ST. Why not share the secrets of good health? The physician's role in health promotion. JAMA 1983; 249:3181.
7. Russell MA et al. Effect of general practitioner's advice against smoking. Br Med J 1979;2:231.
8. Yanowitz FG. Epilogue: a "systems" view toward the 21st century. In: Yanowitz FG, ed. Coronary heart disease prevention. New York: Marcel Dekker, 1992.
9. AACVPR Guidelines for cardiac rehabilitation programs. Champaign, IL: Human Kinetics, 1991.
10. Balady GJ, Weiner DA. Risk stratification in cardiac rehabilitation. J Cardiopulmonary Rehabil 1991;11:39.
11. American Heart Association. An active partnership for the health of your heart. AHA, Dallas, TX: 1990.
12. Leon AS et al. Exercise conditioning component. J Cardiopulmonary Rehabil 1990;10:79.
13. Oldridge NB. Compliance and exercise in primary and secondary prevention of coronary heart disease: a review. Prev Med 1982;11:56.
14. Ferreri JP. Successful strategies for facility planning. Atlantic Business January 1985, p. 46.
15. Yaglou CP. Temperature, humidity, and air movement in industries: the effective temperature index. Am J Physiol 1927,50.439.
16. Vogel JA, Rock PB, Jones BH, Havenith G. Environmental considerations in exercise testing and training. In: American College of Sports Medicine, ed. Resource manual for guidelines for exercise testing and prescription. Philadelphia: Lea & Febiger, 1993.
17. American Heart Association. Exercise standards book. Dallas, TX: AHA, 1979.
18. American Heart Association Task Force on Assessment of Cardiovascular Procedures (Subcommittee on exercise testing). Special report: guidelines for exercise testing. A report of the

American College of Cardiology. J Am Coll Cardiol 1986;8:725.

19. American College of Sports Medicine. Guidelines for exercise testing and prescription. 4th ed. Philadelphia: Lea & Febiger, 1991.

20. Franks BD. Physical warm-up. In: An analysis and evaluation of modern trends related to the physiological factors for optimal sports performances. Claremont, CA: National Coaches Conference, 1976.

21. Foster C, Dymond DS, Carpenter J, Schmidt DH. Effect of warm-up on left ventricular response to sudden strenuous exercise. J Appl Physiol 1982;53:380.

22. Kraus H, Raab W. Hypokinetic disease. Springfield, IL: Charles C Thomas, 1961.

23. Barnard RJ et al. Cardiovascular response to sudden strenuous exercise—heart rate, blood pressure and ECG. J Appl Physiol 1973;34:833.

24. McArdle WD, Katch FI, Katch VL. Exercise physiology: energy, nutrition and human performance. 3rd ed. Philadelphia: Lea & Febiger, 1991.

25. Benson H, Alexander S, Feldman CL. Decreased premature ventricular contractions through the use of relaxation response in patients with stable ischemic heart disease. Lancet 1975;2:380.

26. Benson H et al. Decreased blood pressure in borderline hypertensive subjects who practice meditation. J Chron Dis 1974;27:163.

27. Benson H et al. Decreased blood pressure in pharmacologically tested hypertensive patients who regularly elicited the relaxation response. Lancet 1974;1:289.

28. Franklin BA. The role of electrocardiographic monitoring in cardiac exercise programs. J Cardiac Rehabil 1983;3:806.

29. Meyer GC. Telemetry electrocardiographic monitoring in cardiac rehabilitation: How long? How often? In: Hall LK, ed. Cardiac rehabilitation: Exercise testing and prescription. Jamaica, NY: Spectrum, 1984.

30. Fardy PS, Doll N, Williams M. Monitoring cardiac patients: how much is enough? Phys Sports Med 1982;10:146.

31. Ryan M, Lown B, Horn H. Comparison of ventricular ectopic activity during 24 hour monitoring and exercise testing in patients with coronary heart disease. N Engl J Med 1975;292:224.

32. Simoons M, Lap C, Pool J. Heart rate levels and ventricular ectopic activity during cardiac rehabilitation. Am Heart J 1980;100:9.

33. DeBusk RF et al. Exercise training soon after myocardial infarction. J Am Coll Cardiol 1979; 44:1223.

34. Williams MA, Fardy PS. Limitations in prescribing exercise. Cardiovasc Pulmon Tech 1980;8:33.

35. Haskell WL. Cardiovascular complications during exercise training of cardiac patients. Circulation 1978;57:920.

36. Van Camp SP, Peterson RA. Cardiovascular complications of outpatient cardiac rehabilitation programs. JAMA 1986;256:1160.

37. Borg G. The perception of physical performance. In: Shephard RJ, ed. Frontiers of fitness. Springfield, IL: Charles C Thomas, 1971.

38. Borg GA. Perceived exertion: A note on "history" and methods. Med Sci Sports 1973;5:90.

39. Hackett TP, Cassem NH. Psychological adaptation in convalescence in myocardial infarction patients. In: Naughton JP, Hellerstein HK, Mohler IC, eds. Exercise testing and exercise training in coronary heart disease. Orlando, FL: Academic Press, 1973.

40. Heinzelmann F. Social and psychological factors that influence the effectiveness of exercise programs. In: Naughton JP, Hellerstein HK, Mohler IC, eds. Exercise testing and exercise training in coronary heart disease. Orlando, FL: Academic Press, 1973.

41. Franklin BA. Motivating and educating adults to exercise. JOPER June 1978, p. 13.

42. Golding LA. Programs of exercise—program organization. In: Morse RL, ed. Exercise and the heart. Springfield, IL: Charles C Thomas, 1972.

43. Adams TD, Edgington CE. The physician's role in promoting physical activity. In: Yanowitz FG, ed. Coronary heart disease prevention. New York: Marcel Dekker, 1992.

44. Fardy PS. Effects of two years' exercise in patients with diagnosed coronary artery disease. Med Sci Sports 1980;12:100.

45. Fardy PS et al. A comparison of changes between post myocardial infarct and post bypass surgical patients following three months exercise training. Med Sci Sports 1979;11:101.

10

LONG-TERM CARDIAC REHABILITATION

LONG-TERM PROGRAMS IN cardiac rehabilitation are generally identified as phases III and IV. Patients who exit phase II should enter immediately into

TABLE 10.1. Objectives of Long-Term Programs

1. To improve and maintain physical fitness.
2. To monitor heart rates, blood pressures, electrocardiograms, and signs or symptoms that are potential contraindications for exercise.
3. To provide professional supervision for exercise.
4. To prevent recurrences and complications of coronary heart disease.
5. To promote the importance of a lifetime commitment to physical activity and healthy lifestyles.
6. To introduce new exercise activities.
7. To teach skills for self-monitoring and self-awareness.
8. To provide a smooth transition from structured, closely supervised, and monitored phase II programs to those that are less monitored, supervised, and structured.
9. To continue with educational and behavioral goals consistent with phases I and II.
10. To provide the foundation for safe and effective home-based programs.

the long-term program. Low-risk patients who did not participate in phase II are also good candidates. Phase III usually lasts from 6 to 24 months and generally includes both clinical supervision by an exercise professional or nurse and intermittent ECG monitoring. The primary goals are to improve physical fitness, promote a feeling of well-being, and reduce the risk of a recurring event.

Phase IV is an ongoing long-term program beyond phase III that generally does not include clinical supervision or ECG monitoring. The goals of phase IV include continued improvement and maintenance of fitness, and the program may include both cardiac patients and healthy adults. It is not always necessary to enter phase III prior to IV. The professional staff decides which program is more appropriate.

OBJECTIVES

The objectives of long-term programs are outlined in Table 10.1.
These objectives are consistent for all programs. Other objectives may be appropriate according to the needs of the target population.

ELIGIBLE CANDIDATES

The following subjects are eligible for long-term programs:

1. Patients with coronary artery disease (CAD) as discussed in Chapter 9
2. Patients with CAD risk factors
3. Healthy individuals who are interested in enhancing physical fitness

The focus is on primary prevention for healthy subjects and for those with risk factors and no pathology and on secondary or tertiary prevention for patients with diagnosed CAD. Patients with other cardiovascular diagnoses might also be eligible. The professional staff decides which patients are appropriate.

PATIENT REFERRAL

Patients with a history of CAD require a documented physician referral similar to that required for entrance to phase II. The referral form includes clinical background information to enhance safety and benefit and to assist in the development of the exercise prescription (Fig. 10.1). The physician should seize on this opportunity to take a proactive position that strongly urges the patient to participate. The role of the physician can have a powerful influence on the patient and ultimate success of the program (1–3).

Self-referral is possible for healthy individuals. A form should be developed that would include the subject's objectives, interests, and limitations, as well as medical and lifestyle history. Individuals with risk factors may be physician- or self-referred according to their level of risk.

ORIENTATION TO THE PROGRAM

An orientation session similar to that preceding phase II is recommended to familiarize the subject and significant family and friends with the program. For example, if dietary counseling is an integral part of the long-term program, then the individuals who are responsible for food selection and preparation are urged to attend. Orientation sessions may be scheduled for individuals or for small or large groups. Individual or couple sessions are preferred but may be too time consuming. Specific objectives of the orientation are outlined in Table 10.2.

SCOPE OF THE PROGRAM

The scope of long-term programs requires careful consideration and planning and must be developed within the constraints of the budget for facilities, equipment, personnel, and programs. The socioeconomic status of prospective clientele must be carefully considered when establishing the fee structure. Because long-term programs are usually paid for out-of-pocket, family income is an important factor in the patient's decision of whether to participate (4, 5). A detailed written description of the program should be available to interested parties and

---

REFERRAL FORM
(to be completed by physician)

Patient's Name_____ Date_____
                    Last   First   Middle Initial

Address_____ _____
             Street   City   State   Home Telephone

Birth Date_____ Age_____ Spouse's Name_____

Insurance Company_____ Policy No._____

Diagnosis: _____Bypass Surgery   _____Myocardial Infarct
                  _____Cardiac Patient   _____Angioplasty
                  _____Symptomatic Coronary Artery Disease (Angina)
Other:_____ Explain_____

Specific Cardiac Information_____

Other Limitations_____

Date of Most Recent Hospital Admission_____

Medications	Dosage	Frequency	Date Prescribed	Physician Prescribing

Please fill in information below if possible:
Date of Examination_____
1. Urine: sp. gr._____ Alb._____ Glucose_____ Micro._____
2. Complete blood count: Hbg_____ Hct_____ WBC_____ Diff._____
3. ECG, 12 lead (enclose copy)_____
4. Blood pressure: Systolic R_____ L_____ Diastolic R_____ L_____
5. Cholesterol _____mg%; HDL _____mg%; LDL _____mg%; Triglycerides _____ mg%
6. Exercise Stress Test Results (enclose, if available)

Impression of above information_____

Signed _____, M.D.

Type or Print:

Name of Physician_____
Address_____
Phone_____

FIGURE 10.1. Referral form.

include the program's objectives, procedures, and cost. Table 10.3 outlines considerations of a long-term program.

Facilities

Most long-term programs are conducted in facilities that can accommodate a variety of activities and include space for games, aerobic exercise, walking and

TABLE 10.2. Objectives of Orientation

1.	Introduce the professional staff and demonstrate their competence.
2.	Provide a pleasant atmosphere that will allow people to feel at ease with the program's objectives and procedures.
3.	Provide a tour of the facility.
4.	Demonstrate the use of equipment.
5.	Discuss the content of the program.
6.	Discuss the importance of establishing individual objectives based on needs, interests, and background.
7.	Provide an opportunity for questions and interaction with the professional staff.
8.	Encourage patient sign-up.

TABLE 10.3. Consideration of a Long-Term Program

1.	Budget
2.	Facilities
3.	Equipment
4.	Personnel
5.	Exercise programs
6.	Program evaluation
7.	Ancillary programs (e.g., educational, behavioral, and home-based)

jogging, resistance exercise, and swimming. Community centers, school and university gymnasiums, YMCAs, and Jewish Community Centers are examples of typical long-term facilities. Long-term programs are only occasionally conducted in phase II facilities because the space is seldom sufficient to accommodate large numbers and the objectives are not the same. There are exceptions when phase II and long-term programs coexist, which allows for ease of supervision and improved compliance with some patients (6). Generally, these exceptions are unique situations where small numbers participate. Detailed guidelines for facilities have been developed by the American College of Sports Medicine (ACSM) (7), American Association of Cardiovascular and Pulmonary Rehabilitation (AACVPR) (8), and the American Heart Association (AHA) (9).

Community facilities are often preferred over a hospital location, which is more associated with treatment of acute illness. For some patients, however, a hospital based program provides greater security and appeal. Because the hospital-based program usually has limited space, phase III and phase II may coexist.

The amount of space, type of structure, and shape of the facility partially dictate the activities that are offered. The minimal size that is recommended for phases III and IV is large enough for a basketball court, providing sufficient room for jogging and walking, not more than 20 laps to the mile. A smaller area can become congested and increases the possibility of musculoskeletal injury from frequent turns. Weather permitting, outside facilities should be considered. Being outdoors can be pleasant, uplifting, and help the patient to realize that exercise is not limited to environmentally controlled facilities. Outdoor areas such as a running path need to be carefully marked and supervised. Cross-country jogging should be led by professional staff and incorporate the "buddy system" so that a patient is never alone. The long-term program facility should also include space for meetings, educational classes, and social events. Long-term facilities are also discussed in Chapter 7.

Equipment

The equipment that is selected for long-term programs should provide a variety of exercise options and when possible meet specific patient needs. For example, bicycle ergometers, rowers, and arm ergometers that are mostly used in phase II may also be incorporated into the long-term program for select patients. Equipment requirements for long-term programs are outlined in Table 10.4. The AHA, ACSM, and AACVPR also provide guidelines for equipment (8–10).

Selecting equipment and facilities for long-term programs should also consider the needs of the patient population. For example, programs for healthy individuals or those with CAD risk factors but no clinical pathology are structured differently from programs with high-risk, post–myocardial infarction (post-MI), or post-cardiac surgery (CABG) patients. Subjects at low risk can participate in a wider variety of physical activities, require less supervision, and do not need ECG monitoring. High-risk individuals require more structure, closer supervision, and a more tightly controlled environment. Several months of intermittent ECG monitoring is recommended for high-risk patients. Occasional monitoring is appropriate for all patients as the procedures are relatively simple, inexpensive, and unobtrusive. The variety of activities can be increased and

TABLE 10.4. Equipment Suggestions for Long-Term Exercise Programs

1.	Aerobic exercise devices, ergometers, treadmills, rowers, cross-country ski machines, stair climbers
2.	Resistance exercise devices, free weights, isokinetic machines, variable resistance machines
3.	Equipment for recreation and sport activities
4.	Monitoring equipment, portable ECG monitoring, and DC defibrillator
5.	First aid and emergency equipment
6.	Audio-visual equipment and educational materials
7.	Computers and software packages

monitoring decreased as the clinical status of the patient improves. Healthy subjects do not require monitoring.

Personnel

The ACSM and AACVPR have taken a leading role in developing standards for personnel in cardiac rehabilitation and prevention programs (8, 9). Additional information on personnel is found in Chapters 7 to 9, as well as other references (8, 11–13).

The long-term community-based program is supervised by exercise professionals who are able to interpret ECG rhythms, certified in cardiopulmonary resuscitation, and able to respond to cardiac emergencies. In some instances, especially with programs that are designed for high-risk patients, nurses and physicians may share in supervision. Advanced cardiac life support certification and a basic knowledge of exercise physiology are recommended for all professional staff responsible for the care of patients with diagnosed CAD.

The exercise leader must understand how to apply the principles of exercise physiology and kinesiology, must be able to lead exercises, and must be able to communicate effectively. Academic training is usually in physical education or an appropriate allied health science. The program's participants can also be excellent group leaders once they are familiar with the basic principles of exercise and have sufficiently improved their fitness. Patient leaders also serve as role models, establish a level of achievement to which other patients can aspire, and are excellent motivators.

Another source of exercise leaders can be students from colleges and universities that offer allied health professional preparation programs, that is, health, physical education, recreation, physical therapy, and nursing. Often these institutions have internship programs that require practical experiences. The responsibilities of a typical student intern include leading and assisting exercises, supervising games and recreational activities, exercise testing, recordkeeping, patient monitoring, preparing newsletters, and some aspects of program management.

There is less clinical need to supervise healthy individuals or low-risk patients. However, professional supervision helps to ensure correct mechanics of exercise, reduce the incidence of injury, enhance benefit, and improve adherence. Additional health professionals are recommended to complement the exercise leader and include nutritionists, psychologists, health educators, and behavioralists. Because coronary artery disease is a multi-factorial problem, it requires multidisciplinary and interdisciplinary intervention.

Budget and Finances

Several arrangements for payment are common in long-term programs. The amount, schedule, and method of collection should be provided in a written

369

agreement prepared by the provider and signed by the consumer. The most common method of payment is a membership fee that is usually paid by the client to the exercise center on a quarterly, semiannual, or annual basis. A regular financial statement should be given to the provider. Occasionally, the provider assumes responsiblity for billing and reimburses the exercise center on a scheduled basis. It is often necessary to subsidize the cost of phase III and IV programs to make them affordable to the patients especially when located in low- or low-middle-income neighborhoods. Otherwise only clients who are well-off will participate. On average, fees for long-term programs are between $10 and $20 per session. Records must be maintained meticulously. Information on reimbursement is found elsewhere (14, 15). Budget and finances are also discussed in Chapter 7.

Evaluation

The program must be evaluated objectively and the staff held accountable. The evaluation should include health and fitness benefits, patient satisfaction, program efficiency, fiscal responsibility, and patient safety.

Health and Fitness Benefits

Health and fitness benefits are objectively measured to ascertain that expectations are met on an individual or group basis. The results help to determine whether the program needs to be modified.

Patient Satisfaction

Client satisfaction should be assessed regularly by personal interview or written questionnaire. The latter, if anonymous, is less likely to have biased results. Long-term adherence depends on a high level of patient satisfaction.

Program Efficiency

Logistical considerations are constantly evaluated to ensure that the program operates efficiently. Patient flow, costs, and general operations should be well planned and organized to maximize cost-effectiveness. Factors such as time management, facility and equipment utilization, class organization, growth patterns, referral records, safety procedures, and patient records have to be analyzed. Long-range cost-effectiveness is important as it may provide a good financial rationale to support programs that do not appear to be cost effective (16).

Fiscal Responsibility

The financial objectives of the program should be delineated at the outset. The staff should be aware of financial expectations; that is, whether the program can operate at a loss, be expected to break even, or be profitable. Operating at a loss may be acceptable to an administrator if there are other tangible benefits. Financial reports should be provided to the staff and discussed each month.

Patient Safety

A vigilant watch is maintained over program safety. Precautions are taken (*a*) to prevent and (*b*) to respond to untoward events. Equipment and personnel must be regularly tested to ensure that the program is safe. An emergency plan is adopted with responsibilities assigned to each member of the staff. Emergency procedures should be practiced at least twice a year and include an occasional mock emergency.

The evaluation documents the value of the program. Undocumented claims of success are not advised and often are insufficient in the present-day climate of public health awareness, fiscal responsibility, and safety consciousness.

Patient Evaluation

The patient evaluation is similar to phase II and should include physical, physiologic, psychosocial, lifestyle, and risk factor measurements. The individual patient's program should be based largely on the evaluation. The benefits are determined by comparing results at entrance and exit. Additional information on evaluation, including examples of forms, is provided in Chapters 4 and 5.

Exercise Prescription

The exercise prescription is derived from the results of the individual evaluation and personal interview. Activity interests, personal goals, and physical limitations are obtained during the patient interview and help in selecting the most appropriate modes of exercise and designing the prescription. The use of individual goal contracts may be helpful for some individuals. The procedures used in prescribing exercise are described in Chapter 6.

The results from the graded exercise test help to determine the intensity of training. A conservative level of effort, for example, 70% of maximal heart rate (MHR), is recommended for patients who did not participate in phase II. The target heart rate (THR) is based on the most recent exercise test. The beginning THR is usually 80 to 85% MHR for patients having completed phase II and is usually progressed gradually until 85% MHR when training adaptation is normal. The THR may be increased to 85 to 90% MHR for healthy individuals and select patients in long-term programs (17–19). Low-risk cardiac patients or healthy subjects entering a long-term program are started conservatively if they have not been in phase II or a low-level preliminary program. The same principles of exercise prescription apply, although progression may be more rapid when no disease is present. The rate of progression must also consider physical

371

condition, age, musculoskeletal limitations, and other factors that affect training intensity.

Training specificity is also important in planning patient goals. Some activities and training techniques are chosen to meet specific needs. Training specificity is discussed in Chapter 6.

In some instances exercise intensity is prescribed using the Borg scale ratings of perceived exertion (RPE) (20). The Borg scale is particularly useful with patients who have difficulty in counting their heart rate, those on negative chronotropic medications, and transplant patients. Considerable practice is recommended before ratings of perceived exertion are accurate and consistent (21). The Borg scale is illustrated and discussed in Chapter 6.

Exercise Training

The exercise prescription is the basis of the training program. Individual training sessions consist of the exercise prescription incorporated into a regimen of warm-up, training stimulus, and cooldown.

A 10– to 15–minute warm-up precedes training and consists of general exercises that increase body temperature and circulation and specific exercises that consider individual musculoskeletal needs and limitations. For example, sit-ups and other back exercises are often included as part of warm-up as they help prevent low-back injuries in adults.

The training stimulus primarily consists of rhythmical, aerobic activities that are undertaken to improve cardiovascular fitness. Exercise is performed continuously or intermittently, maintaining the THR for 20 to 30 minutes, three or four times a week. The training program should include a variety of lifetime activities that can be supervised safely. There is no best mode of exercise, although walking and jogging are popular because no additional equipment is necessary, facility requirements are minimal, and they are of low-level skill. Rowing, bicycling, and swimming are also excellent and popular, but require special facilities and equipment. Upper-extremity exercises are important in long-term programs because of training specificity (22). Arm testing is suggested as a part of the exercise prescription (23–25).

Five to 10 minutes of low-level exercise is recommended as a cooldown. The physiologic mechanisms of warm-up and cooldown have been discussed in Chapter 6.

Resistance Training

Resistance exercises have been shown to be safe, as well as beneficial, for cardiac patients (26–32). Contraindications for resistance exercise are presented in Table 10.5 (8, 11, 33). If the patient has been cleared for resistance training, then circuit training with resistive machines has been shown to be popular, safer, easier to learn, and perhaps more beneficial than free weights (27, 28,

TABLE 10.5. Contraindications for Resistive Exercise Training

Absolute Contraindications

1. Unstable ischemia or angina
2. Uncontrolled complex dysrhythmias or dysrhythmias that worsen with exercise
3. Uncompensated congestive heart failure
4. Severe or symptomatic aortic stenosis
5. Ventricular tachycardia at workloads of < 6 METS
6. Individuals with severely depressed LV function (EF < 30%)
7. Individuals with severe 3-vessel or left main disease (nonsurgically treated)
8. Exertional hypotension (> 15 mm Hg)
9. Exercise capacity < 6 METS with ischemic horizontal or down-sloping ST depression ≥2.0 mm and/or angina during exercise
10. Recent complicated MI or recurrent/persistent ischemic symptoms after cardiac event
11. Known history of unrepaired cerebral, thoracic, abdominal, or LV aneurysm
12. Active or suspected myocarditis or pericarditis
13. Thrombophlebitis or intracardiac thrombi
14. Third-degree or advanced AV block
15. Resting systolic BP > 200 mm Hg and/or resting diastolic BP > 105 mm Hg
16. Previous episode of ventricular fibrillation or cardiac arrest that did not occur in the presence of an acute ischemic event or cardiac procedure
17. A medical problem that the physician believes may be life threatening or that warrants contraindication
18. Orthopedic problems that would prohibit resistive exercise
19. Acute systemic illness or fever
20. Severe restrictive or obstructive lung disease
21. Acute episodes of joint inflammatory or degenerative disease (i.e., bursitis, arthritis, gout)

33–35). Circuit weight training (CWT) has been shown to improve muscle strength and endurance, which enables the cardiac patient to participate in a wider range of activities and reduce the potential for musculoskeletal discomfort and injury, while providing added fun and satisfaction. Specifically, circuit weight training has been shown to improve strength, lean body mass, flexibility, and cardiovascular endurance (27, 28, 33, 34) and perhaps to increase bone mineral content, reducing the possibility of osteoporosis with aging (35).

TABLE 10.5. Cont.

Relative Contraindications

1.   Excessive blood pressure rise with resistive exercise: systolic pressure $\geq$ 220 mm Hg or
     diastolic pressure $\geq$ 110 mm Hg
2.   Changing pattern or new development of angina pectoris
3.   Congenital heart disease
4.   Cardiomyopathy
5.   Uncontrolled metabolic diseases (i.e., diabetes)
6.   Neuromuscular, musculoskeletal, or rheumatoid disorders that are exacerbated by exercise
7.   Valvular heart disease
8.   Exercise-induced ST-T wave changes > 2 mm from baseline ECG at heart rate < 135 bpm
9.   Failure to comply with resistive exercise prescription
10. Survivors of cardiac arrest and/or those who have had 2 or more myocardial infarctions
11. Recent coronary artery bypass grafting or other cardiac surgery (< 12 weeks)
12. Functional capacity < 6 METS on follow-up graded exercise test
13. Multiple, severe, initial thallium defects and/or multiple areas showing thallium redistribution
14. Stable congestive heart failure
15. Presence of AICD
16. Resting systolic BP $\geq$ 160 mm Hg and/or resting diastolic BP $\geq$ 100 mm Hg

Designing a circuit weight training program requires consideration of the following:

- Amount of resistance at each station
- Number of repetitions
- Time for completion at each station
- Rest interval between stations
- Number of stations
- Number of circuits to be completed

These variables are illustrated in Table 10.6 (33). Circuit weight training is suggested on alternate days, 2 or 3 days per week. Resistance should be established between 30 and 60% of 1 repetition maximum (RM) or at a level of resistance that can be completed comfortably with 12 to 15 repetitions per station (36, 37). Patients should avoid straining to complete a circuit. Rest intervals should be from 30 to 60 seconds between stations. Each training session should last from

TABLE 10.6. Circuit Weight Training (CWT) Parameters for Cardiac Patients

CWT Parameter	Cardiac Recommendations
Resistance	30-60% of 1 RM or low to moderate weight loads
Repetitions	8-20
	10-15 most often recommended
Exercise duration	20-30 minutes
Number of stations	5-18
Number of circuits/sets	1-3
	Depends on patient fitness level and time allotment for resistive exercise
Rest interval between stations	≥30 seconds
	Potential for greater improvement in cardiovascular endurance with shorter rest intervals
	Greater HR/BP recovery with longer rest intervals and less risk of cardiovascular complications
Speed of muscle contraction	Lift to a count of 2, lower to a count of 4
	Complete limb flexion/extension
Placement of CWT session	After the aerobic phase
	Ensures adequate warm-up, less risk of musculoskeletal injury, and prioritizes aerobic phase
Frequency	Alternating 2-3 days/week
Progression	Increase resistance once 10-15 reps can be performed comfortably (RPE 11-13)
	Increase sets depending upon time allotment for session, fitness level, and fatigability of the participant
Specificity	All major muscle groups
	Exercise large muscles before small muscles

20 to 30 minutes. Added resistance is appropriate when 12 to 15 repetitions can be completed easily at a RPE of 12 to 13 (36). Initially, the patient should attempt one set of exercises and gradually build up to three sets. Resistance exercise may have to be discontinued with the appearance of contraindications (Table 10.7) (11, 33, 38). A comprehensive review of resistance training for cardiac patients is currently in press (33).

Aquatics Exercise

Aquatics programs are gaining in popularity and appear to be a safe alternative to land-based exercise (39, 40). Water exercises are less stressful on bones and joints than weight-bearing activities. Swimming and water exercises that are

TABLE 10.7. Criteria for Termination of a Resistive Exercise Session

1.	Fatigue or weakness
2.	Lightheadedness, confusion, ataxia, pallor, cyanosis, dyspnea, nausea, or any peripheral circulating insufficiency
3.	Onset of angina with resistive exercise
4.	Exertional hypotension ($\geq$ 15 mm Hg drop in systolic blood pressure during lifting from resting baseline)
5.	Excessive blood pressure rise during lifting: systolic $\geq$ 220 mm Hg or diastolic $\geq$ 110 mm Hg
6.	Inappropriate bradycardia (decrease in heart rate > 10 beats/min) during resistive exercise
7.	Symptomatic supraventricular tachycardia or other exercised-induced complex supraventricular dysrhythmias
8.	ST changes ($\geq$ 2 mm) horizontal or downsloping from rest
9.	Ventricular tachycardia (3 or more consecutive PVCs)
10.	Exercise-induced LBBB
11.	Frequent (> 30% of the complexes), complex, or R-on-T PVCs
12.	Onset of 2nd- and/or 3rd-degree AV block
13.	New onset or aggravation of preexisting orthopedic or muscular problem that would prohibit continuation of the resistive session
14.	Failure to comply with exercise prescription, proper lifting technique, and/or appropriate log recording (i.e., recording of physiologic parameters, amount of resistance, number of repetitions)
15.	Discomfort related to past surgery (i.e., CABG, ilial bypass, rotator cuff)

performed in a horizontal position enhance venous return and augment stroke volume by reducing the effects of gravity. The cooling effect of water also decreases the risk of thermal overload as compared to land exercise in hot and humid conditions.

The water temperature recommended for cardiac rehabilitation ranges from 26 to 33°C (80 to 92°F) (41). Temperatures at the lower end of the range are better for dissipation of heat, whereas those at the upper end may be more comfortable for the majority of patients, especially those with peripheral vascular disease where vasodilation from increased water temperature would be helpful in alleviating possible discomfort.

Aquatics exercise includes a wide variety of physical activities that vary in intensity from low to high. Limited data are available on the actual energy cost of most activities in cardiac patients. Activities that are recommended include water walking (with and without the use of arms), swimnastics, water aerobics, aqua stepping or step aerobics, swimming that incorporates a variety of strokes, and water games such as volleyball (41–43).

As with other types of exercise, the activity prescription is individually based following ACSM guidelines (11). The intensity of exercise can be estimated by heart rate, as well as by ratings of perceived exertion, although the latter may not be as accurate with water exercise (41). Exercise heart rates can be determined from bicycle ergometer or treadmill tests (44–46), although upper body testing might be considered for a program that consists mainly of swimming that incorporates upper body work. The frequency and duration of exercise adhere to ACSM guidelines, three times a week, 20 to 30 minutes per session.

Long-term health and fitness benefits require that exercise be performed regularly. Games, recreational sports, and innovative activities are an opportunity for fun and camaraderie that help to ensure long-term adherence (47, 48). Some activities may be modified for safety reasons. Physical condition should be improved before participating in recreational games.

Recreational games may require special planning. Racquet sports, for example, should be preceded by a program of general conditioning and clinical assessment, including ECG monitoring with portable telemetry during actual play. Another recommendation is for a member of the professional staff to play and control the flow of the game. Doubles play is suggested.

Home-Based Exercise

Although most individuals prefer supervised exercise, unsupervised activity is sometimes the only option. Patients at low risk have demonstrated that home exercise can be safe and effective (49). Low risk has been defined as absence of recurrent chest pain, heart failure, or life-threatening arrhythmias and a symptom-limited exercise test at 3 to 6 weeks after infarction (50). The exercise leader is responsible for making unsupervised programs safe and beneficial (51–53). Additional safety suggestions for cardiac patients who exercise alone are (a) undertake a thorough examination (Chapters 3 to 5) that will enable the professional staff to design an individualized program, (b) join a supervised program if possible for a minimum of 2 weeks to assess the patient's readiness for unsupervised and nonmonitored activity. Even a few sessions of monitoring enhances safety (54) and reduces patient anxiety. Supervised exercise also provides an opportunity for the professional staff to evaluate exercise techniques and probably lessens the chance of sustaining musculoskeletal injury.

Some form of ECG monitoring is recommended for home programs. Electrocardiograms can be recorded on small, easily portable tape recorders that are transmitted by telephone to the cardiac rehabilitation center. An alternative method enables "real-time" ECG transmission over the telephone. Transtelephonic monitoring has been shown to be feasible and effective (55). Interpretation and feedback should be provided immediately. The patient needs to be taught how to palpate the pulse to ensure adherence to the target heart rate. If a supervised program is not available for periodic visits, then an alternative system is required to maintain frequent patient contact. Exercise record forms are used and regularly mailed to the cardiac rehabilitation center for subsequent review and discussion with the patient. A schedule of patient visits should be established with the personal physician to encourage long-term adherence. Periodic, supervised exercise and ECG-monitored classes are arranged at the rehabilitation center to assess the patient's progress, to update the exercise program, and to evaluate the patient's clinical status.

Monitoring and Supervision

Although the risk of a fatal event during cardiac rehabilitation is small (56, 57), occasional ECG monitoring is suggested in long-term programs for patients at increased risk. Low-risk patients can exercise safely without monitoring (49). Monitoring can be performed with telemetry, a standard electrocardiogram recorder with monitor-scope, or see-through defibrillator paddles. With defibrillator paddle monitoring, the paddles serve as electrodes (Fig. 10.2) enabling rhythm strips to be obtained quickly. Rapid determination of ECG tracings is extremely important, as a delay of only 30 seconds can significantly decrease heart rate, reduce myocardial oxygen demand, and lessen the likelihood of significant ECG changes. Monitoring equipment should have the capability for a 1–cm/mV calibration signal and 12–lead electrocardiography to document abnormalities observed in paddle-obtained records and to compare with prior 12–lead tracings. The disadvantage of the one-unit see-through paddles system

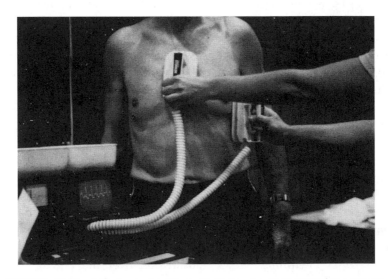

FIGURE 10.2. Monitoring with defibrillator-monitor-recorder system.

TABLE 10.8. Guidelines for Unsupervised Exercise

1. A physical examination, including an exercise test, should precede vigorous physical activity. This is advisable for everyone and is essential for inactive persons over 40 years of age, those with diagnosed heart disease or risk factors, persons with a family history of premature heart disease, or those who have been sedentary for a long time.
2. Realistic training objectives should be formulated.
3. An exercise prescription should be developed to meet the individual's needs.
4. Exercise sessions should adhere to accepted principles of physical conditioning.
5. Periodic reassessment, including upgrading the exercise prescription, should follow.

---

is that burns can be caused if the surface of the paddles gets scratched, and the wires are more likely to break because of frequent use. However, if the equipment is used and stored properly, these problems are unlikely. Long-term programs are staffed by professionals who can recognize and respond to emergencies.

Low-risk patients and healthy subjects are generally not monitored and require fewer precautionary considerations. Some programs are conducted individually at home, or at a nearby community location. If a supervised program is convenient, then the patient is encouraged to attend for a few sessions at the beginning of the program to ensure compliance and safety of the exercise prescription. Guidelines for unsupervised exercise have been described elsewhere (52, 53, 58, 59) and are summarized in Table 10.8.

Individual Progress

Individual progress is closely monitored. Comprehensive evaluations, such as those discussed in Chapters 3 to 5, are recommended annually or semiannually to assess the effectiveness of the program and to update the exercise prescription. Regular progress reports are discussed with the patient and significant others and sent to the referring physician. These reports are useful for motivation and establishing goals for the future.

If the person is not in a supervised program, then the information can be obtained through daily activity diaries that are mailed or provided to the patient at the time of the exercise test. Self-addressed and stamped envelopes should be provided for ease of return to the program center. Instructions are given for completing forms, including a date for return (e.g., the first of each month). Keep the instructions simple (Fig. 10.3).

Name_____

Address_____ Tel. Number_____

_____

Patient Diagnosis_____

Entered Program_____ Current Phase_____

Patient Adherence_____

Attitude Toward Program_____

Heart Rate at Rest_____ During Exercise _____ Recovery____

Blood Pressure at Rest_____ During Exercise_____ Recovery____

Electrocardiogram at Rest_____

Electrocardiogram During Exercise_____

Untoward Events_____

Summary of Changes:	Initial Results	Most Recent
Total Cholesterol	_____	_____
HDL	_____	_____
LDL	_____	_____
Triglycerides	_____	_____
Body Weight	_____	_____
Body Fat	_____	_____
Changes in Fitness_____		

Date_____ Program Director_____

Date	Time	Resting	Heart Rate Immediate Recovery During Exercise	Distance Covered	Duration of Exercise	Comments

FIGURE 10.3. Home recording.

MOTIVATION AND COMPLIANCE

Long-term adherence is a prerequisite for success. Unfortunately, the history of compliance in health intervention programs is not encouraging. Recidivism rates for exercise and other lifestyle programs range as high as 87% (60, 61) with the average about 50% (55, 56) in the initial 6 to 12 months. The current number of dropouts is unacceptable among cardiac patients who should be highly motivated to alter their living habits. Numerous studies have been undertaken to identify factors related to poor adherence (61–64).

380

MOTIVATION
Opinion and attitude
Therapeutic
Instructors
Variation
Aerobic
Team approach
Involvement
Objective testing
Noncompetitive

FIGURE 10.4. Motivational possibilities. (Used with permission of Neil Oldridge, PhD, Mt Sinai Hospital, Milwaukee, WI.)

Variety
Aerobic
Relaxing and Recreative
Individualized
Attitude
Therapeutic
Isotonic
Noncompetitive and fun

FIGURE 10.5. Attributes of a good exercise program. (From Oldridge NB. What to look for in an exercise leader. Phys Sports Med 1977;5:85.

A number of lifestyle and psychosocial variables are associated with poor adherence, and other important factors will most likely be identified. Lifestyle factors include cigarette smoking, blue collar employment, and physical inactivity (63, 65, 66). Psychosocial traits account for almost half of the reasons for program dropouts (61–63, 67, 68) and include depression, hypochondriasis, anxiety, introverted behavior, low self-esteem, lack of interest, poor motivation, and family problems. Other variables that affect adherence include location of the facility, cost, strenuousness of exercise, injuries, and lack of sociability (69, 70). Psychosocial factors, personal convenience, and family lifestyle appear to represent the major impediments to exercise compliance (61, 62, 65–67, 71–73) and are summarized in Table 10.9.

Numerous attempts (64, 74, 75), including enlisting spousal approval (76), have been made to improve adherence. Oldridge uses the words motivation and variation to summarize a list of variables that promote better attendance and decreased dropout rate (64, 77) (Figs. 10.4 and 10.5). Additional information is provided by Oldridge (77) and Franklin (62, 78). Motivational strategies, program modifications, and personnel guidelines (12, 64, 79) are summarized that enhance interest in and enthusiasm for exercise, as well as long-term program compliance (Tables 10.10 to 10.12). It is also necessary to develop adherence strategies for unsupervised programs. Gettman (53) proposes the following suggestions:

TABLE 10.9. Variables Predicting Exercise Dropout

Personal Factors	Program Factors	Other Factors
• Smoker	1. Inconvenient time/location	1. Lack of spousal support
• Inactive leisure time	2. Excessive cost	2. Inclement weather
• Inactive occupation	3. High-intensity exercise	3. Excessive job travel
• Blue collar worker	4. Lack of exercise variety, e.g., running only	4. Injury
• Type A personality	5. Exercises alone	5. Job change/move
• Increased physical strength	6. Lack of positive feedback or reinforcement	
• Extroverted	7. Inflexible exercise goals	
• Poor credit rating	8. Low-enjoyability ratings for running programs	
• Overweight and/or low ponderal index	9. Poor exercise leadership	
• Poor "self-motivation"		
• Depressed		
• Hypochondriacal		
• Anxious		
• Introverted		
• Low ego strength		

From Franklin BA. Exercise program compliance: improvement strategies. In: Storlie J, Jordan HA, eds. Behavioral intervention in obesity. Jamaica, NY: Spectrum, 1984.

TABLE 10.10. Motivational Strategies

1.	Minimize injury with a moderate exercise prescription.
2.	Emphasize exercising in a group.
3.	Emphasize variety and fun in the exercise program.
4.	Include modified recreational games in the conditioning format.
5.	Provide music during workouts.
6.	Incorporate effective behavioral and programmatic techniques in the conditioning program.
7.	Establish a regular workout schedule.
8.	Use fitness testing periodically to assess training results.
9.	Provide progress charts to record exercise achievements.
10.	Recruit spousal support in promoting the exercise program.
11.	Recognize individual accomplishments through a system of rewards.
12.	Be sure that the exercise leader is capable.

TABLE 10.11. Responsibilites of the Exercise Leader

Meet the requirements of the exercise test technician.

Interpret metabolic data obtained on the participant.

Execute the exercise prescription under guidelines established by the physician and the program director.

Educate the participant concerning exercise.

Evaluate the participant's response to exercise.

Interact and communicate with all personnel involved in the exercise program.

Source: American College of Sports Medicine. Guidelines for exercise testing and prescription. 4th ed. Philadelphia: Lea & Febiger, 1991.

1. Teach the individual how to correctly start an exercise program.
2. Provide some supervision in the early stages.
3. Have the individual report on his or her participation every 2 weeks.
4. Encourage the use of a home program because it may be more convenient.

Gettman found that improvement from unsupervised exercise was the same as that following supervised exercise if these suggestions were followed. Similar results were obtained from other home programs with comparable instructions (49). Motivation and compliance are complex issues. Much has been written about them, although many more studies are needed. Other sources are also suggested (80–83).

TABLE 10.12. Behavior Strategies of the Good Exercise Leader

1. Show a sincere interest in the participant.
2. Be enthusiastic in your instruction and guidance.
3. Develop a personal association and relationship with each participant.
4. Consider the various motives underlying exercise participation (e.g., health, recreation, social, personal image) and allow for individual differences.
5. Initiate participant follow-up (e.g., written notes or telephone calls) when several unexplained absences occur in succession.
6. Participate in the exercise session yourself.
7. Honor special days (e.g., birthdays) or accomplishments (attendance, personal achievements) with rewards (e.g., certificates, shirts, trophies).
8. Attend to orthopedic and musculoskeletal problems.

SUMMARY AND CONCLUSIONS

A lifetime commitment to healthful living, including regular physical activity, is the ultimate goal of cardiac rehabilitation. The most important long-term objective of exercise is to improve cardiovascular fitness, although strength, muscle endurance, and flexibility are also significant. After physical fitness has been satisfactorily improved, the long-term objective shifts to maintenance. When planning the long-term program, consider equipment, facilities, personnel, content, finances, evaluation, and home-based programs. Training sessions are based on an exercise prescription that includes intensity, frequency, duration, and mode of activity. Intermittent monitoring and clinical supervision is recommended for high-risk patients but is not necessary for low-risk subjects. Various suggestions are made to enhance motivation and adherence.

REFERENCES

1. Dismuke SE, Miller ST. Why not share the secrets of good health? The physician's role in health promotion. JAMA 1981;249:3181.
2. Adams TD, Holbrook JH. The physician's role in promoting physical activity. In: Yanowitz FG, ed. Coronary heart disease prevention. New York: Marcel Dekker, 1992.
3. Yanowitz FG. Epilogue: a "system's" view toward the 21st century. In: Yanowitz FG, ed. Coronary heart disease prevention. New York: Marcel Dekker, 1992.
4. Oldridge NB, Ragowski B, Gottlieb M. Use of outpatient cardiac rehabilitation services: factors associated with attendance. J Cardiopulmonary Rehabil 1992;12:25.
5. Muller C. Review of twenty years of research on medical care utilization. Health Serv Res 1986; 21:129.
6. American College of Sports Medicine. Resource manual for guidelines for exercise testing and prescription. 2nd ed. Philadelphia: Lea & Febiger, 1993.
7. American College of Sports Medicine. In: Sol N, Foster C, eds. ACSM's health fitness facility standards and guidelines. Champaign, IL: Human Kinetics, 1992.

8. American Association of Cardiovascular and Pulmonary Rehabilitation. Guidelines for cardiac rehabilitation programs. Champaign, IL: Human Kinetics, 1991.

9. American Heart Association. Guidelines for cardiac rehabilitation centers. Los Angeles: AHA, Greater Los Angeles Affiliate, 1982.

10. American Heart Association. Exercise standards book. Dallas: AHA, 1979.

11. American College of Sports Medicine. Guidelines for exercise testing and prescription. 4th ed. Philadelphia: Lea & Febiger, 1991.

12. American College of Sports Medicine. Resource manual for guidelines for exercise testing and prescription. 2nd ed. Philadelphia: Lea & Febiger, 1993.

13. Howley ET, Franks DB. Health fitness instructor's handbook. 2nd ed. Champaign, IL: Human Kinetics, 1992.

14. Meyer GC. Overview of insurance—obtaining and maintaining coverage in cardiovascular rehabilitation. In: Hall LK, Meyer GC, eds. Cardiac rehabilitation: exercise testing and prescription. Vol 2. Champaign, IL: Human Kinetics, 1988.

15. Smith LK. The real politik of rehabilitation. J Cardiopulmonary Rehabil 1990;10:307.

16. Shephard RJ. Exercise in secondary and tertiary rehabilitation: costs and benefits. J Cardiopulmonary Rehabil 1989;9:188.

17. Ehsani AA. Mechanisms responsible for enhanced stroke volume after exercise training in coronary heart disease. Eur Heart J 1987;8 (Suppl G):9.

18. Selvester R, Camp J, Sanmarco M. Effects of exercise training on progression of documented coronary arteriosclerosis in men. Ann NY Acad Sci 1977;301:465.

19. Ehsani AA, Biello DR, Schultz J, Sobel BE, Holloszy JO. Improvement of left ventricular contractile function by exercise training in patients with coronary artery disease. Circulation 1986; 74:350.

20. Pandolf KB. Advances in the study and application of perceived exertion. Exerc Sport Sci Rev 1983;11:118.

21. Bayles CM, Metz KF, Robertson R, Goss FL, Cosgrove J, McBurney D. Perceptual regulation of prescribed exercise. J Cardiopulmonary Rehabil 1990;10:25.

22. Franklin BA, Hellerstein HK, Gordon S, Timmis GC. Exercise prescription for the myocardial infarction patient. J Cardiopulmonary Rehabil 1986;6:62.

23. Quinn TQ, Kertzer R, Olney WB. Physiologic responses of patients with cardiac disease to arm, leg, and combined arm and leg work on an air-braked ergometer. J Cardiopulmonary Rehabil 1992;12.244.

24. Sala R, Laitinen LA. Comparison of arm crank exercise with leg ergometry in the evaluation of patients with past myocardial infarction. J Cardiopulmonary Rehabil 1992;12:174.

25. Wermuth E, Olund C, Pease MO, Hanson PA. Comparison of arm and leg exercise testing to predict cardiovascular responses to simulated work tasks in stable cardiac patients. J Cardiopulmonary Rehabil 1990;10:317.

26. Kelemen MH, Stewart KJ. Circuit weight training—a new direction for cardiac rehabilitation. Sports Med 1985;2:385.

27. Kelemen MH, Stewart KJ, Gillilan RE, Ewart CK, Valenti SA, Manley JD, Kelemen MD. Circuit weight training in cardiac patients. J Am Coll Cardiol 1986;7:38.

28. Kelemen MH. Resistive training safety and assessment guidelines for cardiac and coronary prone patients. Med Sci Sports Exerc 1989;21:675.

29. Franklin BA, Bonzheim K, Gordon S, Timmis GC. Resistance training in cardiac rehabilitation. J Cardiopulmonary Rehabil 1991;11:99.

30. Ghilarducci LEC, Holly RG, Amsterdam EA. Effects of high-resistance training in coronary artery disease. Am J Cardiol 1989;64:866.

31. Sparling PB, Cantwell JD, Niederman RK. Strength training in a cardiac rehabilitation program: a six-month follow-up. Arch Phys Med 1990;71:148.

32. Stewart KJ. Resistive training effects on strength and cardiovascular endurance in cardiac and coronary prone patients. Med Sci Sports Exerc 1989;21:678.

33. Verrill DE, Ribisl PM. Resistive exercise training in cardiac rehabilitation. In: Fardy PS, ed. Training techniques in cardiac rehabilitation. Champaign, IL: Human Kinetics, 1995.

385

34. Gettman LR, Pollock ML. Circuit weight training: a critical review of its physiological benefits. Phys Sports Med, 1981;9:44.
35. Conroy BP, Kraemer WJ, Maresh CM, Dalsky GP. Adaptive responses of bone to physical activity. Med Exerc Nutr Health 1992;1:64.
36. Berra K et al. Guidelines for cardiac rehabilitation programs. Champaign, IL: Human Kinetics, 1991.
37. American College of Sports Medicine. Guidelines for exercise testing and prescription. 4th ed. Philadelphia: Lea & Febiger, 1991.
38. Fletcher GF, Froelicher VF, Hartley LH, Haskell WL, Pollock ML. Exercise standards—a statement for health professionals from the AHA. Circulation 1990;82:2286.
39. Porcari JP, Fernhall B, Wilson PK. Aquatics programming in cardiac rehabilitation. In: Fardy PS, ed. Training techniques in cardiac rehabilitation. Champaign, IL: Human Kinetics, 1995.
40. Fernhall B, Congdon K, Manfredi T. ECG response to water- and land-based exercise in patients with cardiovascular disease. J Cardiopulmonary Rehabil 1990;10:5.
41. Fernhall B, Manfredi TG, Congdon K. Prescribing water-based exercise from treadmill and arm ergometry in cardiac patients. Med Sci Sports Exerc 1992;24:139.
42. Gleim GW, Nicholas JA. Metabolic cost and heart rate responses to treadmill walking in water at different depths and temperatures. Am J Sports Med 1989;17:248.
43. Magder S, Linnarson D, Gullstrand L. The effect of swimming on patients with ischemic heart disease. Circulation 1981;63:979.
44. Heigenhauser GF, Boulet D, Miller B, Faulkner JA. Cardiac output of post-myocardial infarction patients during swimming and cycling. Med Sci Sports 1977;9:143.
45. Thompson DL, Boone WT, Miller ES. Comparison of treadmill exercise and tethered swimming to determine validity of exercise prescription. J Cardiac Rehabil 1982;2:363.
46. Boone WT, Thompson DL. Reproducibility of tethered swimming in exercise prescription research. Am Corr Ther J 1983;37:23.
47. Franklin BA, Oldridge NB, Stoedefalke KG, Loechel WE. On the ball: innovative activities for adult fitness and cardiac rehabilitation programs. Carmel, IN: Benchmark Press, 1990.
48. Inbar G, Wallace JP, Carter S, Koester W, Rink LD. Use and risks of volleyball in cardiac rehabilitation programs. J Cardiopulmonary Rehabil 1990;10:455.
49. DeBusk RF, Houston N, Haskell W, Fry G, Parker M. Exercise training soon after myocardial infarction. Am J Cardiol 1979;44:1223.
50. DeBusk R, Pitts W, Haskell W, Houston N. Comparison of cardiovascular responses to static-dynamic efforts and dynamic effort alone in patients with chronic ischemic heart disease. Circulation 1979;59:977.
51. Fardy PS. Home-based cardiac rehabilitation. Phys Sports Med 1987;15:89.
52. Williams RS et al. Guidelines for unsupervised exercise in patients with ischemic heart disease. J Cardiopulmonary Rehabil 1981;3:213.
53. Gettman LR, Pollock ML, Ward A. Adherence to unsupervised exercise. Phys Sports Med 1983; 11:56.
54. Fardy PS, Doll N, Williams MA. Monitoring cardiac patients: how much is enough? Phys Sports Med 1982;10:146.
55. Pratt CM et al. Clinical benefits of transtelephonic ECG transmission to monitor home exercise programs in coronary heart disease patients. Med Sci Sports Exerc 1983;15:120.
56. Haskell WL. Cardiovascular complications during exercise training of cardiac patients. Circulation 1978;57:920.
57. Van Camp SP, Peterson RA. Cardiovascular complications of outpatient cardiac rehabilitation programs. JAMA 1986;256:1160.
58. DeBusk RF, Haskell WL, Miller NH. Medically directed at-home rehabilitation soon after clinically uncomplicated acute myocardial infarction: a new model for patient care. Am J Cardiol 1985;55:251.
59. Kasch FW, Boyer JL. Adult fitness: principles and practices. Palo Alto, CA: National Press Book, 1968.
60. Dishman RK. Compliance/adherence in health-related exercise. Health Psychol 1982;1:237.

61. Oldridge NB. Compliance with exercise programs. In: Pollock ML, Schmidt DH, eds. Heart disease and rehabilitation. 2nd ed. New York: John Wiley, 1986.

62. Franklin BA. Exercise program compliance: improvement strategies. In: Storlie J, Jordan HA, eds. Behavioral intervention in obesity. Jamaica, NY: Spectrum, 1984.

63. Oldridge NB. Compliance with cardiac rehabilitation services. J Cardiopulmonary Rehabil 1991; 11:115.

64. Oldridge NB. Cardiac rehabilitation exercise programme: compliance and compliance-enhancing strategies. Sports Med 1988;6:42.

65. Oldridge NB, Streiner D. Health belief model as a predictor of compliance with cardiac rehabilitation. Med Sci Sports Exerc 1990;22:678.

66. Oldridge NB, Rogowski B. Prediction of attendance in cardiac rehabilitation. Med Sci Sports Exerc 1989;21 (Suppl):56.

67. Conroy RM, Cahill S, Mulcahy R, Johnson H, Graham IM, Hickey N. The relation of social class to risk factors, rehabilitation, compliance and mortality in survivors of acute coronary heart disease. Scand J Soc Med 1986;14:51.

68. Conroy RM, Mulcahy R, Graham IM, Reid V, Cahill S. Predictors of patient response to risk-factor modification advice after admission for unstable angina or myocardial infarction. J Cardiopulmonary Rehabil 1986;6:344.

69. Miller P et al. Personal adjustments and regimen compliance 1 year after myocardial infarction. Heart Lung 1989;18:339.

70. Giese H, Schomer HH. Life-style changes and mood profile of cardiac patients after an exercise rehabilitation program. J Cardiopulmonary Rehabil 1986;6:30.

71. Andrew GM et al. Reasons for dropout from exercise programs in post-coronary patients. Med Sci Sports Exerc 1981;13:164.

72. Oldridge NB et al. Predictors of dropout from cardiac exercise rehabilitation. Am J Cardiol 1983; 51:70.

73. Oldridge NB. Compliance and dropout in cardiac exercise rehabilitation. J Cardiopulmonary Rehabil 1984;4:166.

74. Oldridge NB. Efficacy and effectiveness: critical issues in exercise and compliance. J Cardiopulmonary Rehabil 1984;4:119.

75. Oldridge NB, Jones NL. Improving patient compliance in cardiac rehabilitation; effects of a written agreement and self-monitoring. J Cardiopulmonary Rehabil 1983;3:257.

76. Daltroy LH, Godin G. The influence of spousal approval and patient perception of spousal approval on cardiac patient participation in exercise programs. J Cardiopulmonary Rehabil 1989; 9:363.

77. Oldridge NB. What to look for in an exercise leader. Phys Sports Med 1977;5:85.

78. Franklin BA. The role of electrocardiographic monitoring in cardiac exercise programs. J Cardiopulmonary Rehabil 1983;3:806.

79. King AC, Martin JE. Exercise adherence and maintenance. In: American College of Sports Medicine. Resource manual for guidelines for exercise testing and prescriptions. 2nd ed. Philadelphia: Lea & Febiger, 1993.

80. Gale JB et al. Factors related to adherence to an exercise program for healthy adults. Med Sci Sports Exerc 1984;16:544.

81. Dishman RK, Ickes W. Self-motivation and adherence to therapeutic exercise. J Behav Med 1981;4:421.

82. Blumenthal JA et al. Physiological and psychological variables predict compliance to prescribed exercise therapy in patients recovering from myocardial infarction. Psychosom Med 1984;44: 519.

83. Dishman RK. Prediction of adherence to habitual physical activity. In: Nagle FJ, Montoye HJ, eds. Exercise in health and disease. Springfield, IL: Charles C Thomas, 1981.

11

CARDIOVASCULAR DISEASE PREVENTION STRATEGIES

PREVIOUS CHAPTERS DISCUSSED the pivotal role of exercise training in the prevention and management of individuals with known or suspected cardiovascular disease. The origins of cardiac rehabilitation in the 1950s were focused on the role of physical activity after myocardial infarction primarily as a means to restore function and confidence in patients with advanced atherosclerosis. The scientific basis of cardiac rehabilitation was derived from studies of the adverse physiologic and emotional effects of prolonged bed rest and the role of exercise in reversing those effects. In the early years of cardiac rehabilitation little was known of the potential for slowing, halting, or even reversing the process of atherosclerosis. With advances in our understanding of atherosclerosis that have accumulated over the last 40 years, cardiac rehabilitation has expanded its scope to include a comprehensive package of prevention strategies. The role of exercise in combating the deleterious effects of prolonged bed rest has become less important because prolonged bed rest is no longer an inevitable consequence of hospitalizations for cardiovascular disease. Exercise training, however, continues to provide the foundation for comprehensive cardiovascular disease prevention because of the known beneficial effects of exercise on the underlying atherosclerotic disease processes.

This chapter considers prevention strategies other than exercise that are usually included in a comprehensive cardiovascular disease prevention program. The focus is on assessment and management of the major coronary disease risk factors: hyperlipidemia, cigarette smoking, hypertension, and diabetes mellitus. Interventions that are discussed include lifestyle restructuring, behavioral techniques, and pharmacologic treatments. Although the emphasis is on the management of patients already in cardiac rehabilitation (i.e., tertiary-prevention), many of the treatment strategies are just as applicable to programs of primary and secondary prevention. The topics for discussion in this chapter are important to health care workers interested in all aspects of cardiovascular disease prevention.

HYPERLIPIDEMIA

For many years the "cholesterol hypothesis" was the raging controversy among health care professionals, as well as the general population. The hypothesis stated that atherosclerosis was *caused* by increased levels of cholesterol in the blood, and that the increased cholesterol in the blood was *caused* by a diet rich in cholesterol and saturated fat. As with many simple theories of disease causation, the scientific evidence relating cholesterol to mechanisms of atherosclerosis, and especially to coronary artery disease, turned out to be much more complicated than was originally thought. Although the full elucidation of the cholesterol hypothesis has yet to be realized, the evidence is sufficiently compelling to conclude that hypercholesterolemia is *one* of the major causes of atherosclerotic cardiovascular diseases (1). Furthermore, data largely obtained during the 1980s, showing that the treatment of hypercholesterolemia prevents atherosclerotic complications, are equally compelling (2–4). For these reasons it is necessary for those working in coronary disease prevention and cardiac rehabilitation programs to be familiar with the current guidelines for detection and treatment of hypercholesterolemia and related lipid disorders.

The recommendations presented in this section are, in part, based on the most recent guidelines of the National Cholesterol Education Program (NCEP) Expert Panel on Detection, Evaluation, and Treatment of High Blood Cholesterol in Adults published in 1993 (5). These guidelines represent the second report of the Adult Treatment Panel and are the result of a careful review of the recent literature by a consensus group of experts sponsored by the National Heart, Lung, and Blood Institute of the National Institutes of Health. The first NCEP report was published in 1988 (6) and resulted in a significant increase in public awareness and changes in physician practices regarding the diagnosis and treatment of hyperlipidemias. The second report updates and further refines the recommendations for cholesterol management based on an individual's cardiovascular risk status.

Coronary Heart Disease (CHD) Risk Status As a Guide to Treatment

Table 11.1 identifies the coronary risk factors other than hypercholesterolemia that should be considered before deciding on a particular course of lipid-lowering therapy. This is especially important in choosing a treatment strategy for persons who have yet to develop clinical heart disease (i.e., primary or secondary prevention). The identification of relatively low-risk individuals such as premenopausal women or young adult men with hypercholesterolemia but no other risk factors should delay the initiation of drug therapy. Cholesterol-lowering treatments are only effective in lowering mortality in patients with an initial high risk of CHD death (7). The intensity of treatment, therefore, should depend on the individual's risk status with the most aggressive interventions

TABLE 11.1. Coronary Risk Factors Other Than Hypercholesterolemia (5)

Positive Risk Factors

- Age in years:
  – Male ≥ 45
  – Female ≥ 55 or prematurely menopausal without estrogen replacement therapy
- Family history of premature CHD (definite MI or sudden death before age 55 in first-degree male relative, or before age 65 in first-degree female relative).
- Current cigarette smoker
- Hypertension (BP ≥ 140/90 mm Hg, or taking antihypertensive medications)
- HDL-C (< 35 mg/dl)
- Diabetes mellitus

Negative Risk Factors

- HDL-C ≥ 60 mg/dl

reserved for patients with the highest risk for future CHD events. Clearly, individuals who already have advanced atherosclerotic disease of the coronary or peripheral arteries are at highest risk for future complications and deserve the greatest attention. For patients without clinical manifestations of CHD the presence of two or more *positive* risk factors listed in Table 11.1 also identifies a moderately high-risk status. The new guidelines take high-density lipoprotein cholesterol (HDL-C) into the risk assessment equation; low HDL-C (<35 mg/dl) is considered a positive risk factor, whereas high HDL-C (≥60 mg/dl) is a *negative* risk factor and serves to cancel out one of the positive risk factors. In general, a net balance of two or more positive risk factors from Table 11.1 identifies a higher risk individual who needs more aggressive cholesterol-lowering interventions.

Classification of Hyperlipidemia

The current recommendations for the general population are to measure serum total cholesterol (TC) and HDL-C in all adults beginning at age 20 or older and repeating at least once every 5 years (5). Contrary to popular belief, these tests can be obtained in the nonfasting state. Table 11.2 indicates the initial classification of the patient's status based on these measurements. Figure 11.1 illustrates the NCEP management suggestions for adults without evidence of clinical coronary heart disease based on the initial classification and risk assessment. If TC is <200 mg/dl *and* HDL-C is ≥35 mg/dl, the person should be provided with general recommendations for maintaining good health and advised to repeat these lipid measurements within 5 years. If TC is borderline

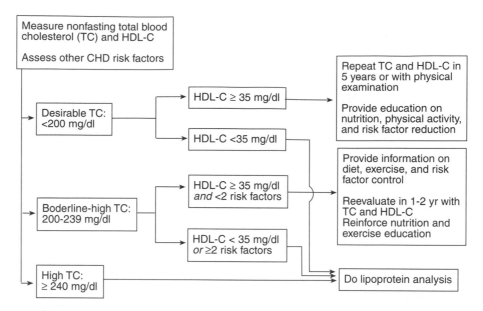

FIGURE 11.1. NCEP guidelines for classifying adults without evidence of clinical CHD (5). Follow-up recommendations are based on the results of total cholesterol and HDL-C levels.

TABLE 11.2. Initial Classification Based on Total and HDL-C Levels (5)

	Cholesterol Level	Initial Classification
Total Cholesterol	<200 mg/dl	Desirable blood cholesterol
	200–239 mg/dl	Borderline-high cholesterol
	≥ 240 mg/dl	High blood cholesterol
HDL Cholesterol	< 35 mg/dl	Low HDL cholesterol

high (200–239 mg/dl) but HDL-C is ≥35 mg/dl, the person should be advised to have repeat lipids in 1 to 2 years and encouraged to maintain prudent dietary and exercise habits. If HDL-C is <35 mg/dl or if TC is ≥240 mg/dl, the person should undergo a fasting lipoprotein analysis and follow the guidelines illustrated in Figure 11.2. Individuals with borderline high cholesterol *and* two or more positive coronary risk factors should also have a lipoprotein analysis.

The fasting lipoprotein analysis includes TC, HDL-C, and triglycerides. Very low density cholesterol (VLDL-C) is calculated as triglycerides/5, as long as the triglycerides are <400–500 mg/dl. From these values LDL cholesterol (LDL-C) is calculated by the following formula:

$$LDL\text{-}C = TC - (HDL\text{-}C + VLDL\text{-}C)$$

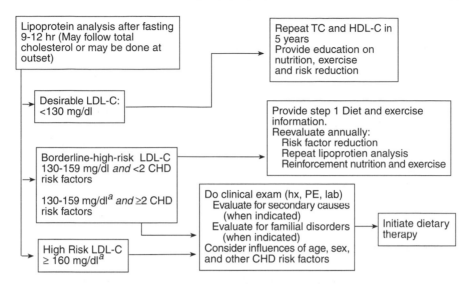

*a*On basis of average of 2 determinations. If the first two LDL-C test results differ by >30 mg/dl, a third test should be done within 1-8 wk and average of the three tests used.

FIGURE 11.2. NCEP guidelines for treatment and follow-up of adults without evidence of clinical coronary heart disease based on LDL-C levels and coronary risk factors (5).

If triglycerides are >500 mg/dl, however, the equation is inaccurate and LDL-C must be measured directly (expensive and time consuming).

The *desirable* LDL-C level is <130 mg/dl; *borderline high-risk* LDL-C is 130–159 mg/dl; *high-risk* LDL-C is ≥160 mg/dl. Treatment and follow-up suggestions for individuals without clinical evidence of coronary disease are indicated in Figure 11.2. Those with desirable levels of LDL-C should be advised to follow a healthy lifestyle and have their lipids repeated within 5 years. Persons with borderline high-risk LDL-C levels *and* fewer than two risk factors should be given diet and exercise instructions and followed annually. Borderline high-risk patients with two or more risk factors and those with high-risk LDL-C levels should undergo further workup to evaluate for secondary causes of hyperlipidemia and to assess the family history for familial hyperlipidemic disorders. Before embarking on an expensive workup and treatment regimen, however, it is wise to repeat the lipoprotein analysis and average the two determinations. If the two LDL-C values differ by more than 30 mg/dl, a third test should be obtained within 1 to 8 weeks and the average of the three tests used for further treatment decisions. This is done to avoid long-term diet and possible drug regimens for a single spurious laboratory value.

For patients with known coronary heart disease or other advanced atherosclerotic vascular disease, classification should be based on one or more fasting

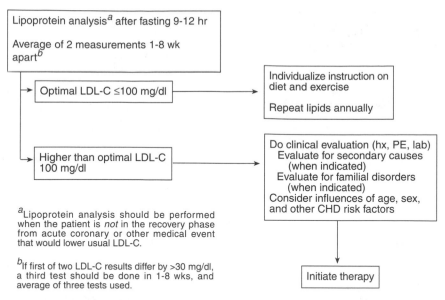

FIGURE 11.3. NCEP guidelines for classification, follow-up, and treatment of patients with known coronary heart disease or other advanced atherosclerotic vascular diseases (5).

lipoprotein analyses as illustrated in Figure 11.3. For these high-risk individuals *optimal* LDL-C levels are defined as ≤100 mg/dl; anything above this is called *higher than optimal* and should be further evaluated and treated as suggested in the figure. It must be emphasized that patients with known atherosclerotic diseases deserve the most aggressive management to slow, halt, or reverse the process of disease and minimize their risk for future complications. This is very important for those working in cardiac rehabilitation because patients recovering from recent cardiovascular hospitalizations are often extremely motivated to change their adverse lifestyles.

Table 11.3 summarizes the treatment recommendations and the LDL-C goal after therapy for the various subgroups defined in Figures 11.1, 11.2, and 11.3. Drug therapy should only be considered after dietary therapy has failed to achieve the desired LDL-C goal.

Dietary Therapy

Two diets have been formally proposed by the NCEP (5). The *step I diet* is recommended for the general public, as well as for most individuals initiating therapy for hyperlipidemia (Table 11.3). The dietary goals are to reduce the intake of saturated fat and cholesterol and to reduce the caloric intake in patients who are overweight. The diet consists of limiting the total fat intake to 30% of total calories or less, the saturated fat to 8 to 10% or less, and the cholesterol to <300 mg/day. Carbohydrates should be increased to 50 to 60% of

TABLE 11.3. Treatment Decisions Based on LDL-Cholesterol Level (5)

Patient Category	Initiation Level	LDL Goal
Dietary Therapy		
Without CHD *and* < 2 risk factors	≥ 160 mg/dl	<160 mg/dl
Without CHD *and* ≥ 2 risk factors	≥ 130 mg/dl	<130 mg/dl
With CHD	> 100 mg/dl	≤100 mg/dl
Drug Treatment		
Without CHD *and* < 2 risk factors	≥ 190 mg/dl	<160 mg/dl
Without CHD *and* ≥ 2 risk factors	≥ 160 mg/dl	<130 mg/dl
With CHD	≥ 130 mg/dl	≤100 mg/dl

TABLE 11.4. Recommendations for Reducing Saturated Fat Intake

Fish-Meats-Poultry		Dairy Products	
Choose	Decrease	Choose	Decrease
• Fish	• Fatty cuts of beef, pork, lamb	• Skim milk or low-fat milk (1-2%)	• Whole milk (4%)
• Shellfish	• Spareribs	• Low-fat yogurt and cheeses	• Whole-milk yogurt, cottage cheese, other cheeses
• Poultry without skin	• Organ meats	• Sherbet	• Cream, half-and-half
• Lean cuts of beef, pork, lamb	• Processed meats (bacon, etc.)	• Sorbet	• Ice cream
• Veal	• Sardines, roe		• Sour cream

total calories, and protein should make up 15% of total calories. Physicians and other health professionals should be knowledgeable in prescribing this diet to their patients. Several excellent cookbooks are also available and have the advantage of providing interesting recipes (8, 9). General recommendations for reducing saturated fat intake are listed in Table 11.4.

The step II diet is more restrictive and is recommended to those who fail to achieve the desired LDL goal listed in Table 11.3. Further reductions in saturated fat intake to <7% of total calories and cholesterol to <200 mg/day are required in this diet. Because of the restrictive nature of the step II diet, it is recommended that a registered dietitian or other qualified nutritionist be involved in meal planning and patient education.

How long should a patient remain on the step I diet before progressing to the step II diet? This depends on the individual's risk for coronary disease and the response to the step I diet. In general, a fall in LDL-C of 20 to 30 mg/dl can be expected within 3 to 6 months of step I dietary intervention. If after 6 months the target LDL-C goal is not reached, the low- to moderate-risk patient should begin the step II diet. For patients with known coronary or other atherosclerotic disease, on the other hand, the NCEP recommends that the step II diet be started immediately (5). If the desired LDL goals are not met within 2 to 3 months, drug therapy should be strongly considered.

For patients without atherosclerotic disease who are at low or intermediate risk, the step I diet should be initiated and the total cholesterol measured in 4 to 6 weeks and again in 3 months. It is not necessary to monitor fasting lipid fractions in these patients since for most patients total cholesterols of 240 and 200 mg/dl correspond to LDL-cholesterols of 160 and 130 mg/dl, respectively. Once the patient has achieved the desired total cholesterol, continued monitoring should be done quarterly for the first year and twice yearly thereafter. If the goal cholesterol is not reached, however, the patient should receive dietary consultation and be considered for the step II diet. For primary prevention the NCEP recommends a minimum of 6 months of intensive dietary counseling and therapy before considering drugs. For very low risk patients (e.g., premenopausal women and men <35 years of age without risk factors) drug therapy should be postponed indefinitely unless LDL-C levels are >220 mg/dl.

For patients who are overweight it is important to emphasize the need for weight reduction and exercise training along with appropriate dietary recommendations. Both of these are often necessary to lower triglycerides and raise HDL-C. Exercise training recommendations are discussed in Chapter 6. Strategies for weight reduction are discussed in several recent publications (10–12).

Drug Therapy

The initiation of drug therapy for primary prevention in patients without coronary disease continues to be controversial, although there are considerable data to justify such an intervention in high-risk individuals (2–4). Arguments against drug therapy include the cost of medications, adverse side effects, and uncertainties about long-term safety. The NCEP recommendations for starting drug therapy are listed in Table 11.3 except in very low risk individuals discussed previously (5). Similar LDL-C goals as for dietary therapy are recommended.

The major drugs for consideration include the bile acid sequestrants or resins (cholestyramine and colestipol), nicotinic acid (niacin), and the hydroxymethylglutaryl-coenzyme A (HMG-CoA) reductase inhibitors (the "statins"). Other second-line drugs that are used in certain situations are gemfibrozil and probucol. Table 11.5 lists the available drugs and dosages (13). Estrogen replacement therapy for postmenopausal women is also an important treatment option in this population, and this will be further discussed in a later section (14–16). The following sections briefly describe the major lipid-lowering drug classes.

Bile Acid Sequestrants

The bile acid sequestrants, cholestyramine and colestipol, have a long and successful track record as safe and effective agents. They are especially useful in patients with isolated LDL-C elevations. These drugs bind cholesterol-containing bile salts in the intestines, decreasing their reabsorption and increasing their excretion in the stool. Because the resins are nonabsorbable, they do not have systemic side effects and are therefore quite safe. The drugs are supplied as flavored or unflavored powders, which are mixed with fluids or other foods (e.g., apple sauce) to increase palatability. The starting dose of cholestyramine is 4 g before a main meal, progressing to 4 to 8 g two to three times a day before meals. For colestipol the initial dose is 5 g before a main meal, progressing to 5 to 10 g two to three times a day before meals. Local gastrointestinal side effects, including bloating, flatulence, and constipation, however, may limit their use in some patients. The addition of dietary fiber or psyllium laxatives (e.g., Metamucil) may decrease symptoms of constipation and contribute to the cholesterol lowering effects. The resins are also effective agents in combination with other drugs such as niacin, the statins, or gemfibrozil.

Nicotinic Acid (Niacin)

Nicotinic acid is a vitamin B agent that is very effective in lowering LDL-C and triglycerides, as well as increasing HDL-C. The drug primarily works by interfering with lipid metabolism in the liver. The starting dose is 100 to 250 mg twice daily after meals, progressing slowly to 1 to 2 g two to three times a day after meals. An unpleasant cutaneous flushing sensation is the most common side effect of the higher doses and often limits its use. The flushing phenomenon is mediated by prostaglandins and can be minimized by taking an aspirin tablet 30 to 60 minutes before the niacin dose. The flushing usually becomes less of a problem with continued use. Other side effects include gastrointestinal distress, liver function abnormalities, hyperglycemia, and hyperuricemia. Although a sustained release preparation is available with fewer side effects, there may be increased liver toxicity with its use (17). Nicotinic acid is very inexpensive and effective. For these reasons it is important to educate patients regarding its use and side effects.

HMG-CoA Reductase Inhibitors (Statins)

These drugs inhibit the rate-limiting enzyme in the synthesis of cholesterol by the liver. They are the newest, most expensive, and best tolerated of the lipid-lowering drugs. Their predominant effect is lowering of LDL-C levels; slight

397

TABLE 11.5. Drugs for Treatment of Hyperlipidemia (13)

Drug	Usual Dose	Cost/month	Mechanism	Comments
Cholestyramine (Questran or Questran Light)	2 scoops bid (1 scoop = 4g); increase gradually	$80	Binds intestinal bile acids, indirectly depleting liver of cholesterol; upgrading of hepatic LDL receptors.	Adding psyllium helps prevent constipation. Decreases absorption of digoxin, thiazides, coumadin, thyroxin.
Cholestyramine (Cholybar)	1 bar = 1 scoop or 4g	$139	As above. Occasionally useful alternative to powders.	Least preferred form of bile acid sequestrants in children.
Colestipol (Colestid)	2 scoops bid (1 scoop = 5 g)	$75	As above.	Unflavored. Tends to be slightly more gritty.
Niacin (Nicotinic acid)	1 g tid; increase gradually	$12-18	Mainly decreases VLDL synthesis; some increase VLDL removal rate. Decreased hepatic cholesterol synthesis.	Flushing is mediated by prostaglandins and is blocked by 1 aspirin an hour before taking. Time release forms may be more hepatotoxic.
Gemfibrozil (Lopid)	60 mg bid	$53	Increases lipoprotein lipase activity with increased VLDL and chylomicron removal rates. ApoA1 synthesis increased.	Usually well tolerated. Useful in types IIb, IV, V/I, III. Reduced CHD risk in men with low HDL.

TABLE 11.5. Cont.

Drug	Usual Dose	Cost/month	Mechanism	Comments
Lovastatin (Mevacor)	20 mg qhs or bid	$55–110	Inhibitor of hepatic HMG-CoA reductase. Upregulates hepatic LDL receptors.	Well tolerated. Most effective in combination with other drugs. Can increase warfarin availability.
Pravastatin (Pravachol)	20 mg qhs	$50	Same as lovastatin.	Well tolerated. No interaction with warfarin.
Simvastatin (Zocor)	5-10 mg qhs	$50	Same as lovastatin.	Just released; Check LFTs q 6-12 wks.
Probucol (Lorelco)	500 mg bid	$48	Mechanism of cholesterol lowering unknown. Inhibits LDL oxidation and may be antiatherogenic.	Decreases HDL levels as much as 50%. Usually well tolerated.

399

decreases in triglycerides and increases in HDL-C also occur. Three agents are currently available in this class of drugs: lovastatin, simvastatin, and pravastatin, with different dosing schedules (Table 11.5). In view of their low-side effect profile these drugs are often the preferred choice of lipid-lowering agents by practicing physicians. Because of the possibility of liver toxicity and occasional skeletal muscle toxicity, however, frequent monitoring of liver and muscle enzymes is recommended during the first year of treatment.

Gemfibrozil

Gemfibrozil belongs to the class of drugs called fibric acid derivatives. These drugs reduce VLDL-C synthesis thereby reducing fasting levels of triglycerides in the blood. They also increase HDL-C levels and have a variable effect on LDL-C levels. Accordingly, gemfibrozil is often used in patients with combined hypertriglyceridemia and hypercholesterolemia, especially when associated with low HDL-C levels. In the well-known Helsinki Heart Study (3), a primary prevention trial, gemfibrozil reduced the incidence of coronary heart disease in asymptomatic middle-aged men with combined hyperlipidemia by 34% compared with placebo. Side effects are uncommon but may include mild indigestion, nausea, abdominal pain, and flatulence. Liver and skeletal muscle enzymes should be monitored during initial dosing and periodically thereafter. Gemfibrozil should not be used in combination with niacin or the statins because of the increased risk of liver toxicity from both drug classes.

Probucol

Although probucol is a relatively weak cholesterol lowering agent, it has interesting antioxidant properties that make it potentially useful as an anti-atherosclerotic agent. Recent studies have suggested that the oxidative modification of the LDL molecule in the arterial wall is an important factor in the pathogenesis of atherosclerosis (18). Experimental animal studies suggest that probucol retards the progression of atherosclerosis independent of its cholesterol-lowering effects (19). Although probucol lowers LDL-C, the mechanism of action is not known. There is also an undesirable lowering of HDL-C, the significance of which is unknown. At the present time the exact role of probucol in preventing atherosclerotic progression and lowering LDL-C is uncertain and is awaiting the results of ongoing research.

Other Therapies

Although the emphasis of the NCEP recommendations for the treatment of hyperlipidemia is on diet, exercise, and lipid-lowering drugs, there are several additional strategies that are under investigation. Included in these promising but still unproved therapies are fish oils, antioxidant vitamins, and estrogen replacement for postmenopausal women. There is increasing public interest in these ancillary treatment modalities, and it is important for health professionals to be aware of their potential usefulness.

Fish Oils

Fish oils, technically known as omega-3 fatty acids, may be obtained from high-fat fish products such as salmon, mackerel, herring, and sardines or ingested as liquids (e.g., cod liver oil) or capsules. Pharmacologically, they inhibit triglyceride synthesis in the liver and lower triglyceride levels in the blood (20). They are most useful therefore in patients with very high triglyceride blood levels, especially those at risk for pancreatitis (i.e., triglycerides >500 mg/dl). A disadvantage of these products is they might actually increase LDL-C levels, and their role in hypercholesterolemic patients is questionable. Fish oils in high dosages also have antiplatelet activity and may decrease thrombus formation. This action is potentially useful in reducing the likelihood of coronary thrombosis in the setting of an unstable atheromatous plaque. There may also be an increased bleeding tendency when used in combination with other drugs such as aspirin and coumadin. At the present time there is not sufficient data to make general recommendations regarding the use of these products. It is prudent, however, to encourage increased intake of fish products high in omega-3 fatty acids, but to be cautious of the ingestion of high doses of cod liver oil and fish oil capsules until results from ongoing studies are known.

Vitamins A, C, and E ("ACE" Inhibition)

The concept of "ACE" inhibition as used here is not to be confused with the angiotension-converting enzyme (ACE)-inhibitor class of antihypertensive drugs, but rather the antioxidant effects of vitamins A, C, and E. Antioxidants, or free-radical scavengers, are generating much excitement in the medical community, as well as in the general population. The rationale for the use of these vitamins is based on the growing evidence linking free-oxygen radicals and oxidatively modified LDL to the process of atherosclerosis (18). Antioxidants can potentially inhibit oxidative injury to blood vessels and protect the LDL-C molecule from oxidative modification, thereby slowing the process of atherosclerosis. Although all three of these vitamins have antioxidant properties, vitamin E (α-tocopherol) appears to be the antioxidant of choice in terms of efficacy (21).

Long-term observational studies of over 80,000 female nurses and 40,000 male health professionals, originally free of coronary disease, have shown that subjects with the highest consumption of vitamin E had the lowest rates of coronary disease events during follow-up (22, 23). Although studies such as these do not prove cause-and-effect relationships because they are not randomized, controlled interventions, they have strongly influenced many health professionals, as well as the general public, to take antioxidant vitamins daily.

401

While more scientifically designed clinical trials are now under way, it may take several years before the definitive answers regarding antioxidant therapies are known. Until then, how should the health professionals working in preventive cardiology programs respond to requests about taking these preparations? Daniel Steinberg, a pioneer in the field of atherogenesis and the oxidative-modification hypothesis, urges caution because of the possibility of adverse side effects and toxicities of long-term, megadose vitamin intake by the general population (24). He argues that recommendations to patients be supported by proof of efficacy in at least one valid long-term clinical trial. Table 11.6 indicates the dose ranges and potential side effects of the three antioxidant vitamins that have been used in studies of atherosclerosis, although the minimal effective dosage has not been established (25).

Estrogen Replacement Therapy

CHD is the leading cause of morbidity and mortality in postmenopausal women (26). It has been estimated that a 50–year-old woman has a 46% chance of developing CHD and 31% likelihood of dying from that disease at a median age of 74 years (15). Although the definitive, randomized controlled trials of estrogen therapy in postmenopausal women will not be completed for several more years, there is already compelling evidence from large cohort studies to recommend this therapy for most women (14, 15). The estimated CHD risk reduction from 31 observational studies attributed to estrogen replacement therapy is 44% (27). Because these studies only compared estrogen users to nonusers, possible selection bias and other uncontrolled confounding variables cannot be excluded.

The scientific rationale for estrogen's protective effects in postmenopausal women is not completely understood. It is likely, however, that multiple metabolic and physiologic processes are affected by estrogen. The most likely targets are the blood lipids. Oral estrogens reduce total and LDL-C while increasing HDL-C to a degree that could theoretically account for a 40 to 50% lowering in CHD risk in women (14). One recently reported population-based study also demonstrated an improved lipid profile in postmenopausal women taking estrogens combined with progestins, which was surprising in view of the widely held belief that progestins negated estrogen's protective effects on lipids (16). In addition to these obvious lipid-lowering benefits, estrogens may favorably influence carbohydrate metabolism by lowering blood glucose and insulin levels, decrease blood pressure when elevated, and modulate a variety of other hormonal systems. Studies in primates also suggest that estrogens may decrease or prevent vasoconstrictor responses of atherosclerotic coronary arteries and thereby decrease the risk of transient myocardial ischemia and infarction (28).

The American College of Physicians has published guidelines for counseling postmenopausal women about preventive hormone replacement therapy (29).

TABLE 11.6. Antioxidant vitamins (25)

Antioxidants	US RDA[a]	Dose Ranges[b]	Possible Side Effects
Vitamin A (as β-carotene)	10,000 IU/day	30,000-60,000 IU/cay	Nausea, diarrhea, skin rash, musculoskeletal pain, hair loss, gingivitis, anorexia, liver toxicity
Vitamin C (ascorbic acid)	100 mg/day	1-4 g/day	Kidney stones
Vitamin E (α-tocopherol)	10 mg/day	100-1200 IU/day	Nausea, diarrhea, prolonged QT interval on ECG, decreased HDL-C

[a]Approximate US recommended daily allowance for adults.
[b]Ranges of doses used in antioxidant studies.

For each person the decision to take hormones should be based on an assessment of the potential risks and benefits of such therapy. Potential risks of estrogen therapy include gallbladder disease, thromboembolic complications, endometrial cancer, and breast cancer. The risk of endometrial cancer, however, can be eliminated by progestin cotherapy. Estrogen therapy is contraindicated in women with active liver or gallbladder disease and in women with a history of breast cancer. The potential benefits of estrogen therapy include, in addition to CHD prevention, osteoporosis prevention and the relief of perimenopausal symptoms; for most women these benefits far outweigh the risks.

The recommended dose of estrogen for CHD prevention is 0.625 mg of oral conjugated estrogen or the equivalent once a day and every day without interruption (29). The transdermal estrogen preparations do not have the same beneficial lipid-lowering effects. For women with an intact uterus two regimens of combined estrogen and progestin therapy are suggested: (a) estrogen plus cyclic progestin (e.g., medroxyprogesterone acetate 5 to 10 mg orally per day) for 10 to 14 days each month; (b) estrogen plus continuous progestin (e.g., 2.5 mg medroxyprogesterone acetate orally per day). For women who have had a hysterectomy there is no reason to add a progestin preparation. Although estrogen replacement usually begins soon after menopause, the beneficial effects in terms of CHD prevention and osteoporosis prevention lasts as long as therapy is continued. For these reasons it is recommended that therapy be maintained for many years (e.g., 10 to 20 years or longer) unless complications develop. Older women who stopped estrogen therapy soon after menopause or who never started are also likely to be benefited by estrogen therapy (29).

SMOKING CESSATION

Cigarette smoking is perhaps the single most important modifiable risk factor in the prevention of CHD. It is estimated that smoking is directly responsible for 21% of total cardiovascular mortality or approximately 115,000 deaths annually (27). The good news, according to the 1989 Surgeon General's report, is that the prevalence of smoking has declined from 40% in 1965 to 29% in 1987, although the decline has occurred mostly in men (30). Former smokers, moreover, have a much lower CHD risk than do current smokers, and the improved prognosis occurs within several years of smoking cessation (31). Unfortunately, in women under age 65 the decline in smoking has been minimal, and the proportion of deaths attributed to cigarette smoking has actually increased from 26% in 1965 to 41% in 1985. The estimated risk reduction from smoking cessation in the primary prevention of CHD, based on well-designed observational studies, is 50 to 70% (27). Studies have also shown that smoking cessation after myocardial infarction (i.e., tertiary prevention) can be associated with up to 50% reduction in sudden death and fatal reinfarctions (32, 33).

Physicians and health care workers must be challenged to develop effective smoking cessation programs for their patients who smoke. The following sections review general strategies applicable to most smoking interventions, as well as more intensive programs that are often needed for the hard-core, nicotine-dependent smokers.

Hospital-Based Smoking Cessation Strategies

Patients recovering from acute cardiac events—myocardial infarction, unstable angina, coronary artery bypass surgery, and coronary angioplasty—are likely to be very receptive to behavioral and lifestyle recommendations, including smoking cessation. Unfortunately, many physicians are pessimistic about their ability to achieve long-term success in changing smoking behaviors in their patients (34). This attitude often interferes with their motivation to provide comprehensive smoking cessation instruction to patients in the hospital or in the office setting; thus a vicious cycle of half-hearted efforts leading to poor compliance and more pessimism is likely to ensue. Cummings et al. (35) recently reported a scientific study showing that physicians who were specifically trained to provide smoking cessation strategies to patients had significantly higher rates of long-term smoking cessation than physicians randomly assigned to a control group. This emphasizes the need to provide more training in behavior modification techniques to physicians working in primary care or with heart disease patients.

Hospital-based cardiac rehabilitation programs have long recognized the importance of smoking cessation interventions in their overall planning of phase I and phase II services. Taylor et al. (36) described a successful nurse-administered smoking cessation program for post-MI patients. Patients were provided with smoking cessation literature and were individually counseled about coping strategies to control the temptation to smoke. Following discharge from the hospital, nurses phoned the patients weekly for 3 weeks and then monthly for 4 months to reinforce the smoking cessation strategies. A randomized controlled study comparing this program to "usual care" post-MI patients reported that 71% of smokers in the intervention program quit smoking compared to 45% of smokers in the control group. The cost-effectiveness of this program was reported by Krumholz et al. (37) in a subsequent paper, concluding that the program was more cost-effective in terms of dollars per year of life saved than the use of beta-blockers after MI.

Outpatient-Based Smoking Cessation Strategies

Developing an outpatient smoking cessation program that could be administered in a physician's office practice or in a cardiac rehabilitation program requires several months of planning to organize the clinic environment and educate the staff. The environment should be smoke-free to reinforce the anti-smoking message. Staff involvement is necessary to implement changes that

TABLE 11.7. Elements of Effective Smoking Cessation Programs

- Involve office staff
- Identify all smokers
- Provide a strong smoking cessation message
- Set a firm quit date
- Provide self-help literature
- Anticipate relapse
- Provide for adequate follow-up
- Provide a list of smoking cessation resources

have to be made in recordkeeping and ensure smooth day-to-day program operations. Self-help patient education materials should be available in the waiting room along with antismoking displays. They can be obtained from a variety of local and national sources, including the National Cancer Institute (38), the American Academy of Family Physicians (39), and the American Heart Association and its state affiliates. In addition, a number of excellent antismoking kits have been developed to help health professionals implement their smoking cessation programs (40–42). Table 11.7 lists general elements of effective smoking cessation programs.

Identify All Smokers

All smokers in an office practice or rehabilitation program should be identified and the smoking status indicated in the patient's medical record. An accurate smoking history should include the duration and amount of smoking expressed in pack-years, the brand smoked, reasons for success or failure of previous attempts to quit, the longest period of abstinence, and any withdrawal symptoms. Other family members and significant others who smoke should also be identified and encouraged to participate in the smoking cessation program.

It is also necessary to identify smokers with nicotine addiction because intense withdrawal symptoms may occur within hours of quitting and present a serious obstacle to becoming a nonsmoker. These symptoms include irritability, anxiety, restlessness, impaired concentration, insomnia, fatigue, depression, mouth sores, constipation, chest tightness, and cough. Withdrawal symptoms and signs may persist for several weeks and prevent the successful completion of the smoking cessation program. Table 11.8 illustrates a self-administered questionnaire developed by Fagerstrom (43) that helps identify the nicotine-addicted smoker. A score greater than 7 indicates "high nicotine dependence"; 4 to 7 indicates "medium addiction"; and 0 to 3 indicates "low dependence." Nicotine-dependent patients should anticipate having withdrawal symptoms and be encouraged to take steps to minimize them by using bronchodilators, high-fiber diets, and other behavioral strategies (44).

TABLE 11.8. The Fagerstrom Nicotine Addiction Questionnaire (43)

Question	0 Points	1 Points	2 Points	Score
1. How soon after you wake up do you smoke your first cigarette?	After 30 min	Before 30 min	–	——
2. Do you find it difficult to refrain from smoking in places where it is forbidden?	No	Yes	–	——
3. Which cigarette smoked during the day is the most satisfying?	Any other but the first one	The first one	–	——
4. How many cigarettes per day do you smoke?	1-15	16-25	>25	——
5. Do you smoke more in the morning than the rest of the day?	No	Yes	–	——
6. Do you smoke when you are so ill that you are in bed most of the day?	No	Yes	–	——
7. Does the brand smoked have low, medium, or high nicotine content?	Low	Medium	High	——
8. How often do you inhale smoke from cigarettes?	Never	Sometimes	Often	——
			TOTAL	

Score = 0–3: low dependence.   Score = 4–7: medium dependence.   Score > 7 points: highly nicotine-dependent.

407

A Strong Antismoking Message

A strongly worded antismoking message from a health professional or personal physician describing the dangers of smoking and the benefits of quitting is often sufficient to achieve long-term success. Six-month quit rates of up to 20% have been reported in trials of brief counseling carried out in a physician's office (44). More impressive, however, is the evidence that more than 60% of smokers recovering from acute MI quit after brief smoking cessation advice and remain abstinent for one year or longer (45). The smoking cessation message becomes even more convincing in the presence of other coronary risk factors because of additive adverse effects of these factors on the atherosclerotic process.

The exact wording of the antismoking message may vary from patient to patient depending on the particular clinical situation and the specific needs of individual patients. Some physicians and health care workers may be less enthusiastic and not insist strongly enough because of previous failures with other patients. Others, however, may feel so strongly about this issue that they refuse to provide further care to their cardiac patients who continue to smoke (46). This strategy is likely to be most effective for those patients who are emotionally attached to their personal physicians.

Setting a Firm Quit Date

When a patient has finally agreed to consider smoking cessation, it is important to set a reasonably firm quit date, preferably during a stress-free time in the patient's life. This enables the patient and significant others to prepare for withdrawal symptoms and, perhaps, to arrange for distractions to help minimize these symptoms. This might be a good time for a sedentary smoker to begin an exercise program, which would not only be distracting but would also help prevent the weight gain that inevitably occurs after smoking cessation. A quit date also establishes a strong commitment by the patient to take responsibility for making this most important behavioral change.

Part of the strategy of establishing a firm quit date is the signing of a "contract" between the patient and the health care provider that explicitly commits the patient to quit smoking on a specific date. The contract should include the reasons for stopping and the proposed methods to quit. The health care provider, in turn, commits to following up with the patient by telephone and appropriately timed visits to motivate the patient and help manage withdrawal symptoms. Copies of the contract should be placed in the patient's medical record and given to the patient along with appropriate smoking cessation materials.

Relapse Prevention

The greatest recurrent problem for many smokers who are initially successful in quitting is the high likelihood of relapse. Because this is the major obstacle to long-term abstinence, most comprehensive smoking cessation programs incorporate relapse prevention strategies along with methods to promote maintenance of the smoke-free status. Green et al. (47) identify three important behavioral techniques for averting a relapse: (a) setting up a strong social support network; (b) acquisition of coping skills, and (c) cognitive restructuring.

The social support network usually includes family, friends, neighbors, and co-workers. Encouragement and positive feedback from these individuals is an important adjunct to the patient's smoking cessation efforts. It is also recommended that other smokers in the patient's social network be encouraged to join the program for the benefit of all.

A variety of coping skills have been recommended to help manage those special occasions where relapse is most likely to occur. Shiffman (48) has identified four particularly troublesome scenarios for new ex-smokers to be aware of: (a) following meals at home, (b) drinking alcohol in social environments with other smokers, (c) during stressful situations at work, and (d) during periods of loneliness at home alone. Patients should be taught to recognize these situations and learn how to substitute more healthful behaviors.

Cognitive restructuring is a useful stress management technique for preventing relapse by focusing on changes in self-perception, knowledge, and attitudes. Although not always easy to achieve, health care workers can help patients by enlisting their active participation in the smoking cessation process. Smokers must be motivated to assume more responsibility for their actions. The change from being a passive recipient of medical services to becoming an active participant in the health care process often leads to a new self-image: one of being in control. This is the most important prerequisite to acquiring the knowledge and attitudes necessary to maintain the smoke-free state.

Strategies for Nicotine-Dependent Smokers

Unfortunately many heavy smokers will not respond to the brief intervention strategies just discussed. The awareness of nicotine addiction by health care workers helps alleviate the widely held but incorrect notion that all it takes is willpower to stop smoking. The craving for nicotine by nicotine-dependent smokers who quit cold turkey is often so strong that few are ever successful in managing their withdrawal symptoms. For these smokers more intensive and formal smoking cessation strategies are required. Similar methods that have been successful in the treatment of other chemical dependencies are often used in these smoking cessation programs, including both pharmacologic and non-pharmacologic techniques. Health care workers should be familiar with the various options even though they may not be personally involved in administering them, since they are often asked by patients and their families for information about them.

Pharmacologic Therapies

The major pharmacologic intervention for nicotine-dependent smokers is nicotine substitution therapy. The rationale for this therapy is to minimize the nicotine withdrawal symptoms after smoking cessation by slowly tapering the substituted nicotine dosage. There are several different nicotine preparations and delivery systems for accomplishing this goal.

The first successful nicotine replacement preparation, nicotine polacrilex "gum," became available in the United States in the mid 1980s. When used as an adjunct to comprehensive behavior modification, randomized controlled studies suggested a doubling of quit rate in nicotine-dependent patients (49). Unfortunately, outside of the research environment practicing physicians were less successful using nicotine gum in their office-based practices (50, 51). Success with this product requires meticulous attention to detail when prescribing it to patients. In a sense, the term "nicotine gum" is a misnomer, since the gum is not to be chewed like ordinary chewing gum. Regular chewing causes the released nicotine to mix with saliva that, when swallowed, is not absorbed into the circulation to produce a pharmacodynamic effect. The proper use of the product requires the patient to chew a fresh piece of gum at most only 10 to 15 times to release nicotine and create sufficient alkalinity in the mouth to ensure absorption directly through the buccal mucosa. After several slow chews the patient is instructed to position the flattened piece of gum in the space between the upper molar teeth and the cheek. The gum is left in place for several minutes until the tingling sensation disappears and then chewed slowly to release more nicotine before positioning the gum in a different location between the teeth and the cheek. This process should be repeated several more times over a 30-minute period allowing absorption to take place from other areas of the mouth.

The absorbed nicotine serves as a substitute for the nicotine in cigarettes. Unlike cigarettes, however, where the inhaled nicotine reaches the circulation within seconds, the nicotine absorbed through the buccal mucosa takes 10 to 15 minutes to achieve adequate blood levels. A careful analysis of the patient's smoking behavior prior to initiating therapy with nicotine polacrilex is necessary to design a dosing schedule that best ameliorates withdrawal symptoms. Patients should be instructed to anticipate the nicotine craving by 10 to 15 minutes and to use the gum at that time to allow for the slow absorption into the circulation. In some heavy smokers it often requires up to 30 pieces of gum a day to provide enough substituted nicotine to ameliorate the withdrawal symptoms. Once an initial dosing schedule is established, the patient can be given a schedule for gradually diminishing the daily dosage of drug until full withdrawal is accomplished. This often takes several months during which time the physician should maintain close contact with the patient to monitor progress, assess side effects, and reinforce behavioral strategies.

Many of the difficulties and obstacles associated with nicotine polacrilex have been overcome by the introduction of "user-friendly" transdermal nicotine delivery systems in 1991. The nicotine patches (e.g., Habitrol, Nicoderm, Prostep, Nicotrol) can be prescribed to deliver various doses of nicotine transdermally over a 16- to 24-hour period. The absorption of nicotine into the cutaneous capillary bed produces steady serum levels of nicotine, thus providing relief from withdrawal and craving while, at the same time, avoiding the addictive effects of peak nicotine levels seen with cigarette smoking and nicotine gum. Clinical trials with these products have consistently shown short-term and long-term efficacy in terms of cigarette quit rates (52–54). Safety and efficacy have also been demonstrated in patients with stable coronary artery disease (55).

The transdermal nicotine systems are available in several dose ranges. The highest dose is prescribed initially for 3 to 5 weeks; the lower doses are then recommended for several weeks each before discontinuing therapy. Optimal duration of therapy for most patients is 6 to 8 weeks. Each of the manufacturers of nicotine patches provides detailed instructions for tapering their products along with self-help guides for patients to follow. As with the gum, success rates are likely to be much higher if the nicotine patches are used in conjunction with counseling, support, and behavioral modification strategies. The National Cancer Institute has published "How to Help Your Patients Stop Smoking," which provides detailed recommendations for clinicians to follow when working with smokers (56).

Contraindications to the use of nicotine substitution therapies include (a) the immediate post-myocardial infarction period, (b) uncontrolled cardiac arrhythmias, (c) severe or worsening angina pectoris, and (d) peripheral vasospastic diseases. In addition, the nicotine gum should not be used in patients with active temporomandibular joint disease or if there is orophyaryngeal irritation. Further warnings, precautions, and side effects of each preparation are found in the Physicians' Desk Reference (57).

Nonpharmacologic Methods

A variety of other methods have been suggested to decrease the psychologic dependency of nicotine (58). Adversive methods such as rapid smoking, smoke holding, and smoking to satiation are rarely successful when used alone and are relatively contraindicated in patients with heart disease. Hypnosis and acupuncture are two promising approaches that have varying degrees of success depending on patient motivation, particular methodologies, length of treatment, and incorporation of other behavioral techniques (59).

411

It is important for health care workers to understand that quitting smoking for good is rarely accomplished with the first attempt. Relapse is common, and physicians and other health professionals should have the necessary resources to reinforce the antismoking message. Strategies for supporting smoking abstinence and managing relapse have already been discussed in this chapter. Patients should also be informed about smoking cessation programs in the community such as those sponsored by the American Lung Association and the American Cancer Society.

NONPHARMACOLOGIC MANAGEMENT OF HYPERTENSION

Health professionals working in the preventive medicine arena, including cardiac rehabilitation, should become familiar with "The Fifth Report of the Joint National Committee on Detection, Evaluation, and Treatment of High Blood Pressure (JNC V)," which was published in 1993 (60). These guidelines represent the most up-to-date recommendations for hypertension management and include strategies for both pharmacologic and nonpharmacologic interventions. The JNC V guidelines for detecting, evaluating, and treating hypertension with drugs were discussed in Chapter 3. This section discusses nonpharmacologic therapies (i.e., lifestyle modifications) that should be considered in every hypertensive patient either before or concurrent with drug therapy. In many individuals with mild-to-moderate hypertension careful attention to healthy lifestyles will often achieve the desired blood pressure reduction and obviate the need for antihypertensive drugs. Even when these behavioral changes are not adequate by themselves to successfully manage hypertension, they often make it easier to control hypertension with drugs and minimize the cardiovascular morbidity associated with hypertension.

The lifestyle modifications that have proven value in the management of hypertension include increased physical activity, weight reduction if overweight, smoking cessation, sodium reduction, moderation in alcohol intake, and increased potassium intake (61). Not only are most of these lifestyle changes useful in the treatment of hypertension, but they are also important in the prevention of coronary heart disease, especially in patients with additional coronary risk factors such as hyperlipidemia and diabetes mellitus. Recommendations for exercise training in healthy adults and those with cardiovascular disease have already been discussed in previous chapters. Strategies for smoking cessation are discussed earlier in this chapter.

Weight Reduction

Approximately 35 to 45% of adult Americans are classified as "overweight" based on an increased body mass index, and the prevalence is increasing (62). Excess body weight, especially in an abdominal fat distribution pattern characterized by increased weight/hip ratios above 0.85 in women and 0.95 in men, has been identified as an important independent risk factor for cardiovascular disease (60, 63). Metabolic abnormalities associated with abdominal or truncal obesity include hyperinsulinemia, insulin resistance, noninsulin-dependent diabetes mellitus, reduced HDL-cholesterol, hypertriglyceridemia, and hypertension. These abnormalities have been correlated with increased risk for stroke, myocardial infarction, and premature death (64). In hypertensive subjects who are more than 10% above ideal body weight, loss of weight is clearly associated with reduced blood pressures (65, 66). Weight loss also improves the response to antihypertensive drugs.

The successful management of obesity often requires comprehensive lifestyle restructuring with attention to healthy eating habits, increased physical activity, and psychosocial coping strategies (67). There is no single "best" way to treat obesity. It is beyond the scope of this chapter to review in detail the many different treatment strategies for losing weight. A National Institutes of Health Technology Assessment Conference on *"Methods for Voluntary Weight Loss and Control"* provides an extensive summary of the weight-loss literature along with recommendations for selecting a weight-loss program (68).

The important message for health professionals is that all overweight hypertensives should be started on an individualized, closely monitored weight-loss program that includes caloric restriction, exercise training, and behavioral interventions. For patients with newly diagnosed mild hypertension (i.e., systolic BP of 140 to 159 mm Hg, and/or diastolic BP of 90 to 99 mm Hg) a weight-loss program along with other lifestyle changes should be tried for at least 3 to 6 months before considering drug therapy (60). For obese patients with more severe hypertension weight loss recommendations should be an integral component of an overall comprehensive drug treatment program.

Moderation of Alcohol Intake

Excess alcohol consumption is associated with increased blood pressure and resistance to antihypertensive therapy (60). All patients with hypertension therefore should be asked about alcohol consumption, including the quantity and frequency of wine, beer, and liquor intake. The CAGE questionnaire (Table 11.9) has proven to be useful in identifying patients likely to have a problem with alcohol abuse (69). These individuals should be referred to appropriate consultants or community programs specializing in the treatment of alcoholism. Hypertensives who consume alcohol but do not have an alcohol abuse problem should be advised to limit their daily alcohol intake to 1 oz of ethanol (i.e., 2 oz of 100-proof whiskey, 8 oz of wine, or 24 oz of beer) (60).

Sodium Restriction

Increased sodium in the diet has long been recognized as a contributor to

413

TABLE 11.9. The CAGE Questionnaire (69)

C: "Have you ever felt you ought to **C**ut down on drinking?"

A: "Have people **A**nnoyed you by criticizing your drinking?"

G: "Have you felt bad or **G**uilty about your drinking?"

E: "Have you ever had a drink first thing in the morning to steady your nerves or get rid of a hangover (**E**ye-opener)?"

elevated levels of blood pressure, although not everybody is equally affected by salt intake. Therapeutic trials suggest that moderate sodium restriction can be associated with reductions in systolic and diastolic blood pressures of approximately 5 to 10 mm Hg (70). Most Americans consume more than 150 mmol/day of sodium in their diets. The JNC V recommendations are to reduce sodium intake to less than 100 mmol/day (i.e., <2.3 g of sodium or <6 g sodium chloride) (60).

Potassium, Calcium, and Magnesium

Many studies have looked at the effects of dietary potassium, calcium, and magnesium intake on the development and treatment of hypertension with mixed results. As an example, Siani et al. (71) carried out a randomized, controlled trial on the effects of increased dietary potassium intake on the need for antihypertensive medications in patients with essential hypertension. They showed that after one year, patients who increased their potassium consumption were able to reduce their antihypertensive drugs to less than 50% of their initial therapy. In addition, potassium depletion caused by diuretic therapy is associated with potentially dangerous cardiac arrhythmias and therefore must be corrected by increasing dietary potassium intake or adding potassium chloride supplements.

The role of calcium and magnesium in hypertension management is less certain, but current JNC V recommendations are to at least maintain adequate intakes of these minerals in the diet (60). In general, supplemental intake of these nutrients is not advised unless patients are not able to take in the currently recommended daily amounts (i.e., 3000 to 3200 mg of potassium per day, 800 to 1000 mg of calcium per day, and 350 to 400 mg of magnesium per day). Magnesium deficiency, however, can occur with diuretic therapy, and it is then necessary to replace the magnesium loss with appropriate supplements.

Other Dietary Factors

The JNC V recommends reduction in dietary saturated fat intake primarily because of the adverse role of these fats on the development and progression of atherosclerosis (60). Studies have failed to show that reducing these fats has any important blood pressure-reducing effects (72). The role of caffeine intake in the development and progression of hypertension is also controversial. Although the acute intake of caffeine may temporarily increase blood pressure, this effect is dissipated in a short period. Unless an individual has an excessive sensitivity to caffeine-containing beverages, it is generally not necessary to limit the intake of these products in most hypertensive patients. Finally, the increased intake of garlic and onion to prevent heart disease and hypertension is not based on any definitive scientific data and cannot be recommended at this time (60).

Stress Management, Relaxation, and Biofeedback

It has long been recognized that many individuals react to stressful encounters with increases in blood pressure. The role of stress in the pathogenesis of hypertension is well established from studies in animals, as well as in human subjects. Unfortunately, the value of stress management in preventing hypertension or in lowering blood pressure in hypertensive patients is still controversial.

The Trials of Hypertension Prevention (TOHP) study, a multicenter randomized control trial, evaluated three lifestyle interventions (weight reduction, sodium reduction, and stress management) and nutritional supplements (calcium, magnesium, potassium, and fish oil) in patients with high-normal diastolic blood pressure (73). Only the weight loss and sodium reduction groups had lower systolic and diastolic blood pressures when compared to control subjects. The stress management limb of this study used four techniques of relaxation (slow breathing, progressive muscle relaxation, mental imagery, and stretching) and included cognitive strategies to manage stress perceptions, reactions, and situations. The 236 subjects who practiced these techniques experienced no change in blood pressure compared to a control group during an 18-month follow-up period.

Because of the lack of convincing scientific data on the benefits of stress management techniques, the JNC V does not recommend the use of these therapies in the prevention and treatment of hypertension (60). Further discussion of stress management in the overall prevention of cardiovascular diseases is presented in Chapter 12.

DIABETES MELLITUS

Diabetes mellitus has long been recognized as a major risk factor for the development and progression of atherosclerotic vascular disease, including coronary heart disease. Space does not permit a complete discussion of the pathogenesis, clinical manifestations, complications, and treatment of this prevalent medical problem. It is important, however, for health professionals working in preventive medicine and cardiac rehabilitation to be familiar with the potential for preventing the vascular complications of diabetes in patients with known coronary heart disease or those at risk for developing this disease. The following discussion addresses these issues.

From a clinical perspective there are two major subsets of patients with diabetes mellitus: (*a*) insulin-dependent diabetes mellitus (IDDM), or type I, and (*b*) noninsulin-dependent diabetes mellitus (NIDDM), or type II. The precise definitions for these two groups were established and published by the National Diabetes Data Group in 1979 (Table 11.10) (74). Insulin-dependent diabetes is by far the more serious, though less common form of diabetes. The disease usually begins in childhood or adolescence, and there is a high probability of developing serious renal, cardiovascular, neurologic, and ophthalmologic complications during the long course of the disease. In contrast, NIDDM is a very common disease of adult Americans with a greater potential for prevention and control than IDDM. The estimated prevalence of NIDDM in the United States is 6.6% (75). It is this form of diabetes that is most often seen by health professionals working in preventive medicine and cardiac rehabilitation. Although called "noninsulin-dependent," many type-II diabetics require insulin therapy during periods of illness or when diet, exercise, and oral hypoglycemic agents fail to adequately control blood glucose levels.

Diabetes mellitus significantly increases the risk for cardiovascular disease, especially coronary heart disease, peripheral vascular disease, and cerebrovascular disease. In NIDDM, or type-II diabetes, the risk is increased two to five times that of a nondiabetic (76). It is likely that the pathophysiologic mechanisms for the increased risk of atherosclerosis are caused by the high

TABLE 11.10. Classification of Diabetes Mellitus (74)

Type	Clinical Characteristics	Criteria for Diagnosis
IDDM type I	Ketosis prone; requires insulin for survival; usual onset in youth; absolute insulin deficiency; anti-islet cell antibodies present.	Elevation of fasting blood glucose ≥140 mg/dl on more than one occasion, *or* 75 g oral GTT yields 0.5, 1.0, or 1.5 hr blood glucose *and* 2 hr values ≥200 mg/dl. Polyuria, polydipsia, weight loss, weakness also present.
NIDDM type II	Ketosis resistant; usual onset after age 40; obesity and insulin resistance often present with inadequate insulin secretion.	Same criteria as for IDDM.

IDDM, insulin-dependent diabetes mellitus; *NIDDM*, noninsulin-dependent diabetes mellitus; *GTT*, glucose tolerance test.

prevalence of obesity (especially the abdominal fat pattern), hypertension, hypertriglyceridemia, hypercholesterolemia, and low HDL-C levels seen in this disease. It is especially important to recognize and manage these clinical entities because their successful treatment not only prevents serious cardiovascular complications, but it also improves or reverses the underlying insulin resistance and glucose intolerance associated with the diabetic state.

The initial and most important therapeutic approach to NIDDM is nonpharmacologic. Since more than 85% of type-II diabetics are obese, weight loss should be the preeminent goal. A hypocaloric, balanced diet that is also low in saturated fat and cholesterol should be prescribed. For most obese diabetics the recommended caloric intake can be determined by subtracting 500 calories from the estimated daily weight maintenance caloric requirements (Table 11.11). It often is not possible for these patients to attain their ideal body weight; fortunately, a loss of only 10 to 20 pounds may significantly improve or cure the metabolic abnormalities associated with the diabetic state (77). Because of the importance of dietary management in the control of type-II diabetes and the associated cardiovascular complications, all patients should be referred to dietitians or nutritionists for expert consultation and follow-up. The expected benefits of successful weight loss are improved glycemic control, lower blood pressures, improved lipid profile, and decreased risk of vascular diseases. Unfortunately, long-term weight control is extremely difficult for most individuals, and a high percentage of those who initially lose weight regain their weight within several years (78).

Because of the difficulties of achieving and maintaining weight loss through dietary means alone, the second major therapeutic goal in the treatment of type II diabetes is exercise. All patients should be given an exercise prescription based on their functional status and cardiovascular risk. The basic principles of exercise prescription have been discussed in previous chapters. In addition to the weight loss benefits, exercise training is likely to improve glycemic control,

TABLE 11.11. Calculation of Caloric Requirements for Obese Diabetics

- Desirable body weight (DBW) in pounds (males) = 106 + 6 × (inches over 5 ft)
- DBW in pounds (females) = 100 + 5 × (inches over 5 ft)
- Weight maintenance calories (sedentary adults) = 13 × DBW
- Weight maintenance calories (moderately active adults) = 15 × DBW
- Weight maintenance calories (active adults) = 20 × DBW

Example: 6 ft obese man (moderately active): DBW = 106 + (6 × 12) = 178 lb
Weight maintenance calories = 15 × 178 = 2678 calories
Weight loss diet = 2678 − 500 = 2178 calories

decrease insulin resistance, lower blood pressure, and improve lipid profile. Some diabetics have a peripheral neuropathy, as well as peripheral vascular disease, which increases their risk for foot injuries during exercise. Exercise specialists should be aware of these potential complications when working with diabetic patients, especially those engaging in high-impact exercise activities. Diabetics, especially those on insulin, are also at increased risk of developing hypoglycemia during exercise because of the ease with which glucose is transported into muscle during exercise. Patients beginning an exercise program should be advised to self-monitor their blood glucose concentrations before and after each exercise session and adjust their insulin doses appropriately. Once an exercise program becomes predictable, daily insulin requirements often are modestly reduced. Diabetics who are exercising should also have access to carbohydrate snacks to counteract any symptoms of hypoglycemia that may occur during exercise.

CONCLUSIONS

This chapter has reviewed the current recommendations for identifying and managing the major coronary risk factors that are responsible for most cases of coronary heart disease and associated vascular complications of atherosclerosis. Clearly there are other important factors that account for the wide prevalence of atherosclerotic diseases in our society. Foremost among these is heredity. The mechanisms by which heredity facilitates the development and progression of atherosclerosis, however, are largely through the modifiable risk factors discussed in this chapter. In other words, individuals who are genetically prone to getting atherosclerotic diseases will do so because of the inherited susceptibility of their arteries to the damaging effects of hyperlipidemia, hypertension, cigarette smoking, and diabetes. The implication to health care professionals is that the control or elimination of these major risk factors will significantly lower the risk of vascular diseases in these high-risk individuals and families.

REFERENCES

1. Gotto AM, LaRosa JC, Hunninghake D et al. The cholesterol facts. A summary of the evidence relating to dietary fats, serum cholesterol, and coronary heart disease. A joint statement by the American Heart Association and the National Heart, Lung, and Blood Institute. Circulation 1990; 81:1721.
2. Lipid Research Clinics Program. The Lipid Research Clinics coronary primary prevention trial results. I and II. JAMA 1984;251:351.
3. Frick MHJ, Elo O, Haapa K et al. Helsinki heart study: primary prevention trial with gemfibrozil in middle-aged men with dyslipidemia: safety of treatment, changes in risk factors, and incidence of coronary heart disease. N Engl J Med 1987;317:1237.
4. Consensus Development Conference. Lowering blood cholesterol to prevent heart disease. JAMA 1985;253:2080.
5. Expert Panel on Detection, Evaluation, and Treatment of High Blood Cholesterol in Adults.

Summary of the Second Report of the National Cholesterol Education Program (NCEP) Expert Panel on Detection, Evaluation, and Treatment of High Blood Cholesterol in Adults (Adult Treatment Panel II). JAMA 1993;269:3015.

6. The Expert Panel. Report of the National Cholesterol Education Program Expert Panel on Detection, Evaluation, and Treatment of High Blood Cholesterol in Adults. Arch Intern Med 1988; 148:36.

7. Smith D, Song F, Sheldon TA. Cholesterol lowering and mortality: the importance of considering initial level of risk. Br Med J 1993;306:1367.

8. Connor SL, Connor WE. The new American diet. New York: Simon & Schuster, 1986.

9. Grundy SM, Winston M, eds. American Heart Association. Low-fat, low-cholesterol cookbook. New York: Times Books, 1989.

10. Butler TG, Yanowitz FG. Obesity. In: Yanowitz FG, ed. Coronary heart disease prevention. New York: Marcel Dekker, 1992.

11. Danford D, Fletcher SW, eds. Methods for voluntary weight loss and control. Ann Intern Med 1993;119:641.

12. NIH Technology Assessment Conference Panel. Methods for voluntary weight loss and control. Ann Intern Med 1992,116.942.

13. Hopkins PM. Hyperlipidemia: detection and treatment In: Yanowitz FG, ed. Coronary heart disease prevention. New York: Marcel Dekker, 1992.

14. Barrett-Connor E, Bush TL. Estrogen and coronary heart disease in women. JAMA 1991;265: 1861.

15. Grady D, Rubin SM, Petitti DB et al. Hormone therapy to prevent disease and prolong life in postmenopausal women. Ann Intern Med 1992;117:1016.

16. Nabulsi AA, Folsom AR, White A et al. Association of hormone-replacement with various cardiovascular risk factors in postmenopausal women. N Engl J Med 1993;328:1069.

17. Blum CB. Current therapy for hypercholesterolemia. JAMA 1989;261:3582.

18. Steinberg D, Parthasarathy, Carew TE et al. Beyond cholesterol. Modification of the low-density lipoprotein that increases its atherogenicity. N Engl J Med 1989;320:915.

19. Carew TE, Schwenke D, Steinberg D. Antiatherogenic effect of probucol unrelated to its hypocholesterolemic effects. Proc Natl Acad Sci 1987;84:7725.

20. Yetiv JZ. Clinical applications of fish oils. JAMA 1988;260:665.

21. Jialal I, Grundy SM. Effect of combined supplementation with α-tocopherol, ascorbate, and beta carotene on low-density lipoprotein oxidation. Circulation 1993;88:2780.

22. Stampfer MJ, Hennekens CH, Manson JE et al. Vitamin E consumption and the risk of coronary disease in women. N Engl J Med 1993;328:1444.

23. Rimm EB, Stampfer MJ, Ascherio A et al. Vitamin E consumption and the risk of coronary heart disease in men. N Engl J Med 1993;328:1450.

24. Steinberg D. Antioxidant vitamins and coronary heart disease. N Engl J Med 1993;338:1487.

25. Bays H, Dujovne C. Antioxidants in clinical practice. Choices in Cardiology 1994;8:6.

26. American Heart Association. 1992 heart and stroke facts. AHA Publication 55-0386 (COM). National Center, 7272 Greenville Avenue, Dallas, TX 75231-4596.

27. Manson JE, Tosteson H, Ridker PM et al. The primary prevention of myocardial infarction. N Engl J Med 1992;326:1406.

28. Williams JK, Adams MR, Klopfenstein S. Estrogen modulates responses of atherosclerotic coronary arteries. Circulation 1990;81:1680.

29. American College of Physicians. Guidelines for counseling postmenopausal women about preventive hormone therapy. Ann Intern Med 1992;117:1038.

30. Department of Health and Human Services. Reducing the health consequences of smoking: 25 years of progress: a report of the Surgeon General. Washington, DC: Government Printing Office, 1989 (DHHS publication no. CDC 89-8411).

31. Kuller L, Meilahn E, Townsend M et al. Control of cigarette smoking from a medical perspective. Annu Rev Pub Health 1982;3:153.

32. Salonen J. Stopping smoking and long-term mortality after acute myocardial infarction. Br Heart J 1980;43:463.

33. Wilhelmsen L. Cessation of smoking after myocardial infarction: effects on mortality after ten years. Br Heart J 1983;49:416.

34. Wechsler H, Levine S, Idelson RK et al. The physician's role in health promotion— a survey of primary-care physicians. N Engl J Med 1983;308:97.

35. Cummings SR, Coates TJ, Richard RJ et al. Training physicians in counseling about smoking cessation. A randomized trial of the "Quit for Life" program. Ann Intern Med 1989;110:640.

36. Taylor AB, Houston-Miller N, Killen JD, DeBusk RF. Smoking cessation after acute myocardial infarction: effect of a nurse-managed intervention. Ann Intern Med 1990;113:118.

37. Krumholz HM, Cohen BJ, Tsevat J et al. Cost-effectiveness of a smoking cessation program after myocardial infarction. J Am Coll Cardiol 1993;22:1697.

38. Quit for good. Bethesda, MD: National Cancer Institute. DHHS National Institutes of Health Publication No. (PHS) 85-1824 and 85-2494.

39. AAFP Stop Smoking Program. Patient stop smoking guide. Kansas City, KS: American Academy of Family Physicians, 1987.

40. I quit kit. American Cancer Society, 4 West 35th Street, New York, NY 10019.

41. Freedom from smoking in 20 days. American Lung Association, 1740 Broadway, New York, NY 10019.

42. A lifetime of freedom from smoking. American Lung Association, 1740 Broadway, New York, NY 10019.

43. Fagerstrom KO. Measuring the degree of physical dependence to tobacco smoking with reference to individualization of treatment. Addict Behav 1978;3:235.

44. Prochazka A, Boyko EJ. How physicians can help their patients quit smoking: a practical guide. West J Med 1988;149:188.

45. Bart A, Thornley P, Illingworth D. Stopping smoking after myocardial infarction. Lancet 1974; 1:304.

46. McIntosh HD. Office strategies to reduce the risk of coronary heart disease. J Am Coll Cardiol 1988;12:1095.

47. Green HL, Goldberg RJ, Ockene JK. Cigarette smoking: the physician's role in cessation and maintenance. J Gen Intern Med 1988;3:75.

48. Schiffman S. A cluster analytic classification of relapse episodes. Addict Behav 1986;11:295.

49. Lam W, Sze PC, Sacks HS. Meta-analysis of randomized controlled trials of nicotine chewing gum. Lancet 1987;2:27.

50. Hughes JR, Gust SW, Keenan RM et al. Nicotine vs. placebo gum in general medical practice. JAMA 1988;261:1300.

51. Cummings SR, Hansen B, Richards RJ et al. Internists and nicotine gum. JAMA 1988;260:1565.

52. Fiore MC, Jorenby DE, Baker TB, Kenford SL. Tobacco dependence and the nicotine patch. Clinical guidelines for effective use. JAMA 1992;268:2687.

53. Lee EW, D'Alonzo GE. Cigarette smoking, nicotine addiction, and its pharmacologic treatment. Arch Intern Med 1993;153:34.

54. Transdermal Nicotine Study Group. Transdermal nicotine for smoking cessation. Six-month results from two multicenter controlled clinical trials. JAMA 1991;266:3133.

55. Rennard S, Daughton D, Fortmann S et al. Transdermal nicotine enhances smoking cessation in coronary artery disease patients. Chest 1991;100:5S.

56. Glynn TJ, Manley MW. How to help your patients stop smoking: a National Cancer Institute manual for physicians. Washington, DC: US Department of Health and Human Services (Public Health Service), National Institutes of Health; 1990. Publication NIH 90-3064.

57. Physicians' desk reference. 48th ed. Montvale, NJ: Medical Economics, 1994.

58. Green HL, Goldberg RJ, Ockene JK. Cigarette smoking: the physician's role in cessation and maintenance. J Gen Intern Med 1988;3:75.

59. Health and Public Policy Committee, American College of Physicians. Methods for stopping cigarette smoking. Ann Intern Med 1986;105:281.

60. Joint National Committee on Detection, Evaluation, and Treatment of High Blood Pressure. The Fifth Report of the Joint National Committee on Detection, Evaluation, and Treatment of High Blood Pressure (JNC V). Arch Intern Med 1993;153:154. (Also published by the National

Institutes of Health, NIH Publication No.93-1088, US Department of Health and Human Services, Public Health Service, National Institutes of Health, Bldg. 31, Room 4AO5, Bethesda, MD 20892.)

61. Kaplan N. Management of hypertension. Disease-a-Month, November 1992, p 783.

62. NIH Technology Assessment Conference Panel. Methods for voluntary weight loss and control. Ann Intern Med 1992;116:942.

63. Peiris AN, Sothmann MS, Hoffman RG et al. Adiposity, fat distribution and cardiovascular risk. Ann Intern Med 1989;110:867.

64. Larsson B, Svardsudd K, Welin L et al. Abdominal adipose tissue distribution, obesity and risk of cardiovascular disease and death: 13-year follow-up of participants in the study of men born in 1913. Br Med J 1984;288:4011.

65. Langford HG, Davis BR, Blaufox MD et al. Effect of drug and diet treatment of mild hypertension on diastolic blood pressure. Hypertension 1991;17:210.

66. Schotte DE, Stunkard AJ. The effects of weight reduction on blood pressure in 301 obese patients. Arch Intern Med 1990;150:1701.

67. Butler TG, Yanowitz FG. Obesity. In: Yanowitz FG, ed. Coronary heart disease prevention. New York: Marcel Dekker, 1992.

68. NIH Nutrition Coordinating Committee. Methods for voluntary weight loss and control. Ann Intern Med 1993;119:641.

69. Ewing JA. Detecting alcoholism: the CAGE questionnaire. JAMA 1984;252:1905.

70. Law MR, Frost CD, Wald NJ. By how much does dietary salt reduction lower blood pressure? III. Analysis of data from trials of salt reduction. Br Med J 1991;302:819.

71. Siani A, Strazzullo P, Giacco A et al. Increasing the dietary potassium intake reduces the need for antihypertensive medication. Ann Intern Med 1991;115:753.

72. Sacks FM. Dietary fats and blood pressure: a critical review of the literature. Nutr Rev 1989; 47:291.

73. The Trials of Hypertension Prevention Collaborative Research Group. The effects of non-pharmacologic interventions on blood pressure of persons with high normal levels. Results of the trials of hypertension prevention, phase I. JAMA 1992;267:1213.

74. National Diabetes Data Group. Classification and diagnosis of diabetes mellitus and other categories of glucose intolerance. Diabetes 1978;28:1039.

75. Harris MI, Hadden WC, Knowler WC et al. Prevalence of diabetes and impaired glucose tolerance and plasma glucose levels in U.S. population aged 20-74 yr. Diabetes 1987;36:523.

76. Kannel WB, McGee DL. Diabetes and cardiovascular disease: the Framingham study. JAMA 1979;241:2035.

77. Hadden DR, Montgomery DAD, Skelly RJ et al. Maturity onset diabetes mellitus: response to intensive dietary management. Br Med J 1975;3:276.

78. Wing RR, Jeffery RW. Outpatient treatments of obesity: a comparison of methodology and clinical results. Int J Obes 1979;3:261.

V. FUTURE PERSPECTIVES

12

FUTURE PERSPECTIVES: A VIEW TOWARD THE 21ST CENTURY

IN SPITE OF RECENT downward trends, the major health care issue in our society today continues to be the unnecessary and premature morbidity and mortality from atherosclerotic cardiovascular diseases (1). Although the causes of atherosclerosis are multifactorial and to some extent still unknown, physical inactivity and other adverse lifestyles appear to contribute significantly to the disease burden. The evidence linking these risk factors to coronary heart disease and other vascular manifestations of atherosclerosis is substantial (2, 3). More importantly, the evidence is equally convincing that modification or elimination of adverse behaviors and other coronary risk factors by restructuring lifestyles and pharmacologic management of hypertension and hyperlipidemia can significantly improve clinical outcomes in high-risk individuals (4). Previous chapters in this book have addressed the role of exercise training and other risk factor management strategies applicable to primary, secondary, and tertiary prevention of cardiovascular diseases. In this concluding chapter several different perspectives regarding the emerging roles of health promotion and disease prevention in the practice of medicine will be explored.

THE PUBLIC PERSPECTIVE

The public is clearly aware of the importance of health promotion and preventive medicine in our society. Since the late 1960s there has been a virtual explosion of public interest in physical fitness, leisure-time activities, good nutrition, smoke-free environments, stress management, and other heart-healthy behaviors. Numerous epidemiologic surveys and public opinion polls have been conducted in recent years to assess attitudes and beliefs about fitness and other health behaviors (5, 6). A number of interesting findings and recommendations are of interest to health professionals.

Prevalence of Leisure-Time Physical Activity

In 1980 the U.S. Department of Health and Human Services recommended that by 1990 all adults should participate in "exercise which involves large muscle groups in dynamic movement for periods of 20 minutes or longer, 3 or more days per week, and which is performed at an intensity of 60 percent or greater of an individual's cardiorespiratory capacity" (7). Although there seems to be a general perception that increasing numbers of people are exercising, the data from epidemiologic surveys indicate that fewer than 20% of the adult American population are actually exercising at this level (8). Furthermore, less than 50% of adults exercise at any intensity for more than 20 minutes a day, 3 or more days per week (8).

Why are there so few Americans participating in regular exercise activities? One explanation offered by a group of experts brought together by the U.S. Centers for Disease Control and Prevention and the American College of Sports Medicine is that many people erroneously believe that only *vigorous* exercise training contributes to improved health (9). Because scientific evidence clearly supports the health benefits of *moderate*-intensity physical activity, the expert panel offered the following two recommendations (9):

- "Every American adult should accumulate 30 minutes or more of moderate-intensity physical activity over the course of most days of the week."

- "Because most adult Americans fail to meet this recommended level of moderate-intensity physical activity, almost all should strive to increase their participation in moderate or vigorous physical activity."

There is therefore a need for more public and professional education regarding

426

cardiovascular and other health benefits of moderate exercise, as well as the behavioral techniques for developing and maintaining fitness. For many years the American College of Sports Medicine has been the leader in the development of guidelines for exercise testing and training (10). These guidelines have been widely distributed to health professionals working in cardiac rehabilitation and other preventive medicine programs. It is necessary for public health agencies, recreational organizations, and professional health service groups to work together to disseminate these important recommendations and promote programs in the schools, work sites, and communities that improve the health and fitness of our citizens (9).

The Determinants of Exercise Participation

The U.S. Public Health Service in collaboration with numerous organizations and professionals has established health promotion and disease prevention objectives for the year 2000 (11). Among these *"Healthy People 2000" objectives* are to "reduce to no more than 15 percent the proportion of people aged 6 and older who engage in no leisure-time physical activity" (11). Although some progress is being made in the numbers of adults participating in exercise programs, the percentage of individuals actually engaging in regular exercise activities remains small. Most likely these national exercise and fitness goals will not be met without active intervention by health professionals. The challenge of the 1990s is to develop effective programs that encourage sedentary individuals to adopt and maintain regular aerobic exercise habits. Intervention strategies aimed at preventing dropouts from exercise programs and cardiac rehabilitation are also badly needed.

Dishman et al. (12) have reviewed the scientific literature to better understand the known determinants of and barriers to regular exercise and physical activity. The reasons why people choose to exercise or choose not to exercise are complex and include personal characteristics, environmental factors, and factors relating to the specific exercise activities.

Personal characteristics that may influence exercise behaviors include past and present experiences with exercise programs and other forms of physical activity, health beliefs and attitudes toward exercise, personality characteristics, biomedical traits, and demographic factors (12). Previous participation in sports during youth, for example, may have a positive (or negative) influence on the subsequent exercise behaviors of adults, although other personal or environmental factors sometimes override. In addition, current involvement in adult fitness or cardiac rehabilitation programs is a strong predictor of future participation. Most dropouts from supervised programs occur in the first 3 to 6 months.

Apparent barriers to participation in clinical exercise programs include blue-collar occupations, cigarette smoking, obesity, and type A behavior (12). In addition, individuals who perceive their health to be poor are unlikely to initiate or maintain a regular exercise program. From these observations it appears that those who are most likely to achieve health benefits from adult fitness and cardiac rehabilitation programs are also the most resistant to participating in them.

Knowledge of and beliefs in the health benefits of exercise seem to be less important motivators to continued participation in exercise programs than feelings of enjoyment and a sense of well-being associated with exercise (13). Individuals most likely to adhere to a fitness program are those who feel good about themselves, feel they are in control of their own destinies, and are self-motivators. The perception of self-efficacy or self-confidence is also an important predictor of adherence to physical activities after myocardial infarction (MI). Ewart et al. (13), for example, have shown that treadmill testing 3 weeks after an uncomplicated MI followed by an explanation of results to patient and spouse was associated with improved self-efficacy scores and subsequent maintenance of exercise activities. These data indicate that effective behavioral interventions aimed at improving confidence and a sense of well-being are important motivational tools for maintaining an exercise program.

Both social and physical environmental factors are determinants of participation in adult fitness and cardiac rehabilitation programs (13). Social reinforcement from family members, friends, and other health professionals are all influential in maintaining good exercise habits. Important physical factors include both the perceived convenience of the exercise facility and the actual proximity of the facility to home or work site. Frequently, however, the significance of these factors is biased by a lack of interest in or commitment to exercise, with environmental factors being the excuse for dropping out. Interventions that focus on specific behavioral and cognitive strategies have been successful in increasing the frequency of adherence to exercise programs. Examples of successful strategies include written agreements and behavioral contracts, contingency incentives, self-monitoring and self-reward skills, goal setting, and decision making (12).

There is a great need for additional research on the determinants of exercise habits and the design of optimal intervention programs for ensuring compliance to exercise regimens. It is clear, however, that to be successful, adult fitness and cardiac rehabilitation programs must take into consideration psychosocial, behavioral, and environmental factors that exert influence outside the immediate environment of the exercise facility.

Physical Activity and Age

In the United States the number of adults over age 65 years is increasing faster than any other age group (14). In 1991, for example, there were 31.8 million Americans over age 65; this represents 12.6% of the entire United State population. Conservative estimates predict that by the year 2040, 68.1 million (22.6%) United States citizens will be 65 years old or older. This number may even be higher if current trends in the reduction of cardiovascular disease morbidity and mortality continue.

The general conclusion from cross-sectional population studies is that there is a decline in physical activity with age (5). The decline is steepest during adolescence and early adulthood because of decreasing participation in sports activities after high school and college. Between ages 55 and 65 years, however, the decline seems to level off, most likely because of the increased interest in leisure-time activities associated with retirement. As the percentage of healthy older adults in our society increases because of improved cardiovascular disease outcomes, it is likely that an even greater number of middle-aged and older adults will be exercising in the future. Because of the importance of keeping older adults healthy and functionally independent, health professionals must be challenged to develop and disseminate cost-effective fitness programs applicable to older individuals. In addition, more emphasis should be given to the specific training needs of older individuals, especially those who have physical disabilities and other health problems.

The Public's Changing Health Care Paradigm

For years it was believed that progress through scientific investigations was the key to understanding and eventually controlling all of nature. This has been especially true for the medical sciences. Since the mid-19th century medicine has been driven by the "scientific method" and the search for disease causation and treatment. This is exemplified by the germ theory of disease, which was first applied to tuberculosis; that is, every disease has a single cause (e.g., the tubercle bacillus) and every clinical problem a discrete solution (e.g., specific antibiotics). Not only were physicians and other medical scientists convinced that health could best be achieved by applying the scientific method to eliminate common diseases, but the general public also accepted this dogma.

As a result of the ongoing health care reform process in the 1990s and the economic realities of medical care in the United States, there is beginning to be a shift in emphasis away from specialization and complex technology toward primary care and ambulatory services. Concurrent with this new perspective are changing attitudes, beliefs, and behaviors of the American public, changes that have been characterized by Freyman (15) as a new societal paradigm. According to Freyman,

> the American middle class is moving rapidly toward a new paradigm of health care. Until recently, most Americans were convinced the key to health was conquest of disease through science. Their new belief is more positive: health is a natural state and the key to it lies in lifestyle and the environment.

This awareness is linked to an increased willingness of Americans to assume more responsibility for their health and well-being (16). The health care professions are slowly moving toward this new societal paradigm in an effort to regain public confidence.

THE MEDICAL PERSPECTIVE

The medical profession is also undergoing major changes in its approach to medical care not only in terms of organizational, business, and reimbursement aspects of medicine, but also in its philosophical basis or belief system. Many of these changes are having, and will continue to have, considerable influence on the physicians' role in health promotion, adult fitness, and cardiac rehabilitation. As stated previously, attitudes of health care providers toward issues relating to exercise and other preventive strategies are, in part, shaped by the public's demand for more information on prevention and health promotion.

The national debate about health care reform has brought to the forefront the need for more preventive-medicine services (17). Economic forces are responsible for the increased growth of alternative health care systems such as health maintenance organizations (HMOs) and preferred provider organizations (PPOs). Because of the financial incentives in these plans to keep enrollees healthy and out of the hospital, providers are offering more risk-assessment and health-enhancement services along with more traditional examinations.

Overall, however, there is still a lack of consensus among medical professionals on the importance of preventive health behaviors. Some physicians are reluctant to offer health promotion services because the evidence for many prevention recommendations is still perceived as conflicting and controversial. Paradoxically, these same physicians are often willing to try new drugs and other therapeutic techniques on the basis of only preliminary evidence of efficacy, even with the realization that these unproved therapies may be costly and associated with some risk to the patient. In contrast, the evidence for many preventive health behaviors is actually substantial, and the recommended interventions are inexpensive and essentially without risk. It is also unfortunate that some physicians still believe that health promotion is not their business but rather the business of public health officials and other health professionals (18). In spite of these obstacles there is a growing movement among physicians, hospitals, and other health care organizations to provide services related to risk assessment, disease prevention, and sports medicine.

In patients with known coronary heart disease (CHD) the lack of aggressive risk factor management by the medical community is especially distressing, since the evidence for efficacy of preventive measures is quite strong. Cohen et al. (19) reported that only 35% of CHD patients with hypercholesterolemia were receiving appropriate risk factor counseling or lipid lowering therapy by their cardiologists or referring internists. Referrals to cardiac rehabilitation programs may even be smaller; it is estimated that only 11% of eligible CHD

430

patients are enrolled in such programs (20). Hopefully growing patient awareness and increasing emphasis of preventive services in the current health care
reform movement will improve participation in these programs.

The "Second Medical Revolution": A New Scientific Paradigm for Medicine

Although to some extent the motivation for more preventive services is in response to public demand and economic forces, there is also beginning to be a
"paradigm shift" in the medical sciences away from the traditional "biomedical" approach to disease toward a more inclusive scientific model (21). Thomas
Kuhn, a philosopher of science, first popularized the concept of a paradigm shift
in his seminal work *The Structure of Scientific Revolutions* (22). According to Kuhn,
a paradigm shift occurs whenever the accumulated scientific evidence in a par
ticular discipline is no longer consistent with the beliefs shared by the scientists
in that discipline, and new theories must be conceptualized or invoked to explain the apparent anomalies. A famous example of a paradigm shift in the field
of physics occurred early in the 20th century with Einstein's theory of relativity
and the birth of quantum mechanics. The new theories resolved a number of
anomalies that could not be explained by the older paradigm of classical
mechanics. A paradigm shift in medicine is presently under way because of
the growing consensus that the biomedical model, which views the patient, the
disease, and its treatment in purely mechanistic terms, is no longer adequate to
explain the origins of today's major chronic diseases, let alone offer effective
solutions to them (21, 23, 24).

Although scientific models are rarely the focus of scientists' or clinicians'
attention, they provide the necessary philosophical foundation from which to
structure a particular scientific discipline. In medicine, for example, the traditional view of practitioners and researchers toward health and disease is mechanistic; that is, the body is conceptualized as a complex machine that can only be
studied by analyzing component parts such as cells, tissues, organ systems, and
their many interactions (24). Disease represents a breakdown or malfunction in
one or more of the body's parts, and it is best studied or diagnosed using
anatomic, physiologic, or biochemical methods. The physician's role in treating
disease therefore is to identify areas of malfunction and then to intervene physically or biochemically to correct the abnormalities of structure and function.

From the perspective of the history of medical progress, the biomedical
model has enabled remarkable advances to be made in our understanding of
the *process* by which various diseases or injuries affect the body. The technologies of biomedicine, ranging from molecular biology to sophisticated diagnostic
and treatment procedures, have increased our knowledge of disease-induced
cellular and organ system malfunction to a level of sophistication never before
imagined. And yet, the *origins* of many of today's chronic diseases such as

atherosclerosis and cancer remain largely unknown. What is known, however, suggests that chronic diseases often occur as a result of adverse lifestyles or interactions between individuals and their environments. The reductionist or biomedical approach to disease focuses attention more on mechanisms than on causes. Unfortunately, this often leads to modern medicine's emphasis on expensive technologic solutions to diagnosis and treatment of diseases with little or no attention given to disease origins, prevention, or health maintenance.

Nowhere is this approach more evident today than in cardiovascular medicine, where technology has become the dominant force governing the practice of cardiovascular specialists. In coronary disease, for example, quantitative aspects of the disease process are examined using noninvasive and invasive technologies that permit exact localization of obstructive vascular lesions and their functional consequences. Treatment interventions are then designed to revascularize ischemic myocardium and pharmacologically manipulate other disease manifestations. The recent emergence of "interventional cardiologists" with expertise in the mechanical alteration or removal of atherosclerotic plaque in arteries is a good example of this trend. A leading article in the *Journal of the American College of Cardiology* (April 1989) focuses attention on mechanistic solutions to coronary disease in its title: "Crackers, Breakers, Stretchers, Drillers, Scrapers, Shavers, Burners, Welders, and Melters—The Future Treatment of Atherosclerotic Coronary Artery Disease?" (26). These exciting technologies coupled with the enormous financial rewards to physicians, hospitals, and industry have overshadowed the efforts of some physicians, public health officials, and others to promote disease prevention.

There is a growing awareness among some medical specialists that the technologic solutions to many of today's major health problems are accelerating health care costs far beyond manageable levels. In addition, many of the present solutions to existing, chronic diseases are palliative at best and not curative, with frequent recurrences of disease manifestations and further costly complications. As a result, attention is being shifted toward the study of disease origins and prevention. With this new perspective, however, comes the realization that the biomedical model may no longer be adequate to fully explain these major health problems.

One of the first attempts to conceptualize a new scientific model for medicine was offered by Dr. George Engel. Unlike the biomedical model, which is based on a factor-analytic or reductionist approach that has characterized the Western scientific method for hundreds of years, Engel proposed a "biopsychosocial" model based on general systems theory (24, 25). The biopsychosocial model is not so much a replacement for the older biomedical model but rather an extension of it, adding the psychologic, social, cultural, and ecologic determinants of health and disease to the more traditional biomedical ones. All the biomedical advances of modern medicine, which are based on studies of organ systems, tissues, cells, and subcellular components, are retained in the new model. In a systems approach to the human patient, however, the new model also focuses attention on the individual person as a dynamic living system that is more complex than just the sum of all the parts.

Figure 12.1, reprinted from Engel (24), illustrates the biopsychosocial model as a hierarchy of systems. Each level in the hierarchy is an organized, dynamic system incorporating all systems below it while, at the same time, serving as a component part of each higher level system. The individual person (or patient) in the model is represented by a midlevel system with the traditional biomedical systems below and the more complex social systems above. Unlike the biomedical model, each subordinate system in the hierarchy can be influenced by all the higher level systems, a feature that essentially does away with the

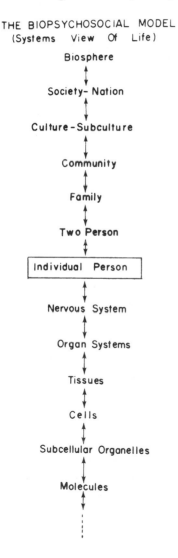

THE BIOPSYCHOSOCIAL MODEL
(Systems View Of Life)

Biosphere
↕
Society-Nation
↕
Culture-Subculture
↕
Community
↕
Family
↕
Two Person
↕
Individual Person
↕
Nervous System
↕
Organ Systems
↕
Tissues
↕
Cells
↕
Subcellular Organelles
↕
Molecules
↕

FIGURE 12.1. Engel's biopsychosocial model. (Reprinted by permission from Engel GL. The biopsychosocial model and medical education. N Engl J Med 1982;306:802.)

outdated concept of "mind-body dualism" introduced by Descartes in the 17th century and a fundamental concept of the biomedical model (27). The biopsychosocial model permits a more realistic appreciation of the role of mental processes (thoughts and behaviors), social supports, and other societal issues in the preservation of health or the development of disease. Furthermore, each system in the hierarchy has distinctive features and interrelationships requiring scientific methodologies unique to that particular level. This has profound implications for medicine since it implies that a multidisciplinary approach, ranging from molecular biologists at one end of the hierarchy to social scientists and ecologists at the other end, may be the only way to truly solve many of today's complex diseases.

Figure 12.2 illustrates how the biopsychosocial model might be applied to the conceptual aspects of CHD. In the classic biomedical approach to atherosclerosis diagnostic studies, treatments, and research investigations have usually focused on the organ system level, tissues, cells, or subcellular components in the progressive downward search for the ultimate molecular and genetic defects responsible for the disease process. In the new model the patient, or whole person, is now the subject of interest, which in addition to numerous host factors and subordinate systems is influenced by all higher level systems. Because the patient is not just a biologic organism in isolation but rather a component part of these higher level systems (i.e., the social and physical environments), it is easy to appreciate the importance of various psychosocial and environmental factors in the development and progression of disease manifestations. The model also facilitates a better understanding of the challenges and eventual solutions to lowering CHD morbidity and mortality by focusing attention on the higher social systems that influence the patient's lifestyle and health behaviors. It is important to appreciate, moreover, that the traditional biomedical issues are not neglected in the model.

Scientific models are, at best, only approximations of reality or truth. The biomedical model has become so ingrained into the belief systems of physicians and medical scientists that its limitations are easily overlooked. The biopsychosocial model appears to be more inclusive and therefore a better approximation of natural phenomena, especially living systems. It too has serious limitations, however, as discussed by Foss and Rothenberg (21) in their book *The Second Medical Revolution: From Biomedicine to Infomedicine*. A philosophical problem occurs when biomedical strategies are combined with psychosocial ones, since only the former are compatible with the prevailing mechanistic paradigm and therefore "scientifically" based (21). The idea that social, psychologic, or behavioral factors might serve as important determinants of health and disease violates fundamental scientific presuppositions. Unlike the levels or systems represented in the biomedical model (i.e., tissues, cells, molecules), psychosocial factors have no physical basis and therefore cannot be re-

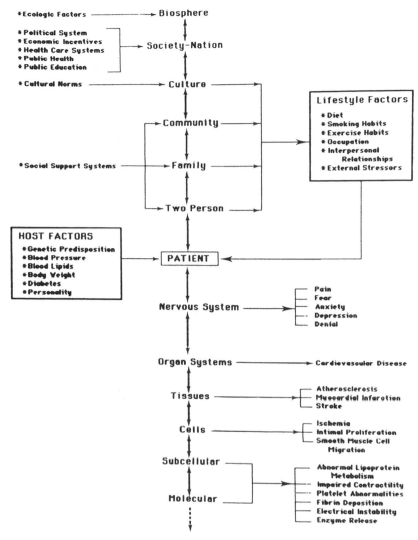

FIGURE 12.2. Application of the biopsychosocial model to the conceptual framework of CHD.

duced to physicochemical terms. They also cannot be placed within the traditional mechanistic definition of patient, disease, or treatment as defined previously. As a result, any application of psychosocial strategies to medical practice must be justified entirely on empirical evidence that these strategies do, in fact, work. Moreover, since these approaches fall outside of biomedicine's scientific boundaries, it is unlikely that they will ever become fully integrated into the mainstream of medical education or practice. Current educational objectives for medical students and physicians in training do not include instruction from disciplines outside the biomedical framework.

435

What is needed is a revised scientific theory that puts existing empirical data on disease prevention (data that fall outside of the biomedical framework) into a legitimate scientific context. In fact, the articulation of such a revision based on 20th century "postmodern" sciences (e.g., relativity and quantum mechanics, information theory, complexity, and others) is already under way and is seriously challenging the dominant biomedical paradigm (21). A fundamental feature of the new theory, one that has far-reaching implications for medicine, is the concept of *self-organizing systems*. Although taken from general systems theory and thermodynamics, this concept is applicable to all complex systems, including the human patient. According to Foss and Rothenberg (21), self-organizing systems differ from simple mechanistic ones by exhibiting the properties of (*a*) *self-renewal*—"the ability to continuously renew and recycle their components while maintaining the integrity of the overall structures," and (*b*) *self-transcendence*—"the ability to reach out spontaneously beyond physical and mental boundaries in the process of learning, developing, and evolving." Anyone working with patients can easily appreciate the importance of these two properties in conceptualizing the process of disease prevention and health maintenance. It is not possible in this brief discussion to present any details of a successor scientific model based on the postmodern sciences. The interested reader will find a stimulating account of this revolutionary thesis in Foss and Rothenberg's book (21).

Although the dominant force in cardiovascular medicine today is still based on the biomedical model with its emphasis on reductionism and mind-body dualism, there is emerging evidence for a "new-wave" movement in medicine concerned with more humanistic issues relating to health and disease and therefore more supportive of preventive health practices and wellness. An expanded medical paradigm based on the postmodern sciences offers an attractive new strategy for incorporating these preventive services into the mainstream of medical care. To be successful, however, it will require radical changes in our system of medical education, with inclusion of courses in the social and behavioral sciences, epidemiology, information theory, ecology, and population biology. These curricular innovations will not be easy to implement, given the enormous influence of the biomedical model on organized medicine. In the current medical environment medical schools, academicians, professional organizations, hospital associations, insurance companies, the pharmaceutical industry, federal agencies, and other organizations all legitimize and profit from the current biomedical model (21). There is room for cautious optimism, however, because increasing emphasis is being given to prevention in the current health care reform movement and the related demand for more primary care physicians.

THE SPORTS MEDICINE PERSPECTIVE

The emergence of recreational and therapeutic exercise in our society has led to a proliferation of professional activities associated with exercise—athletic training, adult fitness, cardiopulmonary rehabilitation, exercise testing, and exercise research—to name just a few. In broad general terms these various activities can be designated as "sports medicine." Unlike other medical specialties, however, sports medicine includes physicians in all specialties, as well as nurses, physical therapists, exercise physiologists, athletic trainers, and many other health professionals.

In reality, sports medicine is much more than a medical specialty, because it encompasses all medically related activities associated with sports medicine. Dr. Allan J. Ryan, one of the founding fathers of sports medicine and long-time editor-in-chief of the journal *Physician and Sportsmedicine*, describes four general categories of sports medicine (28).

The first involves the medical supervision and care of professional and recreational athletes. Included in this aspect of sports medicine are team physicians, orthopedic surgeons, athletic trainers, and other exercise specialists. Services provided by these individuals are primarily directed toward maintenance of or improvement in athletic performance.

A second category of sports medicine concerns the application of exercise training techniques and sports to the physically and mentally handicapped population, also called "adaptive physical education" (28). To some extent this aspect of sports medicine overlaps with physical and rehabilitation medicine, whose practitioners include physical medicine specialists, orthopedic surgeons, neurosurgeons, physical therapists, and nurses. In a broader sense, however, there is a growing interest in promoting recreational and competitive athletic activities for the physically and mentally handicapped outside the institutional setting. Two examples of this "wellness" movement for the handicapped are the popular Special Olympics for mentally retarded individuals, and the increasing number of athletic events organized for wheelchair athletes.

The third focus of sports medicine involves the prescription of exercise for the general population. This is an area that is becoming increasingly important because of the growing public demand for accurate information on exercise. Practically all medical specialties, including pediatrics, obstetrics, family practice, internal medicine, psychiatry, and many others, are beginning to recognize the importance of exercise and are providing patients with information on starting and maintaining exercise programs. In addition, many other health professionals such as exercise physiologists, physical therapists, and nurses are helping the public become more physically active. So-called "sports medicine clinics" are being established all over the country in hospitals, health spas, shopping centers, and recreational resorts. Unfortunately, standards of excellence have not been uniformly followed in setting up and operating these facilities, and as a result there is no way of ensuring that these clinics are providing adequate services. The *Guidelines for Exercise Testing and Prescription*, published by the American College of Sports Medicine (10), has contributed significantly to the development of acceptable standards for exercise prescription, testing, and certification of exercise program personnel. It is expected that as these recommendations get disseminated and incorporated into educational programs for sports medicine specialists that there will be improvement in the quality of programs provided by sports medicine clinics.

The fourth category of sports medicine concerns the therapeutic use of exercise in the treatment and rehabilitation of the sick and injured. Cardiac rehabilitation is the classic example of this aspect of sports medicine, although therapeutic exercise programs also exist for patients with pulmonary disease, arthritis, cerebrovascular disease (stroke), diabetes mellitus, and many other physically disabling conditions. Although physicians are frequently responsible for the overall supervision of these various rehabilitation programs, the day-to-day applications of exercise therapy to patients recovering from illness or injury is usually the responsibility of certified exercise specialists or physical therapists. Explicit behavioral objectives for the training and certification of these exercise personnel have been published by the ACSM (10).

Although not a specialty per se, sports medicine does bring together individuals from many diverse backgrounds who share a common interest in exercise. The ACSM has become the umbrella organization representing the many professional interests of these individuals. Through its committees, its regional and national meetings, and its journal *Medicine and Science in Sports and Exercise*, the ACSM plays an important role in providing scholarly programs and educational materials to the many practitioners of sports medicine. Because of its importance to the overall quality of sports medicine activities across the country, the ACSM needs the continued support of all its members. In addition, individuals who are just starting careers with an emphasis in sports medicine are strongly urged to join the ACSM and contribute to its many activities.

HEART DISEASE REVERSAL: THE FUTURE OF CARDIAC REHABILITATION

For almost 40 years, cardiac rehabilitation has been evolving as a multidisciplinary science and service dedicated to restoring cardiac patients to "optimal physical, social, emotional, psychological and vocational status" (29). During the same period the overall management of patients with cardiovascular diseases, in particular CHD, has improved dramatically.

Whereas in the 1950s acute MI patients remained in bed for weeks at a time, patients today are out of bed soon after hospital admission and home 5 to 7 days post-MI, often with revascularized myocardium. Because of the emphasis on early ambulation and early revascularization, the deconditioning effects associated with prolonged bed rest are generally no longer a problem for most patients. This is also true for patients undergoing surgical revascularization for CHD, because they are ambulated soon after surgery and usually discharged 5 to 7 days later. Financial constraints are leading to even shorter length-of-stays in the hospital. Accordingly, the emphasis in phases I, II and III of cardiac rehabilitation is shifting away from a primary focus on physical reconditioning to a focus more oriented toward modifying the disease process through patient education and behavioral management (30, 31). Of considerable importance to this new emphasis is the concept of atherosclerosis regression or "reversing heart disease" (32).

Evidence for regression of atherosclerosis using aggressive lipid-lowering therapies has been accumulating for over 20 years. Initial studies were done in animals, including nonhuman primates, where atherosclerosis was experimentally induced by dietary means and then allowed to regress by various cholesterol-lowering therapies (33). Early studies in humans focused on peripheral artery disease such as advanced femoral artery atherosclerosis, since it was easier to quantitate angiographic changes in lesion size in these large longitudinal vessels. With advances in quantitative coronary angiography using computerized imaging techniques, a number of well-designed, randomized, controlled clinical trials have now been published that clearly demonstrate the possibility of regression of atherosclerosis (32). In each of the published studies serial coronary angiograms have been used to evaluate changes in lesion size. Patients randomized to various treatment regimens have consistently been shown to have either more regression or less progression of lesions when compared to controls. More importantly, however, has been the evidence that "treated" patients have improved clinical outcomes in terms of reduction in angina frequency, cardiac morbidity, and stress-induced myocardial ischemia compared to controls (32).

While most regression studies in humans used intensive lipid-lowering drug therapies to achieve beneficial outcomes, the Lifestyle Heart Trial carried out by Ornish et al. (34) showed that similar angiographic and clinical outcomes could be achieved by changes in lifestyle alone. Although the study involved small numbers of subjects and suffered from randomization problems, it has attracted considerable media attention and public interest. The intervention received by 22 men and women with advanced CHD included an extremely low-fat (10% calories), low-cholesterol (5 mg/day) diet; moderate aerobic exercise (>3 hours/week); smoking cessation; stress management (stretching, progressive relaxation, meditation and imagery, 1 hour/day); and group support. Nineteen patients were randomized to a control group and were asked to follow their physicians' recommendations about diet, exercise, smoking, and stress. After one year the treatment group had significant improvement in blood lipids, clinical symptoms, and angiographic findings compared to the control group. After four years there was a marked reduction in adverse clinical events in the treatment group and further angiographic improvement compared to controls (35). Ornish and his colleagues are now promoting their "Heart Disease Reversal Program" across the country by establishing satellite hospital-based programs in an effort to reproduce their initial findings and further study the process of atherosclerosis regression.

These impressive regression studies suggest that the optimal care of patients with atherosclerotic vascular diseases should include aggressive lifestyle and pharmacologic interventions to modify risk factors. There is clearly a need for multidisciplinary skills in this endeavor to translate the findings from research studies to clinical practice. It is also apparent that changes in patients' beliefs and behaviors are critical to the success of intensive risk factor modification interventions. This should be within the framework of all future cardiac rehabilitation services. Since exercise training alone is unlikely to significantly alter the progression of atherosclerosis, it is time to move beyond the primary focus of exercise in cardiac rehabilitation toward a more comprehensive program designed to reverse or delay progression of atherosclerotic lesions.

The challenges facing cardiac rehabilitation and other preventive programs now and in the future were articulated by Sullivan et al. (36). Five recent developments were noted that could have a significant impact on the future delivery of preventive services: (*a*) health professionals are becoming increasingly aware that atherosclerosis is a multifactorial disease that can be significantly modified by lifestyle changes and medical therapies designed to reduce risk factors; (*b*) patients are becoming more aware of the importance of good personal health behaviors and adherence to medical therapy to achieve optimal health and control disease; (*c*) multidisciplinary teams, including nurses, exercise specialists, nutritionists, psychologists, and physicians, are being organized to address the prevention needs of patients with atherosclerotic diseases; (*d*) comprehensive risk factor modification programs aimed at reversing heart disease are becoming increasingly available around the country; and (*e*) third-party payers are beginning to reimburse these comprehensive prevention programs. Much remains to be accomplished, however, before effective prevention programs become the standard of care for patients with atherosclerotic cardiovascular diseases.

CONCLUSIONS

Looking ahead toward the 21st century it is clear that there will be remarkable changes in the practice of medicine and the delivery of preventive services. Many important changes are already under way. The current emphasis on "outcomes" research to study the most cost-effective methods for providing high-quality medical services will almost certainly lead to a restructuring of the health care system in this country. The development of medical guidelines for various expensive diagnostic and treatment modalities, including cardiac rehabilitation, is just beginning to affect the way these services are provided. In the future it is very likely that reimbursement for these services will be based on whether appropriate guidelines were followed. The increasing emphasis of managed care and other group health plans will also stimulate the creation of more efficient and cost-effective preventive programs, including cardiac rehabilitation and wellness clinics. For health professionals interested in prevention these are "the best of times," although careful planning is necessary to develop services that are truly cost-effective.

In 1985 the American Association of Cardiovascular and Pulmonary Rehabilitation (AACVPR) was formed to bring together professionals from many disciplines having a mutual interest in cardiac and pulmonary rehabilitation. The purpose of the organization, as stated in the bylaws (37), is as follows: "Recognizing that cardiovascular and pulmonary rehabilitation is a multidisciplinary field, the American Association of Cardiovascular and Pulmonary Rehabilitation is dedicated to the improvement of clinical practice, promotion of scientific inquiry, and advancement of education for the benefit of health-care professionals and the public." In addition to planning regional and national meetings, the AACVPR has designated its official journal to be the "Journal of Cardiopulmonary Rehabilitation." In the ensuing 10 years the AACVPR has contributed substantially to the science of cardiopulmonary rehabilitation and to the education of its members and other interested professionals.

In the future it is anticipated that there will be continued debate and controversy regarding the appropriate roles for preventive and rehabilitative services in the reorganized health care system. It is hoped that professionals working in these disciplines will be sensitive to the issues and challenged by them to provide the scientific basis for the restructuring of existing services that is necessary to best serve the public need.

REFERENCES

1. 1992 heart and stroke facts. American Heart Association, National Center, 7272 Greenville Avenue, Dallas, TX 75231-4596.
2. Stamler J. Epidemiology, established major risk factors, and the primary prevention of coronary heart disease. In: Parmley WW, Chatterjee K, eds. Cardiology. Philadelphia: JB Lippincott, 1993.
3. Grundy SM, Greenland P, Herd A et al. Cardiovascular risk factor evaluation of healthy American adults. A statement for physicians by an ad hoc committee appointed by the Steering Committee, American Heart Association. Circulation 1987;75:1340A.
4. Manson JE, Tosteson H, Ridker PM et al. The primary prevention of myocardial infarction. N Engl J Med 1992;326:1406.
5. Stephens T, Jacobs DR, White CC. A descriptive epidemiology of leisure-time physical activity. Public Health Rep 1985;100:147.
6. Paffenbarger RS, Blair SN, Lee I, Hyde RT. Measurement of physical activity to assess health effects in free-living populations. Med Sci Sports Exerc 1993;25:60.

7. Public Health Service. Promoting health/preventing disease: objectives for the nation. Washington, DC: US Department of Health and Human Services, 1980.
8. US Preventive Services Task Force. Guide to clinical preventive services: an assessment of the effectiveness of 169 interventions. Baltimore: Williams & Wilkins, 1989.
9. American College of Sports Medicine and the US Centers for Disease Control and Prevention. Summary statement: workshop on physical activity and public health. Sports Med Bull 1993;28:7.
10. American College of Sports Medicine. Guidelines for exercise testing and prescription. 4th ed. Philadelphia: Lea & Febiger, 1991.
11. US Deptartment of Health and Human Services. Healthy people 2000: national health promotion and disease prevention objectives. Washington, DC: US Dept of Health and Human Services publication No. PHS 91-50212, 1990.
12. Dishman RK, Sallis JF, Orenstein DR. The determinants of physical activity and exercise. Public Health Rep 1985;100:158.
13. Ewart CK, Taylor CB, Reese LB, DeBusk RF. Effects of early postmyocardial infarction exercise testing on self-perception and subsequent physical activity. Am J Cardiol 1983;51:1076.
14. Reuben DB, Yoshikawa TT, Besdine RW, eds. Geriatric review syllabus supplement. New York: American Geriatrics Society, 1993.
15. Freymann JG. The public's health care paradigm is shifting: medicine must swing with it. J Gen Intern Med 1989;4:313.
16. Brody DS. The patient's role in clinical decision making. Ann Intern Med 1980;93:718.
17. Leaf A. Preventive medicine for our ailing health care system. JAMA 1993;269:616.
18. Dismuke SE, Miller ST. Why not share the secrets of good health? The physician's role in health promotion. JAMA 1983;249:3181.
19. Cohen MV, Byrne M, Levine B et al. Low rate of treatment of hypercholesterolemia by cardiologists in patients with suspected and proven coronary artery disease. Circulation 1991;83:1294.
20. Leon AS, Certo C, Comoss P et al. Scientific evidence of the value of cardiac rehabilitation services with emphasis on patients following myocardial infarction. I. Exercise conditioning component. J Cardiopulmonary Rehabil 1990;10:79.
21. Foss L, Rothenberg K. The second medical revolution—from biomedicine to infomedicine. Boston: New Science Library—Shambhala, 1987.
22. Kuhn TS. The structure of scientific revolutions. 2nd ed. Chicago: University of Chicago Press, 1970.
23. Feinstein AR. The intellectual crisis in clinical science: medaled models and muddled mettle. Perspect Biol Med 1987;30:215.
24. Engel GL. The need for a new medical model: a challenge for biomedicine. Science 1977; 196:129.
25. Engel G. The clinical application of the biopsychosocial model. Am J Psychiatry 1980;137:535.
26. Waller BF. Crackers, breakers, stretchers, drillers, scrapers, shavers, burners, welders, and melters—the future treatment of atherosclerotic coronary artery disease? A clinical-morphologic assessment. J Am Coll Cardiol 1989;13:969.
27. Capra F. The turning point. Science, society and the rising culture. New York: Simon & Schuster, 1982.
28. Roos R. A conversation with Allan J Ryan, MD. Phys Sports Med 1986;14:193.
29. Hellerstein HK, Ford AB. Rehabilitation of the cardiac patients. JAMA 1957;164:225.
30. Blumenthal JA, Califf R, Williams S, Hindman M. Cardiac rehabilitation: a frontier for behavioral medicine. J Cardiac Rehabil 1983;3:637.
31. Levy JK. Standard and alternative adjunctive treatments in cardiac rehabilitation. Texas Heart Inst J 1993;20:198.
32. Blankenhorn DH. Atherosclerosis—reversal with therapy. West J Med 1993;159:172.
33. Malinow MR. Atherosclerosis. Regression in nonhuman primates. Circ Res 1980;46:311.
34. Ornish D, Brown SE, Scherwitz LW et al. Can lifestyle changes reverse coronary heart disease? Lancet 1990;336:129.
35. Ornish D, Brown B, Billings JH et al. Can lifestyle changes reverse coronary atherosclerosis? Four year results of the Lifestyle Heart Trial. Circulation 1993;88(Suppl): I-385(abstract).

36. Sullivan MJ, Cobb FR, Spira JL. Delaying progression of atherosclerosis: a new frontier in cardiology. CARDIO May 1994, p 26.
37. Wilson PK. American Association of Cardiovascular and Pulmonary Rehabilitation. From the president. J Cardiopulmonary Rehabil 1985;304:5.

Index

Page numbers in *italics* denote figures; those followed by "t" denote tables.

445